Our Future Health Secured?

A REVIEW OF NHS FUNDING AND PERFORMANCE

Derek Wanless
John Appleby
Anthony Harrison
Darshan Patel

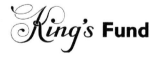

© King's Fund 2007

First published 2007 by the King's Fund

Charity registration number: 207401

All rights reserved, including the right of reproduction in whole or in part in any form.

ISBN 978 1 85717 562 2

A catalogue record for this publication is available from the British Library.

Available from:
King's Fund
11–13 Cavendish Square
London W1G 0AN
Tel: 020 7307 2591
Fax: 020 7307 2801

Email: publications@kingsfund.org.uk
www.kingsfund.org.uk/publications

Edited by Isabel Walker, Eminence Grise
Text typeset by Andrew Haig & Associates, tables and figures by Grasshopper Design Company
Printed in the UK by Hobbs the Printers Limited

Contents

List of figures and tables

About the authors

Derek Wanless has prepared two significant reports for the government on the NHS, *Securing Our Future Health: Taking a Long-Term View* (2002), and *Securing Good Health for the Whole Population* (2004). Also, in March 2006 his report on social care – *Securing Good Care for Older People: Taking a long-term view* – was published by the King's Fund.

He graduated in mathematics from King's College, Cambridge, and then qualified as a member of the Institute of Statisticians and a Fellow of the Chartered Institute of Bankers, of which he was President in 1999. He is a banker, having joined NatWest Group in 1970, and progressing to become its Group Chief Executive from 1992 until 1999. He is currently a Director of Northern Rock plc, Chairman of Northumbrian Water Group, Vice Chairman of the Statistics Commission, and a Member of the Board for Actuarial Standards.

John Appleby is Chief Economist at the King's Fund. John has researched and published widely on many aspects of health service funding, rationing, resource allocation and performance. He previously worked as an economist with the NHS in Birmingham and London, and at the universities of Birmingham and East Anglia as senior lecturer in health economics. He is a visiting professor at the Department of Economics at City University. John's current work includes research into the impact of patient choice and Payment by Results. He is also acting as an adviser to the Northern Ireland Department of Finance and Personnel in respect of the implementation of his recommendations following a review of health and social care services in Northern Ireland.

Anthony Harrison is a Senior Associate of the King's Fund. He has published extensively on the future of hospital care in the United Kingdom, the Private Finance Initiative, waiting list policies and publicly funded research and development.

Darshan Patel was seconded to work on this publication for the King's Fund from the British Dental Association, where he is the Association's economist. He has specialist knowledge of the UK dental market and played an important role in helping to develop the Association's policy, as well as influencing government policy, in the run-up to the reforms of NHS dentistry that took place in April 2006. In 2004 he co-authored the Office of Health Economics publication *The Economics of Dental Care* with Professor Ray Robinson of the London School of Economics.

Darshan holds a Masters in Economics from the London School of Economics and recently completed a postgraduate diploma in health economics from the University of York.

Acknowledgements

During the course of this review many people provided useful insights and comments for which the review team are very grateful. They are:

Deborah Arnott, Sean Boyle, Edward Bramley-Harker, Niall Dickson, Anna Dixon, Jennifer Dixon, Stephen Dunn, Richard Grainger, John Hall, Professor Chris Ham, Duncan Innes, Professor Justin Keen, John Kelly, Professor Klim McPherson, Keith Palmer, Sinead Quinn, Helen Roberts and Clive Smee.

We are also grateful to the British Dental Association for agreeing to second Darshan Patel to the review team.

We would also like to acknowledge that much of the detailed analysis of elective care in Chapter 8 was based on previous unpublished work involving Sean Boyle, Anthony Harrison and John Appleby.

Summary

A major review to examine health care funding needs over the next two decades, led by Sir Derek Wanless, was published by the Treasury in April 2002. *Securing our Future Health: Taking a Long Term View* was commissioned by Gordon Brown, the then Chancellor of the Exchequer, to help close unacceptable gaps in performance both within the United Kingdom and between the United Kingdom and other developed countries. It was the first time such long-term funding projections had been undertaken.

The review outlined three possible spending 'scenarios' for health care up to 2022/3 – *solid progress, slow uptake* and *fully engaged* – each reflecting different assumptions about the effectiveness of NHS performance and the health status of the population. For example, solid progress was a scenario of steady and significant improvement, with public health targets met, performance gaps closed and life expectancy continuing to grow fairly rapidly.

Fully engaged, the most ambitious and resource-efficient scenario, showed NHS spending rising from an estimated £68 billion in 2002/3 to £154 billion (at 2002/3 prices) by 2022/3, representing real growth of 126 per cent; *slow uptake*, the least satisfactory and most expensive scenario, had spending rising to £184 billion – real growth of 171 per cent; while *solid progress*, a scenario of steady improvement, projected a rise to £161 billion – real growth of 137 per cent.

The 2002 review made it clear that spending the recommended amounts would not succeed in transforming the health service unless it was accompanied by radical reform to tackle such underlying problems as excessive waiting times, poor access to services, poor quality of care and poor outcomes. And, while it did not go into detail about the policies the government should pursue to keep spending and performance in line with its assumptions, it did set out in broad terms how health care policy should be developed and included a number of more specific recommendations for policy-makers.

The review's final recommendation was that a further review of future resource requirements should be carried out again, about five years later– that is, in 2007. However, this is one recommendation the government has yet to take forward. Earlier this year the King's Fund asked Sir Derek to lead a team to go some way towards addressing this omission by undertaking a retrospective review of NHS spending five years on from his original report. It builds on the major work the King's Fund commissioned from Sir Derek on the future funding of social care for older people in England in 2006. However, it is not a full-scale, forward-looking review of future funding as was recommended in the 2002 review, and as this report argues there is still a need for such a review. Rather, this latest contribution attempts to provide answers to some pressing questions:

■ did health care resources increase in line with the recommendations of the 2002 review, and what are the prospects for funding up to 2022/3?

- where did the extra money go and what has it achieved in terms of resource inputs (labour and capital), outputs (activity) and, most crucially, outcomes (health benefits and productivity)?

- have the additional resources been used effectively, and if not why not? Have the policy decisions taken since 2002 produced health systems that put the United Kingdom on track for an optimistic future?

- what lessons can be learned to inform similar reviews in future?

The review is divided into two main sections.

Part 1 provides an analysis of NHS funding and its impacts since 2002 and is followed by an assessment of current government health policy and recommendations for the future. It also includes a summary of the findings of the 2002 review and a subsequent publication focusing on the public health aspects of the review's recommendations, *Securing Good Health for the Whole Population: Final Report* (Wanless 2004).

Part 2 presents detailed evidence about what has been spent on the NHS since 2002 and what it has achieved in terms of resources, services, productivity and, crucially, health benefits.

Key findings

The following sections summarise the key findings of individual chapters in Part 2 of the review.

FUNDING: WHAT WAS SPENT

The five years since 2002 have witnessed unprecedented levels of government investment in the NHS – there has been average annual real term growth of 7.4 per cent over the five years to 2007/8. Over that period, real spending on the NHS has risen by nearly 50 per cent – a total cash increase of £43.2 billion – while the proportion of the United Kingdom's gross domestic product (GDP) devoted to health care spending has grown to 9–10 per cent, within striking distance of the European Union average. Chapter 5 of this review examines actual spending in the light of this promise and the funding recommendations of the 2002 review, then goes on to consider funding prospects up to 2022/3.

Total UK and private NHS funding in 2007/8 stands at around £113.5 billion, which takes the UK close to the estimated average EU health care spending in 2007/8. Higher-than-anticipated level of GDP makes the total spend about 0.3 per cent lower as a proportion of GDP than had been assumed. Although the total spend is £2.4 billion higher than assumed by the 2002 review, it is broadly in line with the Wanless recommendations, covering even the most expensive scenario. However, it is important to note that funding in the first five years was the same across all three scenarios, with projected UK spending expected to diverge across the three paths from 2008 onwards.

If, as is widely assumed, NHS funding growth slows to its long-term average of around 3 per cent by the end of the next comprehensive spending review period (2010/11), funding would fall short of the fully engaged spending path by around £7.2 billion, the solid progress path by £9.2 billion and the slow uptake path by £15.2 billion (all at 2002/3 prices). This represents shortfalls of 6 per cent, 7.6 per cent and 12 per cent respectively.

Funding: an overall assessment

Additional UK NHS funding since 2002/3 broadly matched the recommendations of the 2002 review for the first five years of its spending trajectories, taking total health care spend to within striking distance of average European Union spending as a proportion of GDP. Such a rate of increase cannot be sustained indefinitely, but spending would have to increase by at least 4.4 per cent a year in real terms if the NHS were to follow the 2002 review's most optimistic scenario and by more than that in the other scenarios. If funding growth in the health service slows to its long-term average of around 3 per cent by 2010/11, the NHS would fall short of the slow uptake, solid progress and fully engaged spending paths. This would place the United Kingdom near the bottom of future estimates of the average total EU health care spend as a proportion of GDP.

INPUT COSTS: WHY THEY ROSE

NHS funding rose by more than £43 billion in the five years after 2002. Pay and price inflation accounted for £18.9 billion (43 per cent) of the extra investment. Chapter 6 looks at how new employment contracts introduced for virtually all the 1.3 million staff employed by the NHS has contributed to this inflation and considers the impact of the contracts on productivity and other benefits.

The main source of these higher costs has been pay increases arising from three new contracts introduced in the last four years – Agenda for Change (covering all nurses and non-clinical staff) and new contracts for hospital doctors and general practitioners. Consultant pay under their new contract has risen by around 25 per cent, while the new GP contract has boosted average net income by 23 per cent. The cumulative additional cost of Agenda for Change from 2005/6 to 2007/8 has been around £1.8 billion.

Although there is some tentative evidence that these new contracts may have reduced three-month vacancy rates and may be starting to improve productivity among consultants and nurses, there is very little robust evidence so far to demonstrate significant benefits arising from the new pay deals.

Input costs: an overall assessment

Overall, actual increases in input costs in the NHS have broadly matched assumptions made by the 2002 review, with actual pay inflation slightly higher than assumed but non-pay inflation slightly lower. Pay and contract modernisation for all NHS staff groups over the past five years have contributed to higher input costs, with benefits yet to be fully realised. This places the NHS between the slow uptake and solid progress spending paths in terms of input costs.

RESOURCES: INVESTMENT IN STAFF, PREMISES AND EQUIPMENT

The 2002 review echoed and, in some instances, exceeded the commitments of the government's 10-year NHS Plan of 2000 to invest substantially in additional staff, premises, hospital beds, equipment and IT systems. Chapter 7 evaluates progress towards meeting these commitments.

NHS Plan commitments to employ 7,500 more consultants, 2,000 more GPs, 20,000 more nurses and 6,500 more therapists (allied health professionals) by 2006 have been more than achieved, with targets exceeded by 16 per cent, 166 per cent, 272 per cent and 102 per cent respectively. However, the projections of the 2002 review suggest that even *more* staff, particularly in terms of full-time equivalent doctors, will be needed to cope with the predicted increasing demand for care by as early as 2008.

The government seems on track to deliver the NHS Plan targets of building 100 new hospitals and modernising more than 3,000 GP premises. However, it seems unlikely that the 2002 review's more ambitious aspirations to replace one-third of the hospital and community estate by 2022/3 and upgrade the entire primary care estate by 2010/1 will be met. Disappointingly, backlog maintenance increased by a fifth between 2000 and 2005 rather than declining by the one-quarter assumed at the time of the review.

As a result of investment in scanning equipment, around three-quarters of MRI scanners, CT scanners and linear accelerators now in use in the NHS are new, while targets for increased numbers of procedures have been exceeded.

The National Programme for IT (NPfIT) in the NHS is responsible for implementing an integrated care records service, an electronic prescribing system, an electronic appointment booking system and the underpinning IT infrastructure by 2014. The 2002 review identified better use of ICT as key to potential productivity improvements and health gains and recommended a doubling of ICT spend by 2003/4, peaking at around £2.7 billion in 2007/8 in the solid progress and fully engaged scenarios.

Given the well-documented delays that have beset the programme, it is not surprising that actual spending on ICT in England has followed neither the solid progress nor the fully engaged spending trajectories. Actual spending fell short of these projections by around £0.7 billion in 2003/4. Overall, it is estimated to have increased from £1 billion in 2002/3 to £2.3 billion in 2005/6. However, planned spending of just under £2.9 billion in 2006/7 would overshoot both those spending trajectories and so come closer to that assumed in the solid progress scenario.

The fact that actual spending fell short of these projections by around £0.7 billion in 2003/4 reflects the well-documented problems and delays that have beset the NPfIT and have the potential seriously to undermine the productivity gains envisaged by the 2002 review.

Resources: An overall assessment

Additional funding for the NHS over the past five years has enabled the service to invest in substantially increased resources – particularly labour. Staff numbers are at their highest for many years and have exceeded commitments made in the NHS Plan and adopted by the 2002 review. However, the 2002 review estimated that further increases in the number of doctors will be needed before the end of this decade to address anticipated extra demand. There has been substantial replacement and upgrading of buildings but no progress on reducing the maintenance backlog and some way to go on upgrading primary care premises and providing single rooms in hospitals.

Actual spending on modernisation of the NHS ICT infrastructure has followed neither the solid progress nor the fully engaged spending trajectories. And it has not been without its difficulties, with most progress tending to relate to systems that were not originally part of the modernisation plan. The well-documented problems and delays that have beset the

NPfIT have the potential to undermine seriously the productivity gains envisaged by the 2002 review. Future commitment not only to implementing core ICT systems but also to realising patient benefits and productivity gains is vital. The programme needs to be audited comprehensively to ensure that benefits will outweigh costs and to assess the precise impact on future productivity.

Overall, in terms of resources this places the NHS much closer to the solid progress scenario.

OUTPUTS: THE SERVICES DELIVERED

Chapter 8 examines how investment in human and other resources has been translated into activity in terms of hospital services, mental health care, primary care, prescribing and other activities, including NHS Direct, walk-in centres and ambulance services.

Between 1998 and 2005, overall elective (planned) admissions to hospital rose by just over 605,000 – an increase of 11 per cent. A decline of more than 4 per cent in the numbers of people treated as inpatients was more than offset by a 20 per cent increase in the numbers treated as day cases. However, the largest source of overall growth in hospital activity has been an increase in emergency admissions, with a net increase of around 1.6 million (35 per cent) admissions between 1998 and 2005. Attendances at A&E departments remained broadly static between 1987/8 and 2002/3 but have since grown by more than a third to nearly 19 million in 2005/6. These dramatic rises are hard to explain but were probably caused by changes in clinical behaviour and lower A&E waiting time targets, as well as changes in GPs' out-of-hour cover arrangements, which saw PCTs assume responsibility for out-of-hours care in 2004.

Since 2002/3 there has been a reduction in the number of new attendances at maternity outpatient departments, probably reflecting a shift to community-based antenatal care. Similarly, the number of episodes of consultant treatment and admissions related to mental illness fell by 10 per cent and 16 per cent respectively between 1998/9 and 2005/6, also reflecting a shift towards outpatient and/or community treatment. Crisis resolution/home treatment teams and other community-based services designed to manage acute episodes of mental illness were set up between 2001 and 2004, and the evidence suggests these innovations have been effective in reducing hospital admissions.

Attendance figures at GP surgeries – a key activity measure – are not routinely collated by the NHS at national level. The available (limited) data suggests that GP consultations rose by more than a third between the early 1980s and 2005; it stood at around 250 million in 2005. A lack of robust information relating to primary care makes it impossible to estimate activity since 2002/3.

Prescriptions dispensed rose by more than a fifth (135 million items) between 2002 and 2006, with drugs prescribed for cardiovascular conditions – particularly lipid-regulating statins – accounting for the lion's share of the growth but at a lower-than-expected cost. The 2002 review assumed an increase in UK NHS expenditure on lipid-regulating statins from around £700 million in 2002/3 to £2.1 billion by 2010. In fact, although the number of prescriptions for statins dispensed since 2002 has risen by 138 per cent to 39.7 million, the total cost has risen by just 0.3 per cent, with the real cost falling by almost 10 per cent. This is because of a significant increase in the prescribing of low-cost statins, such as simvastatin, which has reduced in cost by almost 90 per cent since 2002. Thus, the actual cost to the NHS of prescribing statins has diverged from the review's projections since 2004, resulting in a cumulative saving.

Calls to NHS Direct seem to have reached a plateau of just under 7 million a year, while NHS Direct Online, launched in 1999, has seen a rapid increase in use and currently receives about 1.5 million visits per month.

By May 2006 there were 75 walk-in centres in England, which cumulatively attracted more than 2.5 million visits in 2005/6.

Although emergency calls on the ambulance service in England nearly doubled to almost six million in the 10 years to 2005/6, the number of planned journeys fell, leading to an overall reduction in ambulance journeys.

Outputs: an overall assessment

With increased resources, the NHS has been able to do more work in most areas. Elective admissions increased by 7 per cent between 2002/3 and 2005/6 and outpatient attendances by 3 per cent. There have also been very large increases in emergency care (+21 per cent) and accident and emergency attendances (+33 per cent). Three-quarters of the 20 per cent increase in prescription items dispensed between 2002/3 and 2006/7 is due to just 10 drugs. Lipid-regulating drugs (statins) account for nearly a fifth of the total increase and are on target for achieving the 2002 review's recommendations at a lower-than-expected cost.

Overall, in terms of outputs, this places the NHS between slow uptake and solid progress.

OUTCOMES AND DETERMINANTS OF HEALTH

The 2002 review's vision was that the health of the population would improve through a combination of better, more responsive health services and changes in health-seeking behaviour. Chapter 9 examines the impact of recent health policy on known *determinants* of health – such as smoking, diet and other lifestyle behaviours; it also considers aspects of the care process that have an impact on health, and general measures of population health.

Broadly speaking, the health of the population has improved, with a fall in overall mortality rates and an increase in life expectancy, although both of these are continuations of long-term trends. It is estimated that by 2022 life expectancy at birth for both females and males is likely to exceed that envisaged in the slow uptake scenario and be marginally higher than for solid progress.

Cancer survival rates have also increased, and infant and perinatal mortality rates have improved a little since 2002, although they remain higher than for many other European countries. Various measures of morbidity, such as longstanding illness, remain unchanged. And inequalities between socio-economic groups, as measured by infant mortality and life expectancy at birth, have grown rather than diminished.

Public health expenditure

The 2002 review estimated health promotion expenditure in England at around £250 million – less than the NHS spends in a day and a half. All three scenarios projected an increase in health promotion spending, with the fully engaged scenario assuming the largest and most rapid rise, doubling to around £500 million by 2007/8. However, it is impossible to track trends in public health or health promotion spending since 2002 as no official figures are kept. Given the lack of accurate information, it is impossible to assess whether the fully engaged aspirations for a doubling in public health spending by 2007/8 have been met.

It is also indicative of the relatively low priority given to public health that, while non-public health medical staff numbers have increased by nearly 60 per cent since 1997, the number of public health consultants and registrars has gone down overall.

Investment in public health is designed to impact on the key determinants of health. A population's health is, of course, determined by many factors, including genetic inheritance, education and welfare services, income, housing and lifestyle choices. While there has been evidence of improvements in some areas, progress in other areas has been slow. Here four key factors are assessed: smoking, obesity, physical activity and diet.

Smoking

Smoking prevention has been successful in general, with England on track to achieve the 2010 targets set out in the government White Paper *Smoking Kills*. However, since the 2002 review, more demanding targets have been set and formalised as a Public Service Agreement (PSA). The 2004 PSA target is to reduce overall adult smoking rates to 21 per cent or less by 2010, with a reduction to 26 per cent or less for routine and manual socio-economic groups. The evidence suggests that England is on track to achieve these headline targets, but large variations between socio-economic groups persist. Progress to date on achieving national smoking targets therefore places England on a solid progress trajectory. Although the tougher targets set since the 2002 review exceed solid progress, they are less demanding than the fully engaged scenario.

Obesity

At the time of the 2002 review, the 1992 White Paper (*Health of the Nation*) target for obesity was for just 6 per cent of men and 8 per cent of women to be classified as obese by 2005. Between 1995 and 2005 the proportion of adult males classified as obese rose by half to 23 per cent of the male population, while the proportion of obese women rose by 42 per cent to around 25 per cent of the female population. Childhood (2–15 years) obesity increased by a similar extent over this period, with the proportion of obese boys and girls rising by 65 per cent and 51 per cent respectively; nearly one in five children are classified as obese. A continuing rising trend in obesity to 2010 is predicted, when some 33 per cent of men, 28 per cent of women, one-fifth of boys and more than one-fifth of girls will be obese. The evidence on obesity is therefore of great concern and while it would be wrong to hold the NHS responsible for this adverse trend, it does mean in terms of achievement that the results are now at a much worse level than even the slow uptake scenario.

Physical activity and diet

Since 1996, the government has recommended that adults should participate in at least 30 minutes of moderately intense activity five days a week. Over a third of men and a quarter of women met these guidelines in 2004, an improvement since 1997. Progress has also been made in increasing children's physical activity. Eighty per cent of pupils in partnership schools – those participating in a national school sports initiative – participate in at least two hours of high-quality physical education and school sport in a typical week – an increase of 11 per cent over the previous year and an improvement on the 2006 target. While progress has been made on salt consumption with rates falling, they remain 50 per cent higher than the recommended 6g per day.

The government is on track with its children's activity targets and may also achieve its interim target for adults, but this will require sustained effort up to and beyond 2011. At best this could be classified as solid progress. This mirrors progress made on diet which is on a solid progress trajectory at best, but is probably somewhere between this and slow uptake.

Process of care

While survey evidence suggests an improvement in patient safety, rates of MRSA infection in hospitals remain high, and other hospital-acquired infections, such as *Clostridium difficile,* may pose an even larger threat in future.

Waiting times for inpatient and outpatient treatment have improved considerably since the last review, although this is unlikely to have had a substantial impact on health outcomes.

Evidence from surveys on patient experiences suggests that the quality of NHS care has been improving over time, particularly in areas of the service that have been subject to co-ordinated action – for example, waiting times and cancer care.

Health outcomes and determinants of health: an overall assessment

The 2002 review's vision was that health would improve through a combination of better and more responsive health care services and changes in health-seeking behaviour. On broad measures, the health of the population has improved. Tackling the causes of ill health is an ongoing long-term task. Continuing reductions in smoking and improvements in levels of physical activity and diet suggest a future close to the solid progress scenario. But over-optimistic targets – such as those relating to obesity – make it difficult to assess engagement levels in relation to the 2002 review scenarios. In addition, tackling recent financial difficulties in the NHS by raiding public health budgets has not been in the long-term interests of the public health of the nation.

Overall, the evidence suggests that the population is a long way short of the fully engaged scenario and is on a path between slow uptake and solid progress.

PRODUCTIVITY: EFFICIENCY AND QUALITY

A crucial issue for the 2002 review, with a significant impact on its funding projections, was the ability to do more (in both volume and quality terms) with each health care pound. Higher productivity offered the potential to restrict growth in the long-term costs of delivering the health care outcomes likely to be sought by 2022.

The 2002 review made an important distinction between two aspects of productivity it assumed would improve over time: those relating to inputs (that is, reductions in unit costs) and those related to outputs or outcomes (that is, improved quality). Chapter 10 attempts to clarify the meaning of productivity, as distinct from efficiency, and goes on to track recent changes in NHS productivity, taking account of quality outcomes as well as unit costs.

It was assumed that under the solid progress and fully engaged scenarios, productivity would improve by 2–2.5 per cent a year in the first decade and 3 per cent in the second. The slow uptake scenario predicted lower productivity improvements of 1.5 and 1.75 per cent a year respectively. The importance of these assumptions becomes evident when they are converted into monetary terms. In the fully engaged and solid progress scenarios, the value of the productivity gains by 2022/3 (at 2002/3 prices) amounts to £46.5 billion – around half of the additional forecast growth in spending over and above the 2002/3 level of £68 billion.

Official measures of NHS productivity are inconclusive and indicate that changes in productivity may have ranged from -7.5 per cent to + 8.5 per cent between 1999 and 2004. The 2002 review's assumptions of annual unit cost reductions of 0.75–1 per cent between 2002/3 and 2007/8 have not been achieved and, broadly, unit costs have increased for all hospital services. Lack of data makes it impossible to draw reliable conclusions about movements in unit costs in mental health and primary care services. However, the cost per prescription dispensed in the community has fallen significantly, largely because of reduced unit costs for lipid-regulating statins, which were available in new generic forms from 2003.

Some attempts to quantify changes in quality over time (in relation to the increased use of statins, for example) suggest significant gains. However, the development of precise measures is hampered by a lack of routinely collected data on changes in patients' health status arising from NHS interventions.

Although indicative measures of quality, such as patient safety, waiting times and satisfaction with the experience of care, suggest improvement, 'hard' measures of quality, valued in monetary terms, are not available to compare with the 2002 review's assumption that the quality of care would improve year on year.

Productivity: an overall assessment
Official measures of NHS productivity provide inconclusive evidence of improvement.

The 2002 review's productivity assumptions of annual unit cost reductions of 0.75–1 per cent between 2002/3 and 2007/8 have not been achieved; broadly, unit costs have increased for all hospital services. Although indicative measures of quality, such as waiting times, and patient satisfaction, suggest improvement, 'hard' measures of quality, valued in monetary terms, are not available to compare with the review's assumption that the quality of care would improve year on year.

Some evidence suggests that the failure to reduce unit costs may have been partially offset by improved quality. However, the NHS has failed to generate the relatively modest improvements in unit cost productivity that might have been expected and were assumed by the 2002 review. Overall, in terms of productivity, this places the NHS closer to the slow uptake scenario.

The policy framework
This section considers whether the health policies that the government has pursued over the past 10 years have supported or hindered the improvements in NHS performance envisaged by the 2002 review. It examines how effective the policy process has been and

whether health policy is moving in the right direction – or whether there is a better alternative. The chapter on policy examines four main routes to improvement, comparing developments in these areas with the recommendations of the 2002 and 2004 reviews, where relevant, and assessing their impact on performance.

The effectiveness of government policy-making in this area has been judged against the government's own criteria for good policy-making, as well as against recommendations made in both the 2002 and 2004 reviews. It is important to note that the 2002 review did not offer a policy blueprint for the government to follow and did not recommend a deviation in policy direction from the NHS Plan. In addition, while the review points to various shortcomings, it must constantly be borne in mind that change does take time and that in many cases it may be too early to tell whether improvements will be realised over the next few years.

Policy development

The New Labour administration that came to power in 1997 initially relied heavily on central direction, with improvements, such as waiting list reductions, enforced through national targets. However, from 2002 a new approach was gradually developed, aiming to:

- reduce central targets and allocate a larger share of NHS budget directly to local purchasers, with incentives to improve performance
- give patients a bigger voice and a greater role in self-care
- promote diversity of supply by introducing independent providers
- improve monitoring arrangements and reduce risks to health.

In broad terms, this new policy framework was in line with the recommendations of the 2002 and 2004 reviews. But how effectively was it implemented – and has it improved NHS performance? The review looks for answers to these questions across a range of policy initiatives, including patient choice, new elective care provision, financial incentives, new commissioning arrangements, personal engagement in health, and Payment by Results.

The review concludes that, although the move away from centralised governance was sensible, implementation of the new framework has been slow and uncertain, with some critical areas, particularly the financial framework, remaining work in progress.

With some initiatives, such as patient choice, not yet fully implemented and others, such as practice-based commissioning, not fully worked out, the new policy framework has had only a modest impact, while targets and central direction have remained the main drivers in the system.

In terms of public health, policy formation has not followed the framework proposed by the 2004 review. Instead, piecemeal, often modest initiatives have continued to emerge.

Organisational change

Since 2002, the government has introduced radical structural changes to the NHS, including abolition of health authorities, creation of strategic health authorities, creation and subsequent re-creation of primary care trusts, introduction of foundation trusts and a strengthening of the regulatory framework.

The new structure embodies a number of the key features proposed in the 2002 review and has a good chance of being more effective than its predecessor; but because it has taken so long to emerge, it remains largely untested with its benefits yet to be realised.

The review also points out that the process of organisational change has been costly, not just financially but in terms of disruption, loss of experienced staff and changes in working relationships both within the NHS and with external organisations.

Service redesign

The NHS Plan of 2000 committed the government to a massive programme of capital investment in hospitals and smaller premises. Other elements of service redesign have included:

- cancer care collaboratives and other learning programmes
- national service frameworks (NSFs)
- initiatives to shift care from hospitals to community settings.

The review concludes that the government was right to make service redesign a key policy objective to improve service quality, costs and access, although it has not yet committed itself to a continuing programme of NSF development as envisaged in the 2002 review.

Question marks remain over the robustness of the evidence for the different types of hospital reconfiguration that are needed to raise quality and about how far hospital services can be transferred to other locations without loss of quality or increased costs. The review emphasises the need for flexibility in the light of uncertainty over the future balance of care, particularly with regards to the government's commitment to the rapid development of new hospitals.

Support programmes

The NHS Plan and the 2002 review recognised that a number of supporting elements were needed to underpin policy and service reforms. These included:

- staff reforms, including large increases in the workforce, changes in role mix and the introduction of new contracts
- implementation of a comprehensive information and communication technology (ICT) programme
- introduction of systematic clinical governance processes to support the improvement of clinical care.

Important flexibilities within the workforce have been achieved, but the reform of the NHS pay structure through three new major pay deals for consultants, GPs and nurses and other non-clinical staff have been costly and has yet to prove itself in terms of improved performance and productivity.

Implementation of the ICT programme has been slow, with its main anticipated benefits not yet achieved. And, although clinical governance now comprises a wide range of policies at individual, service and organisational levels, their specific impact on performance is hard to detect.

How effective has the policy process been?

The review makes two key criticisms.

- Pressure to produce quick results has led to some policies and initiatives being introduced without adequate preparation. For example, policies on the management of long-term conditions were introduced with little prior evaluation; NHS Direct was implemented nationally before the results of pilot studies were available; and the early design of the Payment by Results system took too little account of international experience.

- The government has failed to take full account of the impact of new policies on the system as a whole and to understand how the various elements fit together with each other and with the various resources. These failures were key to the system-wide deficits that emerged from 2004/5 onwards. They are also evident in the shift from hospital to community care, which threatens the economics of acute hospitals.

Is policy moving in the right direction?

The review acknowledges a number of major successes, including:

- identifying more local ways to manage health policy while retaining central direction in key areas

- establishing an improved performance assessment regime with a new regulatory structure, comprising of the Healthcare Commission, Monitor and the Audit Commission, looking stronger than its predecessor

- offering sustained support for self-care and beginning to address the needs of people with long-term conditions

- consistently promoting the need for service redesign and supporting the creation of flexibility in professional roles

- promoting a wide range of measures aimed at improving the quality and cost-effectiveness of clinical care.

The NHS is now in better shape than in 2002 to deliver improved quality and increased productivity, although huge challenges remain around commissioning and choice, competition between providers, the balance between targets, standards and incentives and between central direction and local discretion, and the shift towards local provision of care.

However, the new policy framework deserves only conditional approval at this stage as it will be some time before a clear view can emerge about its effectiveness. And, even if the general direction is right, there can be no guarantee that sufficiently improved performance, in terms of outcomes or productivity, will be achieved at the levels required by the solid progress or fully engaged scenarios of the 2002 review.

The 2007 review identifies two significant issues that the government still needs to get to grips with:
- improved demand management across the NHS as a whole
- full clinical engagement in the process of policy reform.

Is there a better alternative to the current system?

The review concludes that it would be dangerous to embark on further significant change before the new combination of levers to enhance performance has had a chance to prove itself.

The emphasis now should be on developing the new policy framework rather than subjecting it to further fundamental reform. Although changes in policy and practice must continue, structural change should be avoided wherever possible.

The review makes a range of recommendations designed to address some of the problems identified and help take forward policy on health and social care. These are summarised in the following section.

Recommendations

The review includes a number of inter-related recommendations designed to help the government take forward policy on health and social care and address some of the shortfalls identified.

CONTINUE TO ENCOURAGE USE OF RECENT SYSTEM REFORMS TO ACHIEVE THE DESIRED RESULTS

- Commissioners should be encouraged to use available data and processes more effectively to design and monitor outcome-based policies for a range of health service providers. Information should be made available to help local commissioning bodies commission services in the most appropriate ways, incorporating best practice in health and social care.

MONITOR AND ASSESS POLICY AND PERFORMANCE

- Policy-making and implementation has been weak in a number of key respects since 2002. The government needs to strengthen its analytic capacities to monitor the effectiveness of its policies, and be prepared to change direction or pace if policies are unlikely to have the desired impact. In so doing, it needs to take full account of the impact of further change and consider how best to manage any potentially negative effects. In addressing weaknesses, the government must strengthen its capacity to link clinical and service objectives with the resources needed to achieve them.

- Given the potentially high costs of local service reconfiguration, detailed research should be carried out into new models of delivery before they are implemented to assess their impact on patients and their cost effectiveness. Rules about failure of institutions and services that prove unable to generate adequate income as services are reconfigured around them should be clarified before significant commitments are made by local commissioners and providers. It is also recommended that a primary care experiment recommended by the 2004 Wanless review, to assess the benefits of additional resource in information systems, in monitoring risk and in services, be carried out to provide important learning for the future.

- ICT deliverables are critical to many future productivity and service enhancements. However, despite some positive developments, there have been serious criticisms about the implementation of the Connecting for Health programme. Connecting for Health should be subject to detailed external scrutiny and reporting so that forecasts of long-term costs and benefits can be made with more confidence.

PRODUCE REGULAR LONG-TERM RESOURCE ESTIMATES

- There are good reasons for carrying out forecasting exercises on a regular basis, given the long-term nature of many decisions that need to be taken; and the use of scenarios to capture variations in health status, choices and demands makes for a robust approach. The Treasury/Department of Health should establish a mechanism for commissioning and publishing regular independent estimates of the long-term resources likely to be needed for health and social care services either on a five-yearly basis or ahead of each comprehensive spending review. All forecasts should include ranges based on different scenarios, and the forecasting models used in this work should be made publicly available.

- In order to forecast resource requirements it is necessary to define the scope and nature of the health and social care services to be funded. Updated and new National Service Frameworks (NSFs), incorporating costings, resource requirements and research needs, should form the basis of centrally determined standards for health care. The combination of all the NSFs should enable commissioners use a range of local levers to achieve national standards. The meanings of 'comprehensive' and 'high-quality' are not yet defined for social care, and a work programme should be established to fill the huge gap this creates in understanding the long-term financial implications of an ageing population.

- Data that would assist the monitoring of NHS performance remain so limited that some central questions about the relationship between costs and outcomes cannot be answered. The Health and Social Care Information Centre should work with those commissioned to produce long-term resource forecasts, relevant analysts within the Department of Health and the Treasury, and other researchers, to define improvement to health and social care information that could assist the modelling of future spending forecasts.

- Future forecasting of long-term resource requirements in health and social care should pay particular attention to the workforce plans produced by the Department of Health. This will allow for an assessment of whether sufficient staff will be available, able to deliver the volumes of services likely to be needed and also to capitalise on the systems designed to help them produce the required standards of service and efficiency. Full-scale evaluations of the recently introduced staff contracts should be carried out to assist national and local efforts to obtain adequate benefits from them.

MEASURE AND MANAGE PRODUCTIVITY

- Assessment of future productivity is important because public perceptions about how productively resources are used will continue to influence attitudes towards health and social care services. Incentive systems to improve productivity should focus on clinical quality and health outcomes, and the present system of incentives and standards should be progressively developed and refined in the light of experience of their impact. Continuing work into productivity should consider the whole system.

- Although nationwide surveys record the population's self-assessed health status, no equivalent information is collected routinely on NHS patients. Recorded measures of individual health status would aid measurement of productivity and performance as well as helping purchasers and individuals make decisions about prevention, treatment and commissioning. Large-scale trials should be carried out to explore the potential benefits and costs of routinely recording the health status of people treated and advised by all providers working for the NHS.

A framework for public health
- The 2004 Wanless review recommended a conceptual framework to take forward public health in England in a systematic way. It envisaged quantified national objectives for changing the prevalence of all the important determinants of health status for the medium and long term, based on advice from a wide range or organisations and people. This framework was not taken forward and, as a result, health policy has remained focused on short-term imperatives, public health practitioners feel undervalued and significant opportunities have been lost. It is recommended that the recommendations of the 2004 review be now implemented.

Conclusion

The five years since the 2002 Wanless review have witnessed unprecedented levels of government investment in the NHS – real spending has risen by nearly 50 per cent, while the proportion of the UK's GDP devoted to health care spending has grown to 9–10 per cent, within striking distance of the EU average. This rate of funding growth broadly matches the recommendations of the 2002 review for the first five years of its spending trajectories.

The funding increase has helped to deliver some clear and notable improvements – more staff and equipment; improved infrastructure; significantly reduced waiting times and better access to care; and improved care in coronary heart disease, cancer, stroke and mental health. Although difficult to attribute directly to the NHS, life expectancy has also continued to improve.

Our Future Health Secured? concludes that the direction of health care policy now being pursued by the government should be correct to address the key challenges identified in the 2002 review.

However, what is clear is that thus far the additional funding has not produced the improvements in productivity assumed in the 2002 review – costs of providing health services have increased and there is patchy and conflicting evidence on the impact on productivity overall, including little information about community-based care. Hospital activity has increased, but the biggest increase has been in emergency, rather than planned, admissions. In addition, some key measures of the determinants of ill health are below the assumptions of the 2002 review, particularly the unforeseen rise in adult and childhood obesity.

Even with higher productivity and greater engagement by individuals in their own health, funding for health services will need to increase substantially. However, without significant improvements in NHS productivity, and efforts to tackle key determinants of ill health, such as obesity, even higher levels of funding will be needed over the next two decades to deliver the high-quality services envisaged by the 2002 Wanless review. Such an expensive service could undermine the current widespread political support for the NHS and raise questions about its long-term future.

Foreword

The report *Securing our Future Health,* commissioned from Derek Wanless by the Treasury in 2002 has proved to be a seminal work. In part that is because it marked a turning point in attitudes towards the funding of the National Health Service, creating a widespread consensus that health care in this country had been significantly under-resourced for many years. Equally important, it provided the first comprehensive, evidence-based assessment of what funding would be needed to create a sustainable and world class health care system, and ultimately a healthier nation.

The report concluded that over the next 20 years the United Kingdom would need to devote substantially more resources to the health care system to ensure high-quality services capable of meeting public expectations. It also argued that additional funding would have to be matched by fundamental reform to enable those resources to be used effectively.

Over the five years since the publication of the 2002 review, NHS funding has increased by almost 50 per cent in real terms. At the same time, the UK government, which has responsibility for the NHS in England, has pursued a major programme of reform.

Now, five years on, the inevitable questions have started to be raised. Has the government's strategy in England delivered the improvements that were expected? Has the level of funding matched the projections in the 2002 report? Has the pace of reform been sufficient to ensure value for money for the extra investment?

Sir Derek had recommended in the 2002 review that further reviews of future resource requirements should be a regular exercise and that it would be appropriate to carry out such a review after five years. However, this was one recommendation the government has yet to take forward.

Earlier this year the King's Fund asked Sir Derek to lead a team to go some way towards addressing this omission by undertaking a retrospective review of NHS spending five years on from his original report. It builds on the major work the Fund commissioned from Sir Derek on the future funding of social care for older people in England in 2006. However, it is not the full, forward-looking review of the future funding needs of the NHS as originally envisaged by Sir Derek, and this report argues there is still a need for such a review.

Nevertheless, the timing of this report is significant. The huge injections of extra funds year after year will certainly slow from 2008, making it even more important to determine how the additional funding has been used, what it has achieved and, critically, what lessons we can learn for the future.

The funding of health care has been a constant political issue for the past 60 years and is likely to remain so for the foreseeable future. But for now the debate has changed. The traditional explanation that underfunding lay behind underperformance has become less tenable, and as we go forward there is likely to be less discussion about the level of funding and more about whether it is being spent wisely. And that in turn will lead to fundamental questions about the nature of our health care system.

The challenge is a simple one – if we are to sustain a system that is comprehensive, tax funded and free at the point of delivery we will need to be clear about what we want to achieve for this massive investment and be able to demonstrate that is being delivered. We hope this report will be an important contribution to that thinking.

Niall Dickson
Chief Executive
King's Fund

Preface

What health outcomes will be possible in future? What resources will we need to achieve them, in health care and elsewhere? How can we minimise the costs and how do we decide how much is justified? How do we create the flexibility to react when, inevitably, circumstances change? Are we willing and able, both individually and collectively, to meet the cost?

These questions need to be asked repeatedly about our health services and answered with the help of the best information possible. How much of a country's wealth to devote to health care is one of the most important and difficult policy questions for all governments. Pressures to spend more on health care are considerable. Across OECD countries health care spending has nearly doubled over the past 20 years, to around 12 per cent of gross domestic product (GDP). As countries' wealth increases, the spending of choice is on health care.

Historically, the United Kingdom had lagged behind; but the public's desire to spend more on health care was recognised in the political decision taken at the turn of this century to commit to a step change in investment in the National Health Service. An integral part of this commitment was the Chancellor's decision in 2001 to commission a review of future NHS funding to 2022/3.

It was the first time such long-term work on health care funding for the United Kingdom had been carried out. The review (Wanless 2002) showed the need for substantial increases in NHS spending and illustrated the significant variations that could be achieved by better productivity and prevention. A further review (Wanless 2004) explored in more depth how to achieve the public health improvements set out in the most optimistic future spending scenario.

The level of previous (under-) funding had been a focus of discontent about the NHS. But the first review (Wanless 2002) recognised that success could not be guaranteed simply by increasing spending. Radical reform was also vital; and no amount of additional funding would succeed unless such underlying problems as excessively long waiting times, poor access in general, poor quality and outcomes of care were tackled and resolved to the satisfaction of patients and the public.

It is now five years since the original review (Wanless 2002) was published. In that time real spending on the NHS has increased by nearly 50 per cent, and the United Kingdom now devotes around 9–10 per cent of its GDP to all health care spending. The questions this report aims to answer are:
- how has that extra money been spent?
- what has the NHS achieved?
- has government policy promoted effective use of resources?
- what lessons have been learned for the future?

Structure of this report

Part 1 of this report sets out the background, summarises the findings of the two previous reviews (Wanless 2002, 2004), encapsulates the empirical findings described in detail in Part 2, assesses current government health policy and makes recommendations for the future, including a reaffirmation of the importance of conducting regular and detailed assessments of future health and social care resource requirements.

Part 2 presents detailed evidence about what has actually been spent on the NHS since 2002 and what it has achieved in terms of resources, services, productivity and, crucially, health benefits.

Derek Wanless

Part 1 →
Review and recommendations

1 Overview

Introduction

This chapter summarises the objectives and key findings of the 2002 review, set up to consider the resources likely to be needed by the NHS for the next two decades, and a subsequent review focusing on its implications for public health.

It then sets out the rationale for the current review. This was established to look at how the funding increased in line with the 2002 review was spent, what it has achieved in terms of services and health outcomes and what lessons can be learned to inform future reviews.

Closing the gaps: the 2002 review

In March 2001, the Chancellor of the Exchequer commissioned a review to examine future health trends in the United Kingdom and the resources likely to be needed over the next two decades. The government's aim was to close the unacceptable performance gaps both within the United Kingdom and between the United Kingdom and other developed countries.

The terms of reference were:

1. *To examine the technological, demographic and medical trends over the next two decades that may affect the health service in the UK as a whole.*

2. *In the light of (1), to identify the key factors which will determine the financial and other resources required to ensure that the NHS can provide a publicly funded, comprehensive, high quality service available on the basis of clinical need and not ability to pay.*

3. *To report to the Chancellor by April 2002, to allow him to consider the possible implications of this analysis for the Government's wider fiscal and economic strategies in the medium term; and to inform decisions in the next public spending Review in 2002.*

   The report will take account of the devolved nature of health spending in the UK and the Devolved Administrations will be invited to participate in the Review.
   (Wanless 2002)

The review concentrated on the outcomes to be achieved by the health service, and its conclusions were based on the vision (widely supported in consultation) that health services in 2022 should provide better access, higher-quality care in comfortable surroundings and a more patient-centred service, including the availability of greater choice. However, the short-term priorities were to improve safety, increase capacity and reduce waiting times.

TABLE 1: SPENDING PROJECTIONS UNDER DIFFERENT SCENARIOS: OVERALL SUMMARY

	Scenarios		
	Solid progress	**Slow uptake**	**Fully engaged**
Scenario description	Population becomes more 'engaged' with factors to improve their health. Life expectancy increases, health status improves and people have confidence in the primary care system and use it more appropriately. The health service becomes more responsive, with high rates of technology take-up, extensive use of ICT and more efficient use of resources.	There is no change in the level of public engagement. Life expectancy rises, but by the smallest amount of all scenarios. The health status of the population is constant or deteriorates. The health service is relatively unresponsive, with low rates of technology uptake and low productivity.	Levels of public engagement in relation to their health are high. Life expectancy rises considerably, health status improves dramatically and people are confident in the health system and demand high-quality care. The health service is responsive with high rates of technology uptake, particularly in relation to disease prevention. Use of resources is more efficient.
Spending projections	By 2022/3 total health spend (including private spend of 1.2% of GDP) increases to 11.1% of GDP, actual NHS spending rising to £161 billion in 2002/3 prices – 137% real growth on 2002/3.	By 2022/3 total health spend (including private spend of 1.2% of GDP) increases to 12.5% of GDP, actual NHS spending rising to £184 billion in 2002/3 prices – 171% real growth on 2002/3.	By 2022/3 total health spend (including private spend of 1.2% of GDP) increases to 10.6% of GDP, actual NHS spending rising to £154 billion in 2002/3 prices – 126% real growth on 2002/3.

Note: All figures are based on original 2002 Wanless Review; changes in estimates of GDP and economy-wide inflation as measured by the GDP deflator mean that real spend figures have changed.

The resulting report, published in April 2002, set out three possible spending paths for health care up to 2022/3, each derived from different assumptions about the effectiveness of NHS performance and the health status of the population. Detailed assumptions are shown in Appendix 1, pp 251–5. The review also made recommendations about the most effective uses of the extra resources, summarised in Appendix 2, pp 257–9. Its final recommendation was that similar reviews should be carried out periodically.

The business of making such long-term projections is fraught with uncertainty, but there are good reasons for doing so on a regular basis. A long-term perspective is needed to inform many resourcing decisions, such as the number of people to be trained, the skills they will require, the types of building likely to be needed and the information and communication technologies upon which the efficient operation of the whole system will depend.

The 2002 review aimed to help provide greater stability in the funding and delivery of health care. Annual changes in real health care spending had varied substantially over the preceding 40 years and this instability had presented a serious barrier to long-term planning. A long-term view, combined with adequate resources, was expected to help deliver more effective management; for good management depends on clarity about the long-term, strategic direction of the service coupled with the flexibility to respond appropriately to changes as they occur.

The 2002 review identified the following main influences on the resources needed:

- commitments already made to improve the quality of the health service and its consistency in the NHS Plan (Department of Health 2000a) and the National Service Frameworks (NSFs)
- changing patient and public expectations
- advances in medical technologies
- changing health needs of the population
- prices for health services resources, including skilled staff
- productivity improvement that might be achieved.

The review employed three different 'scenarios' in its cost estimates to take account of possible variations in two key factors: the level of public engagement with health and the level of productivity the health service could achieve. Detailed descriptions of these scenarios and their implications for health spending are given in Table 1, opposite. *Solid progress* was a scenario of steady and significant improvement, with public health targets met, performance gaps closed and life expectancy continuing to grow fairly rapidly. Two other scenarios, *slow uptake* (the most expensive and least satisfactory) and *fully engaged* (the least expensive but most ambitious) were devised to illustrate the need for higher or lower long-term patterns of expenditure, as shown in Figure 1, below. The estimates for each scenario showed the level of resources needed first to 'catch up' with best practice and then to ensure the United Kingdom could 'keep up'. Estimates were also made about the levels of human and physical resources needed to deliver a comprehensive and high-quality service.

Spending over the first five-year period was forecast to grow by an average annual real rate of between 7.1 and 7.3 per cent, with little difference between the scenarios because the

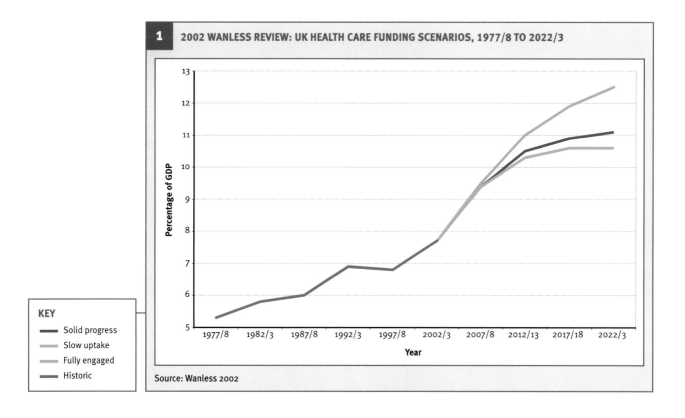

1   2002 WANLESS REVIEW: UK HEALTH CARE FUNDING SCENARIOS, 1977/8 TO 2022/3

KEY
- Solid progress
- Slow uptake
- Fully engaged
- Historic

Source: Wanless 2002

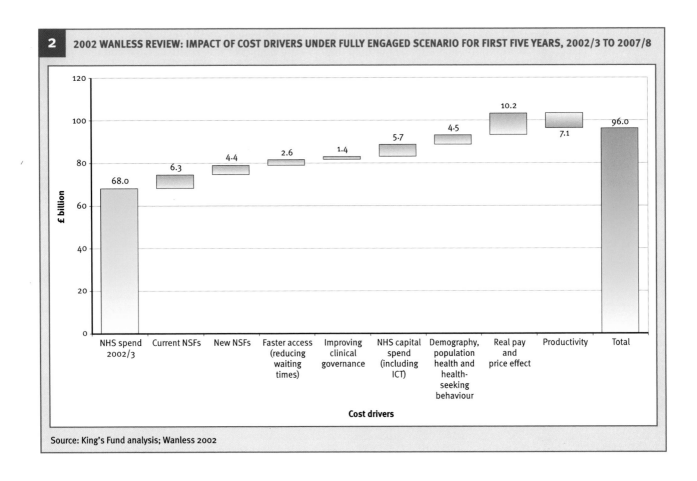

2 2002 WANLESS REVIEW: IMPACT OF COST DRIVERS UNDER FULLY ENGAGED SCENARIO FOR FIRST FIVE YEARS, 2002/3 TO 2007/8

Source: King's Fund analysis; Wanless 2002

forecast was limited by the skilled resources available and set at the upper limit of what could reasonably be spent. Aiming for too-rapid activity growth risked hitting capacity constraints and driving up costs, while aiming too low would mean delaying much-needed improvements in quality and access. Spending growth was predicted to fall in the later years, particularly with the more ambitious scenarios, because it was assumed that 'catch-up' had been achieved and public health improved by better engagement.

Figures 2–4 show the relative importance of the various cost drivers considered by the 2002 review in projecting NHS spending over 5, 10 and 20 years under the fully engaged scenario. These figures have been derived from the results of the modelling exercise undertaken as part of the review's final report and incorporate the review's assumptions about the roll-out of new National Service Frameworks across other disease areas (Wanless 2002).

These 'broad brush' illustrations show that, over the two decades covered by the 2002 review, the factors with the largest impact on the overall increase in projected spending were the new NSFs, increases in real pay for NHS staff and faster access, while productivity improvements produced significant savings. Included in the overall spending estimates for new NSFs were resources devoted to capital spend, to potential pay and price effects and to reducing waiting times. Information was not available to disaggregate the estimated spending on new NSFs into its component parts. The slight fall in projected spending on the original NSFs in 2022/3 is due to lower spending on coronary heart disease as a result of higher spending on preventive measures – particularly statins.

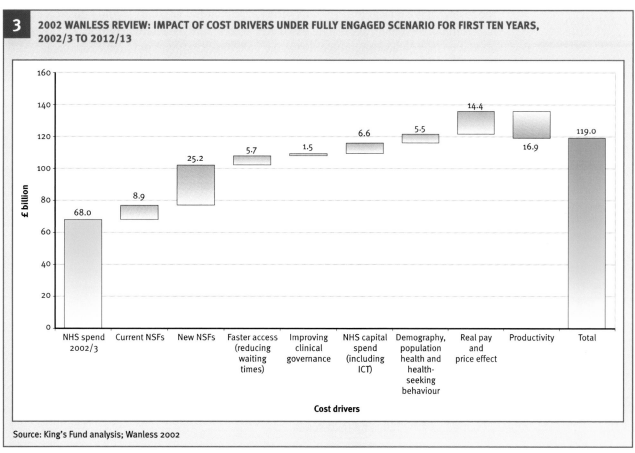

3   2002 WANLESS REVIEW: IMPACT OF COST DRIVERS UNDER FULLY ENGAGED SCENARIO FOR FIRST TEN YEARS, 2002/3 TO 2012/13

Source: King's Fund analysis; Wanless 2002

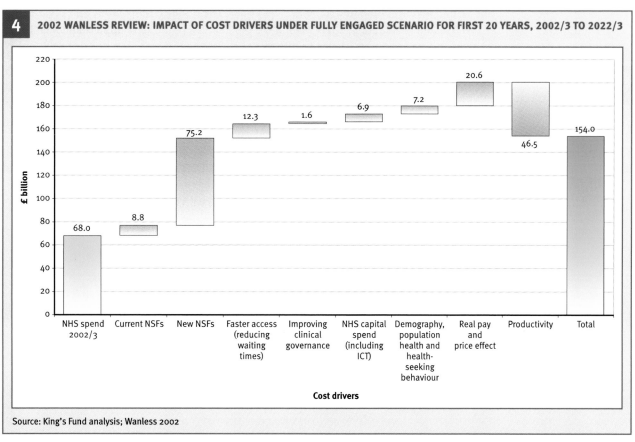

4   2002 WANLESS REVIEW: IMPACT OF COST DRIVERS UNDER FULLY ENGAGED SCENARIO FOR FIRST 20 YEARS, 2002/3 TO 2022/3

Source: King's Fund analysis; Wanless 2002

The review made it clear that spending the recommended amounts would not succeed in transforming the health service unless it was accompanied by radical reform. The review did not go into detail about the policies the government should pursue to keep health spending and performance in line with the assumptions behind its projections; nor did it explicitly endorse all the proposals set out in the NHS Plan (Department of Health 2000a). However, it did set out in broad terms how health care policy should be developed and included a number of more specific recommendations for policy-makers.

Public health and inequalities: the 2004 review

The fully engaged scenario clearly captured the government's preferred future for health care; it was the least expensive but promised to deliver the best health outcomes. Public health and productivity were considered the crucial issues, and in 2003 a further review, focusing on public health in England, was commissioned. The review team was asked to:

- recommend cost-effective approaches to improving public health, preventing ill health and reducing health inequalities in line with the public health aspects of the fully engaged scenario outlined in the first review (Wanless 2002)

- help enlist support from across government and other agencies in addressing these issues

- advise on whether the delivery plan to implement the government's cross-cutting review on tackling health inequalities, and other follow-up action (including national and local public health delivery plans) was consistent with delivering the public health aspects of the fully engaged scenario.

This further review, published in 2004, focused on the public health aspects of the first review's recommendations, set against a historical background of relative public health inaction and a dearth of evidence to inform policy (Wanless 2004). The 2004 review concluded that the key challenges were delivery and implementation, not further discussion. The main threats to future health, such as smoking, obesity and health inequalities, needed to be tackled immediately. Where evidence existed on the cost-effectiveness of public health interventions, it should be used to inform action. Where there was no such evidence, promising ideas should be piloted and evaluated, with appropriate action taken to continue or abandon policy. To achieve the fully engaged scenario would require a step change in effort and achievement.

The review defined public health in very broad terms, with many organisations as well as individuals having important roles to play. Although many of the benefits of such engagement were long term, there were also some immediate and short-term benefits that could reduce demand for health services.

The 2004 review was based on the premise that, although people are ultimately responsible for their own health and that of their children, many need more active support in discharging this responsibility. People have to make up their own minds about whether they wish to be fully engaged in public health, but the government has many levers to influence behaviour. The review produced a framework to aid policy formulation and practical implementation, often at local level.

The review was critical of the way in which targets had been set for key determinants of health, both for the whole population and for important sub-groups. It concluded that quantified national objectives for all the important determinants of health status would aid future resource planning as well as immediate decision-making. The government was recommended to seek advice about what those objectives should be, paying particular attention to those key to reducing health inequalities.

Other recommendations included:

- tackling gaps in activity between the various bodies with a public health role. The crucial relationship between the respective public health roles of NHS and local government had remained difficult because of capacity problems, the impact of organisational changes and the lack of alignment of performance management mechanisms between partners

- creating an adequate workforce capacity, with appropriately broad and changing skill mixes, and with self-care, 'expert patients' and community pharmacists identified as potential improvers of productivity. Information management and technology promised to be a massive driver of change, its high costs partly justified by its potential to identify personal risks

- establishing evidence for the pros and cons of a radical change in primary care.

The overall conclusion of the review was that the activity under way could put England (the nation studied) on course for the solid progress scenario as far as public health was concerned, but a step change would be needed to move to a fully engaged path. The recommendations, listed in Appendix 3, pp 261–2, were designed to create the support for this step change.

The current review looks at what has happened to resources made available for public health since 2004 and how much of the recommended framework has been introduced.

Where the money went: the current review

Both previous reviews pointed to the need for better information and indicated where improvements could be made. In producing this analysis of NHS funding since 2002, the best available information and research has been used. In some areas, however, because of the time it takes to produce evidence – for example, the lag between the health care activity and its impact on population health – the analysis has been constrained by a lack of information. The approach has therefore been to make use of what limited evidence there is to work out whether the policy and organisational shifts since 2002 are consistent with the assumptions and recommendations of the 2002 and 2004 reviews.

This review does not seek either to re-work projections for likely resource requirements to 2022/3 or to extend estimates further into the future. Rather the purpose has been to find out what lessons can be learned and to work these into conclusions designed to assist government in managing our health services and making detailed forecasts.

The key questions arising from the 2002 review for this report are:

- **Funding** Did health care resources increase in line with the recommendations of the 2002 review, and what are the prospects for funding up to 2022/3?

- **Use of resources** Where did the money go, and what has been achieved for the additional NHS investment in terms of resource inputs, outputs and, most crucially, outcomes?

- **Effectiveness** Have the additional resources allocated to the NHS been used effectively and in line with the 2002 review's observations about standard-setting, processes and delivery in the NHS? If not, why not?

- **Policy framework** What have the major decisions taken in these areas since 2002 sought to achieve? What have been the positive effects, the negative impacts and the unintended consequences? Have these decisions produced health and public health systems that put us on track for an optimistic future?

- **Future reviews** What lessons can be learned from this analysis of the actions taken since 2002 to inform similar reviews in future?

Cutting across all these areas are questions about the underlying assumptions made by the 2002 review concerning, for example, future productivity gains, health-seeking behaviour and so on. How realistic do those assumptions look in the light of experience? Have the public health recommendations of the 2004 review been implemented and what progress is England making on the major determinants of health and health inequalities?

The next chapter summarises the large amount of data amassed as part of this review and laid out in more detail in Part 2.

Summary of NHS funding and performance since 2002

Introduction

In the light of the 2002 and 2004 reviews, this chapter summarises and assesses the historical record since 2002, not just in terms of increased NHS funding but the consequence of that increased investment for resources, outputs, outcomes and productivity. The evidence underpinning this chapter is presented in more detail in Part 2 of this review.

While every effort has been made to cover the considerable scope and range of NHS activities, some gaps remain. Furthermore, most of the data relates to England alone. While this bias is unsatisfactory in some respects, it does recognise the inherent problems of comparing four countries with varying health service organisations, definitions of data and trends in reform policy.

A helpful way of reviewing the evidence is by means of a conventional 'production path' (*see* Figure 5, below), starting with a description of financial inputs to the NHS, moving on to how these are converted into resources (such as labour and capital), then to how these combine to produce outputs or activity (such as numbers of patients admitted to hospital) and finally to the outcomes (health) these activities help to produce. This production path also allows for an assessment of changes in productivity – the relationship between resource inputs and outputs.

Funding: how much was spent?

The primary task of the 2002 review was to 'identify the key factors which will determine the financial and other resources required to ensure that the NHS can provide a publicly

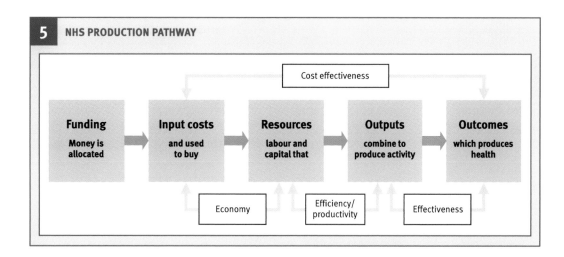

5 NHS PRODUCTION PATHWAY

funded, comprehensive, high quality service available on the basis of clinical need and not ability to pay'. It concluded that the share of national wealth devoted to health care would need to increase substantially to achieve the high-quality comprehensive service desired, at the volumes expected to be demanded. This increase would be modified to some extent by changes in the way services were delivered and by levels of public engagement with health.

The review determined that total real UK NHS spending needed to rise from an estimated £68 billion in 2002/3 to between £154 and £184 billion in 2022/3; at a minimum, this represented real growth of around 126 per cent (see Table 2 below). The first decade of spending was designed to 'catch up' with best practice in other countries, while spending in the second decade was intended to ensure the United Kingdom could 'keep up' with other developed countries. Overall, by 2022/3 total health care spending in the United Kingdom – both public and private – was projected to consume between 10.6 and 12.5 per cent of gross domestic product, depending on the scenario used.

The 2002 review underpinned the announcement by the then Chancellor of the Exchequer, Gordon Brown, in his 2002 Budget that over the five years to 2007/8 the NHS across the UK would receive a 7.4 per cent average annual real-term growth in funding (Brown 2002).

As Table 2, below, shows, although there was a difference in base year spending (where the actual spend in 2002/3 was £66.2 billion compared with the 2002 review's estimated spend of £68 billion), real NHS spending has matched the review's recommendations. This analysis indicates that total UK health care spend in 2007/8 will be around £113.5 billion (at 2002/3 prices), which includes an estimated £17 billion attributed to private health care. As a percentage of UK GDP, total spend on health care in 2007/8 will be around 9.3 per cent, slightly below that recommended by the 2002 review. This reduction is due partly to revised figures for GDP and the GDP deflator (which reduces spending as a percentage of GDP at 2002/3 prices) and partly to a change in the calculation of private spending, which increased its level over that assumed by the 2002 review.

TABLE 2: ACTUAL UK SPENDING ON THE NHS COMPARED WITH 2002 WANLESS PROJECTIONS UNDER DIFFERENT SCENARIOS, 2002/3 TO 2022/3

	Spending (£ billion)[1]						
	2002/3	2003/4	2004/5	2005/6	2006/7	2007/8	2022/3
Projections							
Solid progress[2]	68.0	72.9	78.1	83.6	89.6	96.0	161.0
Slow uptake[2]	68.0	73.0	78.4	84.1	90.3	97.0	184.0
Fully engaged[2]	68.0	72.9	78.1	83.6	89.6	96.0	154.0
Actual	66.2	72.5	78.0	82.9	90.0[3]	96.5[3]	–

Source: Wanless 2002; HM Treasury 2006, 2002a
[1] 2002/3 prices
[2] 2002 Wanless figures for intervening years between 2002/3 and 2007/8 have been interpolated as equal changes between these years.
[3] Figures for 2006/7 and 2007/8 refer to planned spending.

Although the Prime Minister claimed at the time the additional NHS funding was announced that the extra money would bring the United Kingdom up to the European Union (EU) average, this was not a specific recommendation of the 2002 review. The concern of the review was less with comparing spending and more with achieving the sort of health outcomes on which the United Kingdom has historically lagged behind many EU countries. Nevertheless, it is worth noting that if NHS spending reverts to its long-term trend of around three per cent real annual growth, actual spending by 2012/3 would fall short of the fully engaged spending path by around £7.2 billion and by more than this for the other two scenarios. This would place the United Kingdom near the bottom of future estimates of the average total EU health care spend as a proportion of GDP.

For a more detailed analysis of NHS spending since 2002, *see* Part 2, Chapter 5.

FUNDING: OVERALL ASSESSMENT

Additional UK NHS funding since 2002/3 broadly matched the recommendations of the 2002 review for the first five years of its spending trajectories, taking total health care spend to within striking distance of average European Union spending as a proportion of GDP. Such a rate of increase cannot be sustained indefinitely, but spending will have to increase by at least 4.4 per cent a year in real terms on the 2002 review's most optimistic scenario and by more than that in the other scenarios.

Input costs: the impact of the new staff contracts

Real NHS spending – that is, cash spending deflated by a measure of inflation for the economy as a whole (the GDP deflator) – increased by 46 per cent between 2002/3 and 2007/8. However, because of the types of inputs used by the NHS, the sum of changes in its input prices can differ substantially from this broad measure of economy-wide inflation.

The 2002 review assumed that hospital and community health services (HCHS) pay would rise by 2.4 per cent a year in real terms (over and above GDP deflator inflation). With inflation assumed to be 2.5 per cent throughout the 20-year period covered by the review, this implied a nominal increase of 4.9 per cent a year. Pay and prices in the General Medical Services sector were assumed to rise by 2.2 per cent a year in real terms, and for the personal social services sector by 2.3 per cent. These assumptions were made in line with historic averages and did not reflect a judgement about what rates of pay would be required to recruit, retain, motivate and increase the effectiveness of staff. The 2002 review assumed non-pay inflation would average 2.5 per cent a year for the NHS as a whole. Both the pay and price assumptions were common to each of the three scenarios.

However, since 2002 there have been major overhauls of employment contracts for virtually all of the 1.3 million UK NHS staff, and all the new contracts have generated additional costs for the NHS. Of the total £43.2 billion cash increase in UK NHS spending between 2002/3 and 2007/8, it is estimated that £18.9 billion (43 per cent) has been absorbed by higher pay and prices in the NHS; and the main source of these higher costs has been pay increases arising from three new contracts introduced during this period.

Effectively, therefore, this cash increase of over £43 billion has been reduced, after NHS inflation, to around £24.3 billion.

COSTS AND BENEFITS OF PAY MODERNISATION

The government and the 2002 review considered pay modernisation an important tool for improving the recruitment and retention of staff and encouraging flexibility in the workforce, thus enhancing overall capacity and promoting positive changes in the skill mix in the service. However, the costs of the resultant new contracts have been substantial, with few signs so far of improved productivity.

Between 2002 and 2007, pay for hospital and community health staff (around 90 per cent of all NHS staff) increased by about 30 per cent (a real rise of about 15 per cent).

The new consultant contract led to average earnings rising by nearly 27 per cent between 2002/3 and 2005/6 (NAO 2007a). Around a quarter of the rise in the consultants' pay bill in England was due to increased numbers of consultants and the remainder to increases in the *per capita* costs of employment. Similarly, the new general practitioners' contract resulted in significant additional costs, with the average net income of a GP increasing by around 23 per cent between 2003/4 and 2004/5 (The Information Centre 2007a).

Have these contracts and other new pay deals led to increased staff productivity? Crude measures suggest that productivity among nurses and consultants has started to improve, but these need to be interpreted with caution. From 2003/4, emergency admissions per full-time equivalent nurse started to increase, with a similar trend for elective admissions from 2004/5. Furthermore, hospital admissions per whole-time equivalent consultant, which had been falling since 1999/2000, appear to have risen by 2005/6. However, more detailed research into productivity across the whole health service will be needed before more robust conclusions can be drawn.

More generally, there is a dearth of robust evidence of other benefits arising from the new contracts and pay deals. There has been no national evaluation of Agenda for Change, the new national pay and grading system for non-medical NHS staff, and the limited evidence on the impact of the new consultant contract suggests it has yet to deliver value for money (NAO 2007a). The new GP contract is also under scrutiny, with the House of Commons Committee of Public Accounts (2007a) commenting that the preparations for the new out-of-hours service was 'a shambles'. The Health Committee's report (2007) into NHS workforce planning also noted that large pay increases were granted without securing increases in productivity, and that attempts to create a more flexible workforce have had mixed results.

Despite these increased pay costs, combined pay and non-pay NHS inflation between 2002/3 and 2007/8 closely matched the 2002 review's assumptions, with the former slightly higher and the latter slightly lower than had been assumed.

For more detail on input costs since 2002, *see* Part 2, Chapter 6.

Resources: staff, premises and equipment

The 2002 review did not specify in detail all the resources the NHS needed in order to deliver its vision of the health service in 2022/3. However, it did implicitly endorse the commitments of the 10-year NHS Plan (Department of Health 2000a) and in some instances recommended additional investment (Wanless 2002).

The NHS Plan presented a 'shopping list' of staff and other resources expected to be purchased by the extra funding announced in the 2000 budget. The headline investments were:

■ 7,500 more consultants, 2,000 more GPs, 20,000 more nurses and 6,500 more therapists
■ 7,000 extra beds in hospitals and intermediate care
■ more than 100 new hospitals and 500 new 'one-stop' primary care centres
■ more than 3,000 GP premises modernised
■ 250 new scanners
■ modern ICT systems in every hospital and GP surgery.

TABLE 3: COMPARISON OF THE NHS PLAN GROWTH TARGETS WITH ACTUAL WORKFORCE GROWTH[1]

Staff group	NHS Plan target for numbers of new staff 1999–2004	Actual new staff 1999–2004[1]	Variance from NHS Plan target	% increase in new staff 1999–2006
Consultants[2,3]	7,500	7,329	2% under target	41
GPs[4,5]	2,000	3,056	53% over target	16
Nurses[6,7]	20,000	67,878	239% over target	21
Allied health professionals[8]	6,500	11,039	70% over target	27

Source: King's Fund analysis; Information Centre 2007c

[1] Headcount
[2] The number of consultants includes Directors of Public Health.
[3] The NHS Plan target for consultants was achieved in 2005, both in terms of headcount and full time equivalent.
[4] The number of GPs excludes retainers and registrars.
[5] In 2005 the target for GPs was also achieved in full time equivalent terms.
[6] The number of nurses includes practice nurses.
[7] The target for nurses was achieved in terms of both headcount and full time equivalent.
[8] The target for allied health professionals was achieved in terms of both headcount and full time equivalent.

The aim was to achieve most of these commitments by 2004, with the new hospitals delivered by 2010. Did this actually happen?

NHS STAFF

NHS staff numbers have risen considerably since 1999 and by 2006 totalled more than 1.3 million – an increase in headcount terms of over a fifth. Most of the staffing commitments of the NHS Plan were achieved on target, with the target for extra consultants achieved a year late in 2005 (see Table 3, below). By 2006 the workforce targets outlined in the Plan had all been exceeded, particularly for nursing, allied health professionals and GPs.

The 2002 review predicted that the health care workforce might need to increase by almost 300,000 by 2022 and that the then planned increase in the number of doctors would eventually fall well short of demand.

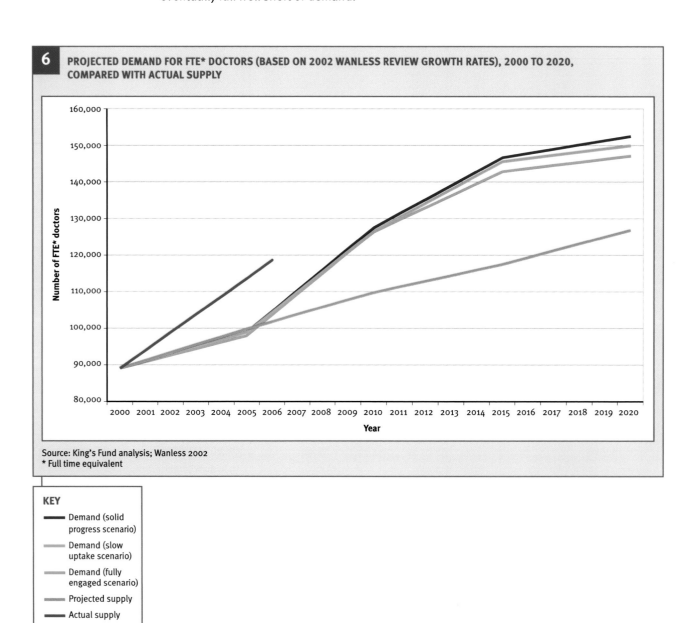

6 PROJECTED DEMAND FOR FTE* DOCTORS (BASED ON 2002 WANLESS REVIEW GROWTH RATES), 2000 TO 2020, COMPARED WITH ACTUAL SUPPLY

Source: King's Fund analysis; Wanless 2002
* Full time equivalent

KEY
— Demand (solid progress scenario)
— Demand (slow uptake scenario)
— Demand (fully engaged scenario)
▬ Projected supply
— Actual supply

Figure 6, opposite, shows that the actual supply of doctors has so far exceeded the original NHS Plan targets. However, it is likely that increasing demand will absorb this excess supply over the next few years.

Sustained slow growth is what is needed to produce further increases in the NHS workforce, with short-term adjustments likely to prove detrimental in the long term.

HOSPITALS AND OTHER PREMISES

The NHS Plan promised that by 2004 there would be 500 new one-stop primary care centres, that 3,000 general practitioner premises would be modernised and at least a quarter of the NHS maintenance backlog cleared. It also promised to build 100 new hospitals by 2010. The 2002 review not only accepted these commitments but went further in suggesting that a third of hospital and community health estates would be replaced by 2022/3, that three-quarters of all beds in new hospitals would be in single en-suite rooms, with a maximum of four beds in other rooms, and that the entire primary care estate would be upgraded or replaced by 2010/1. Have these suggestions been implemented?

Since 1997, 84 new hospitals have replaced existing facilities, with a further 25 under construction (Department of Health 2007a). The Construction Products Association (CPA) reported in late 2006 that 65 new hospitals had become operational since 2000 (CPA 2006). The CPA also found that the commitments on primary care centres and GP premises had been met, albeit after the 2004 deadline (CPA 2005). The Department of Health confirmed in 2007 that over 625 new one-stop primary care centres had been created since 2001, while around 3,000 (or almost one-third) of GP surgeries had been substantially refurbished or replaced (Department of Health 2007a).

The government seems on track to build at least 100 new hospitals by 2010. However, the evidence suggests it is unlikely to achieve the 2002 review's target for single rooms: indeed, the government is still struggling to meet its commitment to single-sex wards.

Similarly, the 2002 review's recommendation that the entire primary care estate be upgraded or replaced by 2010/1 seems unlikely to be met; at the current rate of progress this will not happen until 2016.

A major disappointment has been the failure to shift the maintenance backlog, which has grown rather than shrunk, and in 2005/6 stood at £3.7 billion – an increase of nearly a fifth since 1999/2000 (CPA 2006).

HOSPITAL BEDS

The number of NHS hospital beds in England has been declining for many years. This is partly due to increased use of day surgery, which reduces the need for long stays in hospital, and partly to policy initiatives, such as the commitment to provide more community-based services.

The NHS Plan committed to providing an additional 2,100 general and acute and 5,000 intermediate care beds by 2004. Table 4, overleaf, shows that these promises were fulfilled by 2003/4 and 2005/6 respectively. However, since then the number of general and acute beds has fallen by more than 4,200 and there are now fewer than when the Plan was

TABLE 4: NUMBERS OF GENERAL, ACUTE AND INTERMEDIATE CARE BEDS IN ENGLAND, 1999/2000 TO 2005/6

Year	Number of general and acute beds	Change in the number of general and acute beds since 1999/2000	Number of intermediate care beds	Change in the number of intermediate beds since 1999/2000
1999/2000	135,080	–	4,242	–
2000/1	135,794	714	na	–
2001/2	136,583	1,503	7,021	2,779
2002/3	136,679	1,599	7,493	3,251
2003/4	137,247	2,167	8,697	4,455
2004/5	136,184	1,104	8,928	4,686
2005/6	133,033	-2,047	9,771	5,529

Source: Department of Health 2006d
Note: The figures for intermediate care beds are quarter 2 figures.

published. The overall reduction of around 2,050 general and acute beds between 1999/2000 and 2005/6 is almost entirely due to a decline in geriatric beds.

The 2002 review noted that around 4,200 patients in English hospitals – equivalent to 10 full hospitals – experienced delays in discharge. In 2004, at the review's suggestion, a system of charging, pioneered in Sweden, was introduced to encourage local authorities to speed up the discharge of relevant patients. Although delayed discharges subsequently fell by a third, the longer-term trend shows that this is a relatively small fall compared with the reductions in delayed discharges between 2001 and 2003.

ICT

The 2002 review identified better use of information and communications technologies (ICT) as key to productivity in terms of both reduced costs and better quality; it argued that there was a strong case for rapid investment – but only if this was sure to deliver cost-effective solutions.

The National Programme for IT in the NHS (NPfIT – now Connecting for Health) is responsible for implementing an integrated ICT infrastructure into all NHS organisations in England by 2014. The programme originally had four key deliverables:
- integrated care records service
- electronic prescribing system
- electronic appointment booking system
- the IT infrastructure to support these systems.

The programme has since assumed responsibility for other services, including Picture Archiving and Communications Systems (PACS), the Quality Management and Analysis System (QMAS) and NHSmail.

The total cost of NPfIT is estimated at £12.4 billion (at 2005/6 prices) over the 10 years to 2013/4 (NAO 2006) , and the ICT resources recommended by the 2002 review should be sufficient to cover this cost. Given the well-documented delays that have beset the

TABLE 5: NUMBER OF NHS ACTIVITY CATEGORIES AND ESTIMATED SHARES OF TOTAL NHS SPENDING, 2005/6

Activity	Number of activity categories[1]	Approximate share of total NHS spending	
		(£ billion)[2]	(%)
Elective patients	>500	6.26	9.3
Non-elective patients	>500	8.74	13.0
Outpatients	~300	5.79	8.6
Accident and emergency	9	1.27	1.9
Mental health services	30	5.15	7.6
Primary care prescribing	~200	7.82	11.6
Primary (GMS) care	5	7.70	11.4
NHS Direct calls answered	1	0.10	0.1
NHS Direct online 'hits'	1		
Walk-in centre visits	1	0.005	0.01
Ambulance journeys	1	0.96	1.4
General ophthalmic services	1	0.40	0.6
General dental services	1	1.91	2.8
Others (critical care, audiology services, pathology, radiology, chemotherapy, renal dialysis, community services, bone marrow transplants and rehabilitation)	>100	3.38	5.0
Central budgets[3]		18.00	26.6
Total		**67.49**	**100.0**

Source: Adapted from Department of Health 2004e
[1] Categories for elective, non-elective, outpatients and accident and emergency are measured in health care resource groups. Other categories are a mix of visits, calls and so on.
[2] King's Fund estimates based on National Reference costs (2005/6) (Department of Health 2006e).
[3] This refers to centrally funded organisations (such as the Department of Health itself) and services. There are no routine activity measures to cover this disparate set of budgets.

programme, it is not surprising that actual spending on ICT in England has followed neither the solid progress nor the fully engaged spending trajectories; in fact it is estimated to have increased from £1 billion in 2002/3 to £2.3 billion in 2005/6 (NHS Connecting for Health 2007a). However, planned spending of just under £2.9 billion in 2006/7 would overshoot both those spending trajectories and so come closer to that assumed in the solid progress scenario.

There is as yet no convincing evidence that the benefits will outweigh the costs of this substantial investment. Two factors likely to impact on the 2002 review's productivity assumptions are:

- an apparent reluctance to audit and evaluate the programme
- a structure for NPfIT contracts that risks creating monopolies in various areas of the programme.

Although there has been some progress in modernising the NHS ICT infrastructure, this has generally been in areas (such as PACS) that do not relate to the original four key deliverables.

On the timetable for implementing NPfIT, the House of Commons Public Accounts Committee (2007a) stated that 'The Department is unlikely to complete the Programme anywhere near its original schedule', and that 'At the present rate of progress it is unlikely that significant clinical benefits will be delivered by the end of the contract period'.

SCANNERS AND OTHER EQUIPMENT

Finally, the NHS Plan committed to investing in 250 new scanners by 2004. By April 2006, new and replacement equipment delivered through central programmes included 146 magnetic resonance imaging (MRI) scanners, 135 linear accelerators, 224 computerised tomography (CT) scanners and more than 730 items of breast-screening equipment (Department of Health 2006a). More than seven out of every ten MRI scanners, CT scanners and linear accelerators now in use in the NHS were purchased after January 2000. Between 1999/2000 and 2005/6, the number of MRI and CT examinations performed in England has risen by 91 and 82 per cent respectively, suggesting that the proposed investment has been effectively used.

For more detailed evidence on investment in physical resources, *see* Part 2, Chapter 7.

RESOURCES: OVERALL ASSESSMENT

Additional funding for the NHS over the last five years has enabled the service to invest in substantially increased resources – particularly labour. Staff numbers are at their highest level ever and have exceeded commitments made in the NHS Plan and adopted by the 2002 review. Unfortunately, this has contributed to recent overspending in the NHS. However, the review estimated that further increases in the number of doctors will be needed before the end of this decade (Wanless 2002).

There has been substantial replacement and upgrading of buildings but no progress on reducing the maintenance backlog and some way to go on upgrading primary care premises and providing single rooms in hospitals.

Modernisation of the NHS ICT infrastructure has not been without its difficulties (or its critics), with most progress tending to relate to systems that were not originally part of the modernisation plan. Future commitment not only to implementing core ICT systems but also to realising patient benefits and productivity gains is vital. The programme needs to be audited comprehensively to ensure that benefits will outweigh costs and to assess the precise impact on future productivity.

Outputs: use of NHS services

The NHS produces a considerable range of outputs, whose variety means they cannot easily be added together. Recent productivity measures developed by the Department of Health list around 1,700 specific categories of NHS activity covering primary, secondary, community and other NHS services. In addition, over time the measured units of activity (such as an operation or an outpatient attendance) change in terms of what they deliver in health terms. All of this makes it difficult to calculate trends in total output for the NHS and assess changes in productivity.

Table 5, p 19, lists the NHS activity categories with their approximate costs. The rest of this section explores trends in outputs associated with these activity categories. Despite a lack of published evidence on some outputs, it has been possible to examine activity relating to almost 90 per cent of NHS spending, excluding central budgets.

ELECTIVE AND EMERGENCY ADMISSIONS TO HOSPITAL

In 2005/6 the NHS in England carried out around 12 million elective and emergency interventions in hospitals, representing a rise in total admissions of 22 per cent since 1998/9 and by 14 per cent by 2002/3 (*see* Table 6, below).

Elective admissions

Elective interventions accounted for about half of total admissions to hospitals in 2005/6, having increased by just over 605,000 (11 per cent) since 1998/9 and by just under seven per cent since 2002. Within this overall upward trend, there has been a noticeable change in the type of cases, with inpatient admissions declining by around 90,000 (4 per cent) and day cases increasing by nearly 700,000 (20 per cent) between 1998/9 and 2005/6.

TABLE 6: TRENDS IN HOSPITAL ADMISSIONS, 1998/9, 2002/3 AND 2005/6

Type of admission	Number of admissions			% change 1998/9–2005/6	% change 2002/3–2005/6
	1998/9	2002/3	2005/6		
Elective	5,484,885	5,681,570	6,090,191	11	7
Inpatient	2,070,237	1,974,267	1,979,341	-4	0
% of all elective	*37.7%*	*34.7%*	*32.5%*	*-14%*	*-6%*
Day case	3,414,648	3,707,303	4,110,850	20	11
% of all elective	*62.3%*	*65.3%*	*67.5%*	*8%*	*3%*
Admitted from a waiting list	2,925,708	2,346,259	2,177,190	-26	-7
% of all elective	*53.3%*	*41.3%*	*35.7%*	*-33%*	*-13%*
Booked admission	1,689,940	1,973,735	2,257,707	34	14
% of all elective	*30.8%*	*34.7%*	*37.1%*	*20%*	*7%*
Planned admission	869,237	1,361,576	1,655,294	90	22
% of all elective	*15.8%*	*24.0%*	*27.2%*	*72%*	*13%*
Emergency	4,587,628	5,112,779	6,196,392	35	21
% of total admissions	*45.5%*	*47.4%*	*50.4%*	*11%*	*6%*
Total admissions	10,072,513	10,794,349	12,286,583	22	14

Source: King's Fund analysis; Hospital Episodes Statistics 2007

Over this period nearly a fifth of the net increase in total elective admissions was accounted for by just one health care resource group (HRG): cataract extraction with lens implant, which is now the most common elective procedure. This operation, together with two other interventions (large intestine: endoscopy/intermediate procedures and haematological disorders with minor procedures) account for over 40 per cent of the net increase in elective admissions. Nearly 30 per cent of the net decrease in elective inpatient admissions is accounted for by a reduction in cataract operations, offset by a rapid rise in the number carried out as day cases. Within the top 10 elective HRGs which have grown in number, only cataract extraction, cardiac catheterisation and renal replacement therapy show evidence of a significant switch from inpatient to day care.

Another way of disaggregating elective activity – and one that touches on the government's dominant policy of reducing waiting times – is to examine the sources of patient admissions. Table 6, p 21, shows that virtually all the net increase in elective admissions between 1998/9 and 2005/6 was due to a rise in planned admissions of 786,000 (90 per cent). These cases are not counted as part of the waiting list. Conversely, admissions from the waiting list fell by 749,000 (26 per cent), to some extent offset by a rise of 568,000 (34 per cent) in booked admissions, which *are* counted as part of the waiting list. These trends have continued since 2002/3. There is no obvious epidemiological or clinical reason for the rise in planned admissions; it may be due to changes in clinical behaviour, possibly relating to waiting time targets or changes in the coding of operations.

Emergency admissions

Table 6, above, shows that emergency admissions to hospitals rose by 35 per cent (around 1.6 million) between 1998/9 and 2005/6. Around a quarter of this net increase, which accelerated from 2003/4, was accounted for by just 20 HRGs. Again, there is no obvious epidemiological or clinical explanation for this trend; it was probably caused by changes in clinical behaviour and trusts' admission policies – possibly driven by the need to meet maximum four-hour wait targets in accident and emergency departments.

Maternity-related admissions

There were just over one million maternity-related hospital admissions in 2005/6, a rise of 12 per cent since 2002/3; over this period, the number of NHS hospital deliveries rose by 8 per cent to 593,400 (The Information Centre 2007c).

OUTPATIENT CARE AND REFERRALS

Outpatient care accounts for around 9 per cent of total NHS spending, with more than 45 million attendances every year. In 2005/6 more than one in four people in England had a first attendance at an outpatients department. Since the mid-1990s, total outpatient attendances have risen by 6 million (15 per cent), although since 2002/3 growth has been more modest, at 3 per cent. Since 2002/3 there has been an 11 per cent reduction in first attendances at maternity outpatients departments, probably reflecting a shift towards community antenatal care (Department of Health 2007b).

Since 2000/1 there has been little change in the number of GP referrals. Although total referrals grew by over a fifth between 2002/3 and 2005/6, this was all due to an increase in consultant-to-consultant and other referrals.

ACCIDENT AND EMERGENCY SERVICES

Accident and emergency (A&E) services account for around 2 per cent of NHS expenditure and around 20 million attendances. A&E activity was relatively stable between the late 1980s and 2002/3, with an upward trend in first attendances balanced by a downward trend in follow-up visits. However, after 2002/3 there was a dramatic increase in new attendances, which rose by around 4.8 million (more than 37 per cent) by 2005/6. Explanations for this are likely to lie with changes in the service itself, such as reduced waiting times to meet the four-hour maximum wait target. However, changes in other services, such as GP out-of-hours cover are also likely to have encouraged more visits to A&E.

GENERAL PRACTICE AND MENTAL HEALTH

Attendance figures at GP surgeries are not routinely collated by the NHS at national level. However, General Household Survey data (ONS 2006a) suggests there were around 250 million GP consultations in Great Britain in 2005, a rise of around a third since the early 1980s. A lack of robust information relating to primary care makes it impossible to estimate activity since 2002/3.

Between 1998/9 and 2005/6, the number of consultant episodes and admissions related to mental illness fell by 10 per cent and 16 per cent, respectively. These downward trends are partly due to a policy shift towards outpatient and/or community treatment. Crisis resolution/home treatment teams and other community-based services designed to manage acute episodes of mental illness were set up between 2001 and 2004, and the evidence suggests these innovations have been effective in reducing hospital admissions.

PRESCRIBING

In 2006, 752 million prescription items were dispensed in the community in England, representing a rise of almost 22 per cent since 2002 (Department of Health 2006b). The cost of this prescribing to the NHS in 2006 was £8.2 billion, a rise of 20 per cent since 2002. Of the total net increase of 133.5 million prescription items between 2002 and 2006, three-quarters were accounted for by just 10 drugs, with lipid-regulating drugs accounting for over 18 per cent of the net change.

The 2002 review assumed that over the 20 years from 2002/3 there would be a reduction in prescriptions relating to coronary heart disease (CHD) and stroke for 15–64 year olds, with an overall reduction in prescriptions for this age group in the solid progress and fully engaged scenarios – particularly the latter (Wanless 2002). It is too early to detect any such long-term trend; but it has been found that of the 10 drugs that enjoyed the highest volume increases between 2002 and 2006, six were related to cardiovascular problems.

The review assumed an increase in UK NHS expenditure on lipid-regulating statins from around £700 million in 2002/3 to £2.1 billion by 2010 (Wanless 2002). In fact, although the number of prescriptions for statins dispensed since 2002 has risen by 138 per cent to 39.7 million, the total *cost* has risen by just 0.3 per cent, with the real cost falling by almost 10 per cent. This is because of a significant increase in the prescribing of low-cost statins, such as simvastatin, which has reduced in cost by almost 90 per cent since 2002. Thus, the actual cost to the NHS of prescribing statins has diverged from the review's projections since 2004, resulting in a cumulative saving.

OTHER SERVICES

NHS Direct

NHS Direct has handled more than 36 million calls since it was launched in 1998 and currently receives around half a million calls a month (Department of Health 2006c). NHS Direct Online was launched in December 1999 and the website currently receives around 1.5 million visits per month. The latest usage information, as of February 2007, indicates that the online service has around 24 million visitors each year, with seven million calls made to NHS Direct, while NHS Direct Interactive is available through digital TV to 16 million households.

Walk-in centres

By May 2006, 75 walk-in centres had opened in England, and in 2005/6 more than 2.5 million visits were made, with an average of just over 100 daily visits per centre (Department of Health 2006c). Although one of the aims for these centres was to relieve the pressure on primary care (Department of Health 1999b), a recent study found no evidence that they had improved access to primary care and concluded that their results 'do not support the use of walk-in centres for this purpose' (Maheswaran *et al* 2007).

Ambulance service

The number of ambulance journeys in England fell from around 18 million to 16.5 million in the 10 years to 2005/6, with a current cost of nearly £1 billion. However, over this period the number of calls to the ambulance service in England nearly doubled to almost six million, with the percentage of calls resulting in a response falling from around 90 to 80 per cent. Around three-quarters of ambulance journeys are planned rather than being in response to emergency calls, and it is a reduction in these planned journeys that has accounted for the overall reduction mentioned above.

For more detail on use of NHS services, *see* Part 2, Chapter 8.

OUTPUTS: OVERALL ASSESSMENT

With increased resources, the NHS has been able to do more work in most areas. Elective admissions increased by 7 per cent between 2002/3 and 2005/6 and outpatient attendances by 3 per cent. Virtually all the increase in elective admissions was due to a 22 per cent increase in planned cases, with just a 3 per cent increase in patients admitted from waiting lists (including booked admissions).

There have also been very large increases in emergency care (+21 per cent) and accident and emergency attendances (+33 per cent).

Three-quarters of the 20 per cent increase in prescription items dispensed between 2002/3 and 2006/7 is due to just 10 drugs. Lipid-regulating drugs (statins) account for nearly a fifth of the total increase and are on target for achieving the 2002 review's recommendations at a lower-than-expected cost (Wanless 2002).

Productivity: unit costs and quality

A crucial issue for the 2002 review, with a significant impact on its funding projections, was the ability to do more (in both volume and quality terms) with each health care pound (Wanless 2002). Higher productivity offered the potential to restrict growth in the long-term costs of delivering the health care outcomes likely to be sought by 2022.

The review made an important distinction between two aspects of productivity improvement: those related to inputs – that is, reductions in unit costs – and those related to outputs or outcomes – that is, improved quality.

It was assumed that under the solid progress and fully engaged scenarios, productivity would improve by 2–2.5 per cent a year in the first decade and 3 per cent in the second. The slow uptake scenario predicted lower productivity improvements of 1.5 and 1.75 per cent a year respectively.

The importance of these assumptions becomes evident when they are converted into monetary terms and set against the review's final projections for health care spending up to 2022/3 (*see* Figure 7, below). In the fully engaged and solid progress scenarios, the value of the productivity gains by 2022/3 (at 2002/3 prices) amounts to £46.5 billion – around half of the additional forecast growth in spending over and above the 2002/3 level of £68 billion.

It is important to emphasise that productivity is difficult to measure, not just in the NHS but in many sectors of the economy. As the latest official measures of NHS productivity show (*see* Figure 8, overleaf), there is a wide range of estimates depending on the

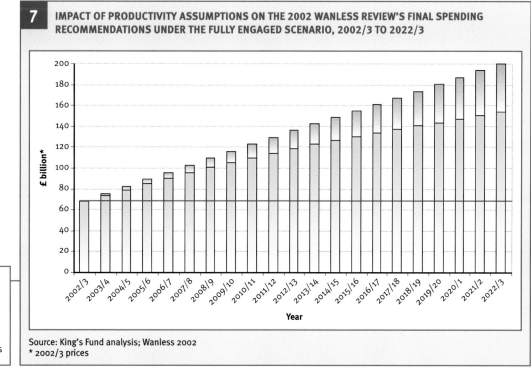

7 **IMPACT OF PRODUCTIVITY ASSUMPTIONS ON THE 2002 WANLESS REVIEW'S FINAL SPENDING RECOMMENDATIONS UNDER THE FULLY ENGAGED SCENARIO, 2002/3 TO 2022/3**

KEY
- Value of productivity assumptions
- 2002 spending recommendations

Source: King's Fund analysis; Wanless 2002
* 2002/3 prices

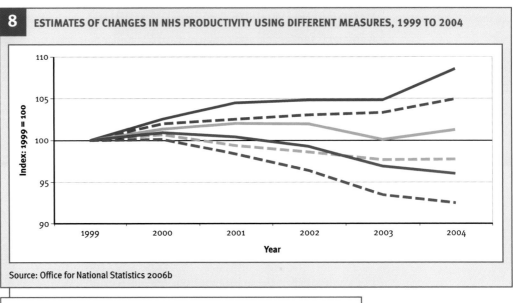

8 ESTIMATES OF CHANGES IN NHS PRODUCTIVITY USING DIFFERENT MEASURES, 1999 TO 2004

Source: Office for National Statistics 2006b

KEY

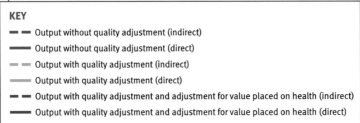

– – Output without quality adjustment (indirect)
—— Output without quality adjustment (direct)
– – Output with quality adjustment (indirect)
—— Output with quality adjustment (direct)
– – Output with quality adjustment and adjustment for value placed on health (indirect)
—— Output with quality adjustment and adjustment for value placed on health (direct)

methods used to measure and value NHS inputs and outputs (ONS 2006b). As Figure 8, above, shows, changes in NHS productivity may have ranged from minus 7.5 per cent to plus 8.5 per cent between 1999 and 2004, depending on the assumptions made.

It is clear from Figure 8, above, that adjusting NHS outputs to reflect (assumed) increases in the value (linked to personal income growth) the public place on NHS products is one way of boosting apparent productivity. However, adjusting the value of NHS outputs in this way is contentious and was not recommended by the 2002 review.

Given the current state of development of official NHS productivity measures, it is probably not sensible to draw definitive conclusions about changes in productivity. At best, and allowing for considerable uncertainty, it could be claimed that productivity improved slightly between 1999 and 2004, largely because of improvements in the quality of outputs.

Triangulation with other performance indicators, such as the average length of stay in hospital, elective day case rates, emergency readmissions and public attitudes to health care, also contributes to an uncertain view of changes in productivity (ONS 2006b). The downward trend in average hospital stays, the upward trend in elective day cases and increased public satisfaction with the NHS suggests increasing productivity. However, the rising trend in emergency readmissions since 2002 leads to the opposite conclusion.

UNIT COST ANALYSIS

While these official indicators provide a rather inconclusive picture of recent trends in NHS productivity, one of the 2002 review's productivity assumptions – that the costs of producing a 'unit' of activity would fall over time – is easier to assess.

The National Reference Cost (NRC) database is the primary source of information about unit costs, extended to cover around £36 billion of activity by 2005/6. Unit costs across five NHS service areas have been examined: elective and emergency services, outpatient services, mental health services and prescribing. Information on the unit costs of primary care is not available due to a lack of routine data.

Table 7, below, summarises changes since 2002/3 in unit costs across various sectors of the NHS.

Elective and emergency activity

Elective (inpatient and day case) and emergency activity accounted for around £15 billion of NHS spending in 2005/6. Between 1998/9 and 2005/6 there was an overall real rise in total spending, most of it due to increases in input costs. Average unit costs rose by 38 per cent, in real terms, over this period, from £849 to £1,179 per case. Of this rise, only 0.3 per cent is estimated to be due to changes in case mix. Real unit costs for elective and emergency activity combined have risen by 10 per cent since 2002/3.

TABLE 7: SUMMARY OF PERCENTAGE CHANGES IN REAL UNIT COSTS OF SERVICES SINCE 2002/3

Services	% change in real unit cost 2002/3–2005/6
Elective admissions	
Elective inpatients	20
Elective day cases	15
Emergency admissions	8
Outpatient attendances	6
Mental health services[1]	
Inpatients (excluding specialist services)	22
Outpatients (excluding specialist services)	22
Domiciliary	33
Secure units	19
Primary care prescribing[2]	-12
Primary (GMS) care	na

Source: King's Fund analysis; National NHS Reference Costs 2007
[1] These services account for around 77 per cent of mental health spend in 2005/6.
[2] The data for prescribing covers the period 2002 to 2006.

Outpatient activity

In 2005/6, total expenditure on outpatient services (excluding mental health) amounted to around £5.8 billion. Trends in the aggregate of first, subsequent and 'undefined' outpatient appointments show that between 1999/2000 and 2005/6 real unit costs increased by 28 per cent. Since 2002/3, real unit costs have risen by 6.1 per cent, although in 2005/6 they actually fell by 3.4 per cent.

General practice and mental health

General practitioner and mental health services account for a significant proportion of the total NHS budget, but no conclusions can be drawn about productivity changes for the former since 2002 because of a lack of routine and consistent data on which to calculate unit costs. However, for mental health the trend in unit costs since 2001/2 appears to have been upwards. NRC data show that for around 77 per cent of mental health spending in England in 2005/6, real unit costs have risen since 2002/3 by between 19 and 33 per cent.

Prescribing

The cost to the NHS of dispensing 752 million prescriptions in 2006 was £8.2 billion. Since 2002 total costs have risen by a fifth. However, the cost per prescription has fallen by around 1.8 per cent, and in real terms by 12 per cent, with much of this accounted for by reduced unit costs for statins between 2004 and 2006.

QUALITY AND PROCESS OUTCOMES

Despite recent attempts by the Department of Health to quantify improvements in the quality of NHS outputs, there is no agreed overall measure of quality. However, there are aspects of care – such as waiting times, safety and patient choice – that can give an indication of quality changes.

Patient safety and clinical negligence

Activities geared to improving patient safety are wide-ranging in the NHS. The 2002 review saw increased time spent by NHS staff on clinical governance as the main driver for improvements in safety. The authors assumed that, by 2010/1, 10 per cent of staff time would be devoted to clinical governance, with the benefits realised relatively quickly. As a consequence of increased time spent on clinical governance, the review predicted (Wanless 2002):

- a 15 per cent reduction in hospital-acquired infections in acute care by 2012/3
- a 10 per cent reduction in other adverse incidents in acute care by 2012/3
- a reduction in the clinical negligence bill obstetrics and gynaecology of 25 per cent by 2005.

A central function of the National Patient Safety Agency (NPSA) is the national reporting and learning system (NRLS), which collates reports of incidents affecting patient safety; but the lack of historical data makes it hard to assess recent changes. It is difficult, therefore, to quantify and assess progress towards the 2002 review's assumptions.

Anecdotal evidence from the Healthcare Commission's annual survey of NHS staff suggests that the situation has been improving (Healthcare Commission 2006a); this showed that the percentage of NHS staff witnessing errors, near misses or incidents that could harm patients, staff, or both, declined between 2003 and 2005.

Information from the NHS Litigation Authority on clinical negligence claims relating to obstetrics and gynaecology is recorded, but the significant time lag between original incidents and final settlement of claims makes it impossible to demonstrate reliable trends in obstetrics and gynaecology between 2002 and 2005.

Hospital cleanliness and hospital-acquired infections
The patient environment action teams (PEAT) reviews have reported progressive improvements in scores for hospital cleanliness in England over the past few years. However, the proportion of hospitals classified as 'poor' or 'unacceptable' more than doubled, from 2.3 per cent to five per cent between 2004 and 2006 (National Patient Safety Agency 2007; NHS Estates 2007).

There are currently no national targets for the hospital-acquired infection *Clostridium difficile (C difficile)* although there are targets to reduce rates of methicillin-resistant *Staphylococcus aureus* (MRSA) by 50 per cent by 2008, compared with 2003/4 (Department of Health, 2004b). The latest progress report by the Health Protection Agency (HPA 2006) suggests little movement towards the MRSA target. The agency reports just over 7,000 MRSA bacteraemia episodes in England during 2005/6 – just 8 per cent fewer than in 2003/4; and its latest commentary (2007) noted 1,542 reports of MRSA bacteraemia between October 2006 and December 2006, representing a 7 per cent decrease on the previous quarter. Mandatory surveillance of *C difficile*-associated disease (CDAD) in people aged 65 years and over has been in place since 2004 and has shown a rise of just over a quarter to 55,681 cases in 2006.

The 2002 review assumed a 15 per cent reduction in hospital-acquired infections (HAIs) in acute care by 2012/3 (Wanless 2002). The government has set more ambitious targets for reductions in MRSA and, although it seems unlikely that these targets will be met, current progress does suggest that a 15 per cent reduction in MRSA incidents in acute care is possible by 2012/3. However, this does not take account of other HAIs, such as *C difficile*, which may pose a larger threat to patient safety in future.

Patient choice
Patient choice of hospital is a key element of the government's health system reforms. Since January 2006, all patients referred by their GP for a specialist consultation at a hospital outpatient department should have been offered a choice of at least four hospitals, including NHS and private; and from 2008 the government intends that all patients needing elective care will be offered the choice of any accredited hospital, public or private, anywhere in England. National patient choice surveys commissioned by the Department of Health have shown progress on the choice agenda (Department of Health 2007c). The fourth survey (relating to referrals made in November and early December 2006) showed an increase in the proportion of patients who recalled being offered a choice of hospital for their first outpatient appointment (41 per cent compared with 30 per cent in the May/June 2006 survey); and 35 per cent of patients were aware before they visited their GP that they had a choice of hospitals for their first appointment, compared with 29 per cent in the May/June survey. Furthermore, 78 per cent of patients who were offered choice were satisfied with the process, with only 5 per cent dissatisfied.

Waiting times

Improving access to health care by reducing waiting lists and waiting times has, arguably, been the dominant NHS policy issue of the last 10 years. The NHS Plan promised that by the end of 2005 no one would wait more than six months on an inpatient list or 13 weeks on an outpatient list. It also promised that no one would wait more than 48 hours for a GP appointment or four hours before being treated in hospital A&E departments. The 2002 review echoed these goals but suggested even shorter waiting times in future, so that by 2022/3 the maximum wait for inpatients and outpatients would be no more than two weeks (Wanless 2002).

Trends in inpatient and outpatient waiting times since 2000 have shown considerable improvement. By April 2007, 40 per cent of outpatients were waiting less than four weeks from GP referral to their first appointment, with a further 30 per cent waiting up to eight weeks. Furthermore, the percentage of patients seen within four hours in A&E rose from around 75 per cent in 2002 to nearly 98 per cent in 2006.

The outstanding waiting time target is the maximum 18-week wait from GP referral to treatment in hospital if needed. The latest departmental milestone is for 85 per cent of trusts to have achieved this target by March 2008 and the remainder by December 2008.

Speed of treatment has important health consequences for some conditions, such as suspected cancer and heart disease (where particularly short waiting time targets have been set); but the impact of reduced waiting times on aggregate patient health (and on overall NHS productivity) may be much less significant. This is partly because most patients are treated well within the target times. Also the effects of waiting are less damaging than might be supposed; for waiting lists do not operate on a simple first-come-first-served basis and patients may move up the queue if, for example, their symptoms deteriorate.

Patient experience and satisfaction

By May 2007, around 1.4 million patients had participated in the national patient survey programme. Analysis of the surveys – which probe patient experience rather than satisfaction – indicates that most patients are very appreciative of their care, particularly in areas of the NHS that have been subject of co-ordinated action as part of national service frameworks or formal targets (Coulter 2005; Picker Institute Europe 2005; The Healthcare Commission 2005a and 2007a).

In 2005 and 2006, 77 per cent of inpatients rated their care as excellent or very good, compared with 74 per cent in 2002. There are, however, some areas of concern to patients, including a lack of involvement with their care, a lack of privacy during treatment and a decline in the perceived cleanliness of hospitals.

The latest British Social Attitudes Survey (Park 2007)) also suggests that general satisfaction with the overall running of the NHS increased in 2005 by comparison with previous years.

For detailed evidence on productivity, *see* Part 2, Chapter 10.

Official measures of NHS productivity provide inconclusive evidence of improvement.

The 2002 review's productivity assumptions of annual unit cost reductions of 0.75–1 per cent between 2002/3 and 2007/8 have not been achieved; broadly, unit costs have increased for all hospital services (Wanless 2002).

Although indicative measures of quality, such as waiting times, and patient satisfaction, suggest improvement, 'hard' measures of quality, valued in monetary terms, are not available to compare with the review's assumption that the quality of care would improve year on year.

Some evidence suggests that the failure to reduce unit costs may have been partially offset by improved quality. However, the NHS has failed to generate the relatively modest improvements in unit cost productivity that might have been expected and were assumed by the 2002 review.

Health outcomes and determinants of health

What justifies the commitment of scarce monetary and human resources to health care services is the restoration of quality of life during illness and, within the limits of the powers of the NHS, the prevention of ill health.

However, as previous sections have shown, while the NHS collects large amounts of data about most of its activities and outputs, there is none about the impact it has on the health status of the patients it treats. This remains a glaring omission that hampers any proper assessment of NHS performance. Second-best information comes from routine data sources recording aspects of the health of the population as a whole, such as life expectancy, rates of cancer survival, and so on. But changes in, say, mortality rates, cannot necessarily be attributed to interventions by the NHS because a wide variety of factors contribute to mortality, often over many decades. The following assessment revisits five measures of health outcome examined in the 2001 Interim Report (Wanless 2001) with links made, where appropriate, to assumptions of the 2002 review.

Self-reported health
The 2005 General Household Survey (GHS) indicated that 59 per cent of the adult population of Great Britain reported their health status as good, 27 per cent fairly good and 14 per cent not good (ONS 2006a). A third of the population said they had a longstanding illness, which was 'limiting' for around a fifth. These statistics have remained largely unchanged since 1998.

Life expectancy at birth
The 2002 review assumed that life expectancy at birth would continue to increase under all three scenarios, with slow uptake associated with the smallest rise (see Table 8, overleaf). Because of evidence that past projections had tended to underestimate future numbers of elderly people, the Government Actuary's Department's (GAD) principal life expectancy assumptions were used for the review's slow uptake scenario rather than the solid progress scenario (Wanless 2002). Solid progress used GAD's 'high' life expectancy

TABLE 8: UK LIFE EXPECTANCY PROJECTIONS IN 2022

Projection	Life expectancy at birth in 2022 (years)	
	Men	Women
2002 Wanless: solid progress	80.0	83.8
2002 Wanless: slow uptake	78.7	83.0
2002 Wanless: fully engaged	81.6	85.5
Latest GAD principal projection	80.3	84.0
Latest GAD low life expectancy variant	79.1	83.3
Latest GAD high life expectancy variant	81.5	84.8

Source: Government Actuary's Department 2006
Notes: The life expectancy data used to produce GAD projections are based on historic mortality rates and projected mortality rates from the 2004-based national population projections.

assumptions, while fully engaged used even more positive assumptions prepared by Eurostat.

In the UK, female life expectancy rose from 79.7 years in 1998 to 80.7 in 2003 (the latest year for which international comparisons have been produced) – an increase of 1.3 per cent (OECD 2007). For males, life expectancy rose by 1.9 per cent, from 74.8 to 76.2 years, over the same period. The UK's performance over this period exceeded that of the EU-15 (population-weighted) average, which rose by 1 per cent for women and 1.7 per cent for men. However, life expectancy still remains lower than in the seven comparator countries identified in the 2001 interim report (Wanless 2001): Australia, Canada, France, Germany, Netherlands, New Zealand and Sweden. The latest GAD principal projections estimate that by 2022 life expectancy at birth for both females and males is likely to exceed that envisaged in the slow uptake scenario and be marginally higher than for solid progress (*see* Figures 9 and 10, opposite).

Infant mortality
Compared with the EU-15 average and comparator countries, the United Kingdom continues to have a poor infant mortality rate (OECD 2007). In 2003 there were 5.3 deaths per 1,000 live births, a reduction of 7 per cent since 1998. However, the EU 15 as a whole saw a 16 per cent reduction, with Greece and Portugal recording reductions of 40 and 32 per cent respectively – although from a higher base. More recent data for the United Kingdom show that infant mortality fell to 5.0 deaths per 1,000 live births in 2006.

Potential life years lost
The United Kingdom also compares unfavourably with comparator countries in terms of potential years of life lost (PYLL) per 100,000 of the population (OECD 2006).Although in 2002, the UK PYLL (excluding self-harm) for males ranked better than the EU-15 average, between 1998 and 2002 it had reduced by only 5 per cent, a rate of decline lower than all comparable countries and the EU 15. For females the PYLL rate in 2002 was higher than for all comparator countries (where data was available) and also higher than the EU-15 average. Furthermore, PYLL data for specific diseases and causes of illness in 2002 suggests that the United Kingdom continues to compare poorly with comparator countries

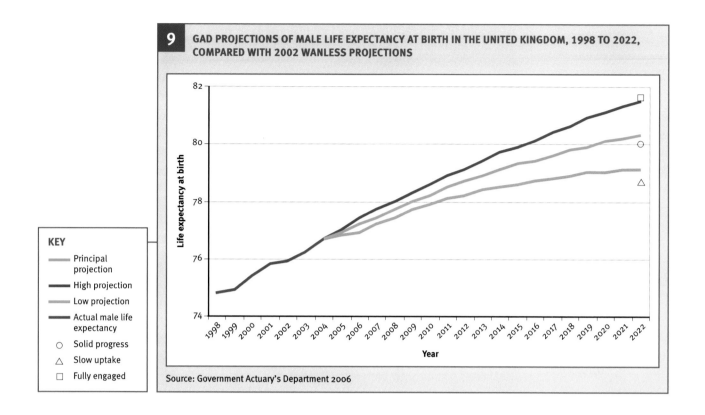

9 GAD PROJECTIONS OF MALE LIFE EXPECTANCY AT BIRTH IN THE UNITED KINGDOM, 1998 TO 2022, COMPARED WITH 2002 WANLESS PROJECTIONS

KEY
— Principal projection
— High projection
— Low projection
— Actual male life expectancy
○ Solid progress
△ Slow uptake
□ Fully engaged

Source: Government Actuary's Department 2006

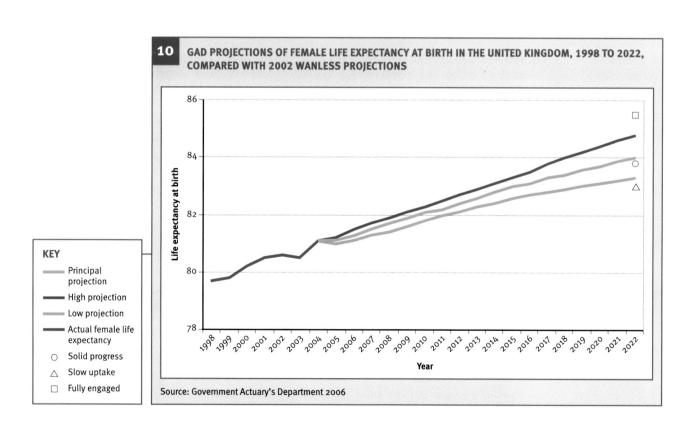

10 GAD PROJECTIONS OF FEMALE LIFE EXPECTANCY AT BIRTH IN THE UNITED KINGDOM, 1998 TO 2022, COMPARED WITH 2002 WANLESS PROJECTIONS

KEY
— Principal projection
— High projection
— Low projection
— Actual female life expectancy
○ Solid progress
△ Slow uptake
□ Fully engaged

Source: Government Actuary's Department 2006

for ischaemic heart, cerebrovascular and respiratory diseases, but performs better for cancer, ranking higher than France and the Netherlands. Data lags mean that information from 2002 onwards is not yet available.

Cancer survival rates

Survival rates for cancer, which account for around a quarter of all deaths in the United Kingdom, have been improving, although they still lag behind those of comparator European countries. The EUROCARE-3 study, based on people diagnosed with cancer between 1990 and 1994, shows that the age-standardised relative five-year survival rate for all cancers in England is notably lower than for France, Germany, the Netherlands and Sweden (Coleman *et al* 2003; Sant *et al* 2003). The five-year survival rate for all cancers in England was 35.9 per cent for males and 46.8 per cent for females. This compares with male survival rates above 40 per cent and female survival rates above 50 per cent in the other comparator European countries.

Despite lower five-year survival rates, England appears to be catching up with other European countries. Between the EUROCARE-2 (Berrino *et al* 1999) and the EUROCARE-3 studies, the English five-year survival rate for all cancers rose by 15.4 per cent for males and 9.6 per cent for females. By comparison with the comparator countries, this improvement was more pronounced for females than males, with improvements in female survival rates significantly better than for Sweden, France and the Netherlands and improvements in male survival rates better than for Sweden and Germany. However, since England started from a lower base than other countries, a larger proportionate improvement might have been expected.

Although this is the latest international comparative information on cancer survival rates, the Office for National Statistics (2007a) has published more recent cancer survival rates for England. Survival rates for eight cancers show a continuing improvement in five-year survival for breast, lung, prostate and stomach cancers. Between 2001 and 2004, five-year survival rates for lung cancer increased by 13.5 per cent for males and 26.3 per cent for females, while the survival rate for stomach cancer has also experienced double-digit growth for both sexes.

However, it is important to point out that the multiple causes of cancer and the long time it takes for disease to develop make it difficult to attribute the latest improvements in many cancer survival rates to activities of the NHS over the past 10 years (and particularly since 2002).

HEALTH DETERMINANTS

An underlying assumption of the 2002 review was that public health and its influence on public engagement was crucial to the funding levels associated with the three scenarios. The solid progress scenario saw public engagement with health determinants achieved in line with prevailing government targets; the fully engaged scenario assumed these targets would be attained more rapidly, while slow uptake predicted that health determinants would remain largely unchanged or follow historical trends (Wanless 2002).

A population's health is, of course, determined by many factors, including genetic inheritance, education and welfare services, income, housing and lifestyle choices. Here four factors are assessed: smoking, obesity, physical activity and diet.

TABLE 9: PROGRESS TOWARDS 1998 WHITE PAPER SMOKING REDUCTION TARGETS, BY GROUP

Group	Percentage of smokers			
	1998 baseline	2005 target	2010 target	Actual 2005
Children	13	11	9	9
Adults	28	26	24	24
Pregnant women	23	18	15	17

Source: Bolling K 2006; Goddard 2006; Information Centre 2006a

Smoking

The adverse health impacts of smoking are well known: more than 1.4 million hospital admissions in England in 2004/5 were related to smoking, and smoking was a factor in around 18 per cent of all deaths in 2004.

At the time of the 2002 Review, the government's smoking targets were formalised in *Smoking Kills: A White Paper on Tobacco* (Department of Health 1998b), with specific targets for adults, children and pregnant women. In England, all of the intermediate (2005) targets were met, while the 2010 targets for children and adults were met in 2005 (*see* Table 9, above).

However, since the 2002 review, more demanding targets have been set and formalised as a Public Service Agreement (PSA). The 2004 PSA target is to reduce overall adult smoking rates to 21 per cent or less by 2010, with a reduction to 26 per cent or less for routine and

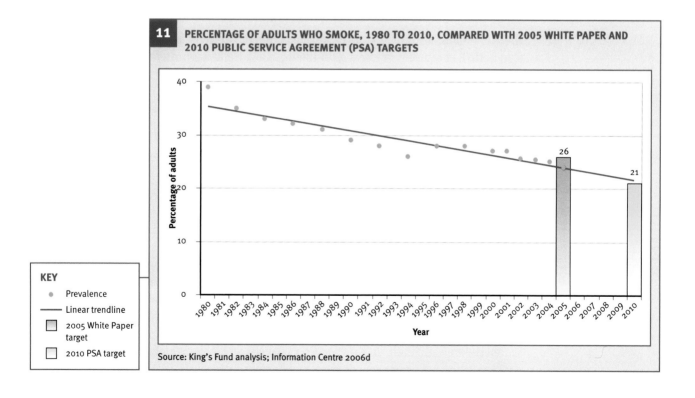

11 PERCENTAGE OF ADULTS WHO SMOKE, 1980 TO 2010, COMPARED WITH 2005 WHITE PAPER AND 2010 PUBLIC SERVICE AGREEMENT (PSA) TARGETS

KEY
- Prevalence
- Linear trendline
- 2005 White Paper target
- 2010 PSA target

Source: King's Fund analysis; Information Centre 2006d

manual socio-economic groups. The evidence suggests that England is on track to achieve these headline targets (*see* Figure 11, p 35), although large variations between socio-economic groups persist. Evidence of progress in reducing these inequalities is weak at best; between 2001 and 2005 there was an 11 per cent reduction in the prevalence of all adult smokers but only a 6 per cent reduction for routine and manual groups. This trend suggests that the 2010 PSA target for these groups may not be achieved.

Progress to date on achieving national smoking targets places England on a solid progress trajectory. While the tougher targets set since the 2002 review exceed solid progress, they are less demanding than the fully engaged scenario.

Obesity

Obesity is estimated to be responsible for more than 9,000 premature deaths a year in England and is an important risk factor for a number of chronic diseases, including heart disease, stroke, some cancers, and type 2 diabetes. At the time of the 2002 review, the 1992 *Health of the Nation* target (which has not been updated) for obesity was for just 6 per cent of men and 8 per cent of women to be classified as obese by 2005 – an exceedingly optimistic target (Secretary of State for Health 1992).

In fact, between 1995 and 2005 the proportion of adult males classified as obese rose by half to 23 per cent of the male population, while the proportion of obese women rose by 42 per cent to around 25 per cent of the female population (The Information Centre 2006b). Childhood (2–15 years) obesity increased by a similar extent over this period, with the proportion of obese boys and girls rising by 65 per cent and 51 per cent respectively; nearly one in five children are classified as obese.

A new PSA target for obesity was established in 2004 to 'halt the year-on-year rise in obesity among children aged under 11 by 2010 in the context of a broader strategy to tackle obesity in the population as a whole'.

The 2006 National Centre for Social Research report, *Forecasting Obesity to 2010* (Zaninotto P *et al* 2006) predicts a continuing rising trend in obesity to 2010, when some 33 per cent of men, 28 per cent of women, one-fifth of boys and more than one-fifth of girls will be obese. Furthermore, the proportion of obese children aged 2–11 is also forecast to rise. The evidence on obesity is of great concern and puts achievement at a much worse level than even the slow uptake scenario.

Physical activity and diet

Increased physical activity and improved diet are important levers for halting the rising prevalence of obesity and combating the other ill effects of sedentary lifestyles.

Since 1996, the government has recommended that adults should participate in at least 30 minutes of moderately intense activity five days a week; the long-term target is to have 70 per cent of adults in line with this recommendation by 2020 and 50 per cent on track by 2011 (Department of Health Strategy Unit 2002). Over a third of men and a quarter of women met these guidelines in 2004, an improvement since 1997 (The Information Centre 2006b).

The children's physical activity PSA target in England is to increase the proportion of school children spending at least two hours a week engaged in 'high quality' sport from 25 per cent in 2002 to 75 per cent in 2006 and 85 per cent in 2008. Progress to date has been encouraging (TNS 2006). The *School Sport Survey 2005–06* found that 80 per cent of pupils in partnership schools – those participating in a national school sports initiative – participate in at least two hours of high-quality physical education and school sport in a typical week – an increase of 11 per cent over the previous year and an improvement on the 2006 target.

So the government is on track with its children's activity targets and may also achieve its interim target for adults, but this will require sustained effort up to and beyond 2011. At best this could be classified as solid progress.

The Department of Health's 2005 publication *Choosing a Better Diet: A food and health action plan* (Department of Health 2005a) set out six dietary objectives for England relating to consumption of fruit and vegetables, fibre, salt, saturated fat, total fat and sugar. Of these, five are recommendations and only one is a target with a timetable for delivery: to reduce average intake of salt to 6 grams per day by 2010. Recent research, using urinary sodium tests, carried out in 2005–6 found that salt consumption in Great Britain is falling but remains 50 per cent higher than the recommended 6g per day (National Centre for Social Research 2006). As with physical activity, progress on diet is on a solid progress trajectory at best, but is probably somewhere between this and slow uptake.

Health promotion expenditure

The 2002 review estimated health promotion expenditure in England at around £250 million – less than the NHS spends in a day and a half. All three scenarios projected an increase in health promotion spending, with the fully engaged scenario assuming the largest and most rapid rise, doubling to around £500 million by 2007/8 (Wanless 2002).

It is impossible to track trends in public health or health promotion spending since 2002 as no official figures are kept. However, some indication of spending can be gleaned from the Department of Health's National Programme Budget Project (NPBP) initiative and also from expenditure on public health campaigns and the size of the public health workforce. NPBP data shows that, between 2003/4 and 2005/6, there was a real expenditure increase of around 16 per cent in its 'healthy individuals' category, while departmental spend on public health campaigns showed only a 1 per cent real increase over this period (Department of Health 2005b, 2006c; Hansard 2007a). A useful development of the NPBP dataset would be to identify public health spending separately.

It is indicative of the relatively low priority given to public health that, while non-public health medical staff numbers have increased by nearly 60 per cent since 1997, the number of public health consultants and registrars has gone down overall. The Chief Medical Officer's 2005 annual report noted that local public health budgets have regularly been 'raided' to find funding to reduce hospital deficits or meet productivity targets. It is hard to disagree with Sir Liam Donaldson's assessment that public health is 'way off' the fully engaged scenario and more in line with slow uptake (Donaldson 2006).

For more detail on health outcomes, *see* Part 2, Chapter 9.

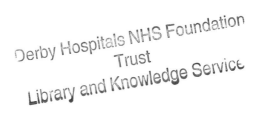

HEALTH OUTCOMES AND DETERMINANTS OF HEALTH: OVERALL ASSESSMENT

The 2002 review's vision was that health would improve through a combination of better and more responsive health care services and changes in health-seeking behaviour.

Assessing the overall contribution of the NHS to improvements in patient and public health is extremely difficult and hampered by the lack of routine information on changes in patients' health status.

On broad measures, the health of the population has improved: overall mortality rates have fallen and life expectancy has increased, although both of these developments are continuations of long-term trends. Cancer survival rates have also increased. Infant and perinatal mortality rates have improved a little since 2002 but are still higher than for many other European countries. And various measures of morbidity, such as longstanding illness, remain unchanged.

Tackling the causes of ill health is an ongoing long-term task. Continuing reductions in smoking and improvements in levels of physical activity and diet suggest a future close to the solid progress scenario. But over-optimistic targets – such as those relating to obesity – make it difficult to assess engagement levels in relation to the 2002 review scenarios. Overall, however, the evidence suggests that the population is on a path between slow uptake and solid progress.

Given the lack of accurate information on public health expenditure since 2002, it is impossible to assess whether the fully engaged aspirations for a doubling in public health spending by 2007/8 have been met. Tackling recent financial difficulties in the NHS by raiding public health budgets has not been in the long-term interests of the public's health.

Implications for long-term resource needs

The models used in the 2002 review necessarily made a great many assumptions. Since then new information has revealed other factors that could impact on long-term expenditure. Official demographic forecasts have caught up with those in the 2002 review's models. Mortality rates have declined over many decades, and if this trend continues the number of older people needing health care could increase much more sharply than was projected in the review.

Lifestyle improvements over the past few years are, on balance, somewhere between slow uptake and solid progress, and productivity improvements are low. Information weaknesses make productivity difficult to position against the 2002 scenarios, but it is difficult to avoid the judgement that it is closer to slow uptake than to the more optimistic scenarios.

New national service frameworks (NSFs) have not been rolled out systematically, nor have existing NSFs been updated in the systematic way proposed in 2002. Of course, new treatments continue to become available and many are cost-effective, but it is not possible to compare their total cost with the equivalent components in the 2002 projections. Yet such comparisons are crucial to forecasting what the delivery of a comprehensive health service would cost.

Neither the NHS Plan nor the 2002 review set out to define a specific path or timeline for improvements in productivity and quality of care; nor, indeed, did the government have a complete 'blueprint' for reform when the Plan was published. Neither of these documents contained a set of specific five-year improvement targets which could provide a baseline for measurement. The comprehensive vision in the 2001 Wanless Interim Report (2001) was set out for 2022/3 not 2006/7.

When the recent trends in prevention and productivity are combined with demographic forecasts predicting a growth in the older population, it is difficult to avoid the conclusion that delivery of comprehensive, high-quality health services could require long-tem resources close to those envisaged in the slow uptake scenario. Such an expensive service would raise questions about the sustainability of current widespread support for the NHS if it continues to be much less efficient than it could be.

The 2002 review emphasised that success would not be guaranteed by simply spending money and concluded that radical reform was equally vital (Wanless 2002). In the light of subsequent performance the urgent need to improve prevention and productivity is even greater.

The next chapter considers whether government policies for the NHS were appropriately designed and implemented or whether some of the shortfalls indicated in this chapter can be attributed to failures on this front. The question is: how much did the government do, in terms of reform and policy implementation, to help realise the aspirations of the 2002 review and create a system that will be able to deliver in the future?

3 The policy framework

The last chapter described improvements in the NHS over the course of this decade. Some of these, such as new hospitals and increased staffing, are the direct consequence of a rapid increase in resources. However, as has been shown, the use made of those resources has not been as effective as was projected in the 2002 review scenarios. It has also been made clear how critical the projected improvements in productivity – including both cost and quality – were to the costings set out in the scenarios.

This chapter considers whether the policies the government has pursued over the past 10 years have supported or hindered the required improvements. It focuses on four main routes to improved performance:

- policy development
- organisational change
- service redesign
- support programmes.

Where appropriate, developments in these areas are compared with the recommendations of the 2002 and 2004 reviews and their impact on performance assessed. Finally, the effectiveness of the policy process is considered and whether alternatives might offer a greater chance of sustained improvement.

Policy development: moving away from central direction

The government recognised from the outset that the process of change had to be actively driven forward. During the 1990s, some significant improvements in performance had taken place, such as reductions in the numbers of patients waiting a long time for admission to hospital following introduction of the *Patient's Charter* (Department of Health 1995b) and shorter hospital stays. But the internal market had exerted only limited impact (Le Grand *et al* 1998) and the Conservatives' final White Paper *A Service with Ambitions* (Department of Health 1996) contained few ideas for ensuring those ambitions were realised.

The approach the New Labour administration initially adopted relied heavily on central direction. Enforcement of the waiting list target – which had formed part of its election manifesto in 1997 – through ad hoc injections of funding and strong central pressure on the local NHS set the pattern for the much larger programme of improvements set out later in the NHS Plan. These too were 'enforced' by the centre through active management via its regional offices. As a result, chief executives were under no illusions about where to focus their attention. The *NHS Implementation Plan* (Department of Health 2001a) made it clear that the process would be overseen centrally and directed by 'clear targets and milestones' set on an annual basis.

However, by 2001, with the publication of *Shifting the Balance of Power* (Department of Health 2001b), the government was already beginning to recognise that the implementation process adopted in 2000 had to be modified; in particular, it accepted that reform could not be entirely directed from the centre, that targets alone were not enough to drive the improvements it was looking for and that having a vast range of targets might be counterproductive.

Delivering the NHS Plan explicitly stated that '...the 1948 model is simply inadequate for today's needs. We are on a journey.... which represents nothing less than the replacement of an outdated system' (Department of Health 2002, p 3). The centralised model was not abandoned, however: key targets remained in place as did other centrally driven programmes, such as National Service Frameworks. However, a different approach was gradually developed alongside these initiatives.

This approach aimed to:

- diminish the role of the centre by reducing the number of centrally imposed targets and allocating a larger share of the NHS budget directly to local purchasers

- employ a variety of incentives to improve local performance and standards for measuring progress, while allowing greater freedoms to local organisations (particularly foundation trusts)

- give patients a bigger say in the operation of the service and a greater role in protecting their own health

- promote diversity in the supply of health care by introducing independent sector providers – including those from the third sector – into areas which had hitherto been largely the preserve of the NHS

- improve monitoring arrangements to aid identification of progress towards quality and service goals as well as service failures

- reduce risks to health.

The underlying logic was as follows:

1. Reducing the role of the centre should release local initiative to pursue local priorities and rebut the charge of micro-management. Nevertheless, some national targets would remain.

2. Setting financial and other incentives should serve to promote specific goals, such as shorter waiting times, and general goals, such as greater efficiency in service delivery, while leaving the precise implementation to local commissioners and providers. Greater freedom from central controls should encourage service innovation and improvement, while national and local standards should set minimum levels of performance, not regulate differences.

3. Giving individuals a greater say in the operation of the service, through choice and other mechanisms, should promote a more user-sensitive service and also put pressure on providers to make service improvements. Engaging people in their own health should reduce demands on professional services and lead to better outcomes.

4. Introducing diversity of supply should create pressure on existing providers to improve their performance, while the resultant innovation might raise quality and produce a better match between users' needs and service provision.

5. Improving monitoring through independent regulators should identify poor performance, while technical support should provide the means to improve.

6. Reducing risks to health should lead to lower demands on health care services.

In broad terms, these policies match those put forward in the 2002 review, which also envisaged an enhanced role for the local NHS, albeit within a framework of some national targets and standards. The review envisaged that pressure to improve performance, in cost and quality terms, would be imposed through incentives rather than direction, with the outcomes systematically monitored. It also envisaged an enhanced role for self-care. Both the 2002 and 2004 reviews emphasised the benefits of risk reduction.

At a general level, the government's new policy framework was in line with the recommendations of the 2002 and 2004 reviews. The key questions are: has that framework been implemented effectively and has it led to improved performance?

IMPACT OF THE POLICY FRAMEWORK

Evidence of the impact of the main strands of policy set out above is very limited and it is not possible to demonstrate with certainty what the contributions of the various elements have been. As the following examples show, what evidence there is suggests that the changes introduced since 2002 have so far had only a modest impact, in some cases because they are not yet fully implemented and in others because they have not been fully worked out.

Patient choice
Patient choice was instituted on a pilot basis as early as 2002 and subsequently expanded nationally and over a wider range of services. The early evidence was encouraging: a significant number of patients did exercise choice and were able to reduce their waiting time.

But as the pilot scheme was rolled out nationally, it became apparent that GPs had not been persuaded of its value and the IT systems required to make it work were behind schedule (National Audit Office 2006). Surveys carried out in 2006 revealed significant numbers of patients who had not been offered choice by their GPs; and of those who were, only a minority exercised their choice in favour of non-local providers (Department of Health 2007u).

No evidence is available about how providers responded when patients did choose to go elsewhere. It is possible that the potential loss of business acted as a spur to improving performance, but there has been no research on this.

New providers of elective care
The Government has repeatedly claimed that introducing new providers has made a decisive contribution to reducing waiting lists and times. Departmental evidence to the Health Committee (House of Commons Health Committee 2006b) acknowledged that this claim could not be substantiated, however, even in the case of cataract surgery, for which

much of the new capacity had been commissioned. Comparison of the time when the new capacity became available with improvement in waiting list performance showed that the latter predated the former. Again, it is possible that the potential loss of business acted as a spur to better performance, but there is no systematic research which supports this.

Financial incentives

The new policy framework is critically dependent on incentives to guide organisations in the desired direction. The main financial instrument used in this way has been Payment by Results, combined with changes to the accounting framework designed to bring about tighter financial management. The limited evidence available on the impact of payment by results suggests that it has had little effect so far (Farrar *et al* 2006).

In line with a recommendation in the 2002 review, *The NHS Improvement Plan* proposed that a system of financial incentives should be introduced to encourage speedier discharge from hospital. The evidence suggests that this has been successful (*see* p 122–3). The number of delayed discharges has been reduced by comparison with other developed countries, where they are still rising. While some long delays still occur, the numbers involved are now much smaller than in 2002.

However, the charging regime cannot take all the credit for this improvement. Delays in discharge were falling before it was introduced and in some areas the charging regime was not applied by mutual agreement between health trusts and local authorities (Godden *et al* 2007). Other changes, such as expanded intermediate care, supported by targeted allocation of funding to health and local authorities, have also contributed to the improvement.

Commissioning

In this key area, the new arrangements – particularly the introduction of practice-based commissioning (PBC) – have only recently been put in place. The case for a merger of primary care trusts (PCTs) into larger units was based on the need to give purchasers greater influence over providers – itself a recognition that the more local structure introduced in 2002 had been largely ineffective. The new PCTs have not been in place for long enough to measure their impact and the same is true of practice-based commissioning: although it has been fully implemented in theory, the budgetary systems to support it are generally not yet in place. The government has claimed (Department of Health 2007g) that PBC has led to a fall in hospital referrals, but there is no systematic evidence as yet on how these or any other benefits are being realised.

Other evidence suggests the NHS has found it hard to institute a successful contracting regime. A report from the House of Commons Public Accounts Committee (2007c) on the introduction of the new contracts for out-of-hours services identified some serious failings in purchasing, for which both the department and local organisations were responsible, and showed that subsequent monitoring (a local responsibility) had not been effective. In addition, some of the resultant services could have been obtained at lower cost, without sacrifice of quality, had purchasing been more effective. Other centrally driven contracts for services, such as high street dental services and independent sector treatment centres (ISTCs) have also performed below expectations. The hoped-for improvements in access to dental care have not been fully realised, and the Department was unable to satisfy the Health Committee that the ISTC programme had provided value for money (Health Committee 2006b).

The general implication to be drawn from these examples is that there was, and probably remains, a lot to learn about how to set and monitor contracts in the more open and diverse environment the government is trying to create (Smith *et al* 2006). There may also be lessons to be learned about possible limitations to centrally imposed contracts.

Personal engagement
The initial focus of this element of policy was the expert patient programme (EPP), which was announced before publication of the *NHS Plan*. The 2002 review built in the cost benefit of improved self-care by using Department of Health estimates that for every £100 spent on encouraging self-care around £150 worth of benefits would be delivered in return (Wanless 2002).

Since 2002, a number of related policies have been introduced to promote self-care. Initial evaluation of the EPP produced favourable results – including a reduction in GP consultations, A&E attendances and outpatient appointments (Department of Health website at: www.dh.gov.uk). However, although the intention to greatly expand the programme was announced in 2005, it was only in 2007 that the organisational foundation was put in place ready for national roll-out in 2008 (Department of Health 2007k).

Other policies, such as health trainers, are too recent or too limited to evaluate. *Supporting People with Long Term Conditions for Self Care: A guide to developing local strategies and good practice* was published as late as 2006 (Department of Health 2006k).

The White Paper *Choosing Health* (Department of Health 2004c) announced a new service – Health Direct – that will provide information on health choices. Health Direct is to be developed as a telephone, internet and digital television service and will also be available to people who do not have home internet access through the government-funded UK Online centres. However, implementation of this service only began in 2007.

In January 2007 the Department of Health and NHS Direct began looking for a local health community to act as 'early adopter' for an NHS Health Direct scheme to provide multi-media advice supporting personal health improvement. The early adopter scheme will be launched by October 2007 and evaluated to inform national roll-out of NHS Health Direct in 2008.

As in other areas, most of these programmes have not been established long enough for their impact to be discernible. In the fully engaged scenario, the impact of increased self-care is assumed to have double the impact that it has in the slow uptake and solid progress scenarios, reflecting a step change in public engagement. In the solid progress and slow uptake scenarios, the 2002 review assumed that increased self-care would result in a switch of 1 per cent of GP activity to pharmacists and a reduction of 17 per cent in outpatient attendances by 225,000 people using self-care. In the fully engaged scenario, the effect of increased self-care is larger, with an assumption of a 2 per cent transfer of GP activity to pharmacists and a reduction of 17 per cent in outpatient attendances among 450,000 people using self-care. These forecasts have yet to be realised.

Although early findings from the expert patient programme, based on self-reported changes, suggested that use of professional services had declined, later work (National Primary Care Research and Development Centre 2007) found very little evidence of this impact. There are also reasons to believe that it may be hard to develop self-care beyond the bounds of an enthusiastic minority (Bury 2007) and whether it offers the financial benefits assumed in the 2002 review (Robertson and Dixon 2007).

The policy journey

In most cases policy development has been incremental. For example, patient choice was initially introduced as a means of shortening waiting times by allowing people to go to hospitals with shorter waiting times. Two years later, choice was being presented as a means of promoting quality and efficiency. This may have reflected original policy intentions, but these were not made explicit in, for example, the NHS Plan.

The decision to procure more elective operations from the private sector was initially justified as a sensible use of spare capacity. Two years later the introduction of new providers was justified in terms of 'contestability' – a spur to innovation and greater efficiency. As with choice, this goal may have been part of the original policy intention, but this was not explicit in the NHS Plan.

Similarly, the introduction of Payment by Results (PbR) was initially explained by the need to support choice: money had to follow the patient. While that justification remains, a prospective tariff set at national average costs automatically introduces an incentive for better performance (at least in terms of reducing costs where these exceed tariff prices), irrespective of whether patients exercise choice. In addition, the centre can put pressure on nearly all providers by including the annual efficiency improvement factor in the national tariff.

By 2005 it was apparent that the initial design of the new reimbursement system was faulty in some key respects. The initial focus was on elective care, with an explicit intention to incentivise hospitals to increase activity (particularly for interventions with long waits). But that was the wrong incentive for emergency admissions, which the government wanted to reduce. Some ad hoc changes to the emergency tariff were subsequently made and, after a rapid review in 2006, the need for a more thorough review has been acknowledged with the publication of a consultation paper (Department of Health 2007s). Now the government accepts that the payment system has to support a wider range of objectives than reductions in waiting times and that what was suitable for elective care did not necessarily support other policies (such as the transfer of care away from acute hospitals) or encourage better services for chronic conditions.

In addition, the government recognised that mistakes were made in the application of the resource accounting and budgeting regime to the NHS. This was introduced from 2001 across the public sector as a whole, but problems with its application within the NHS became quickly apparent (Palmer 2005; Audit Commission 2005). Nevertheless, the government persisted with the regime until 2007 when, after initial suggestions that it had to remain, it decided to withdraw it from trusts (although not PCTs) (Department of Health 2007r). The only obvious effect of the introduction and subsequent withdrawal of this regime was to waste management time and demotivate trust staff obliged to work with this apparently arbitrary and damaging financial system.

In other areas, too, the government has backtracked on its original intentions. The government originally described the internal market as a 'misconceived attempt to tackle the pressures facing the NHS' (Department of Health 1997). Four years later it embarked on the series of measures which led to the creation of both an internal and an external market, and to the explicit use of financial incentives to drive performance.

Throughout this period, the importance of the commissioning function has never been questioned, but its form has been radically changed more than once. In 1997, the government decided to maintain the purchaser/provider split while abolishing fundholding, and in 1998 it announced the creation of primary care groups. In 2002/3 it established new purchasing structures in the form of primary care trusts; but in 2005 it decided that this change had been a mistake and brought about the merger of PCTs into larger units, while simultaneously promoting a practice-based commissioning scheme that embodied some of the features of the fundholding arrangements rejected in its first White Paper.

Even by 2007 implementation of the new framework was far from complete. Although the main elements of the new approach were apparent in 2002, and in some cases earlier, it has taken a great deal of time for the new framework to be fully developed and for its various elements to be worked out into operational policies. The length of time taken and the incremental nature of the reform process have undermined confidence in what was being attempted. The fact that the purchasing side of the NHS has been 'in transition' for nearly two years *may* have contributed to rising deficits during this period; and it has *certainly* made it harder to tackle them.

More fundamentally, however, commissioning is believed to have failed to produce the patient benefits that might have been expected. Reorganisations – even for the right reasons – have interfered with commissioners' ability to get to grips with their main purchasing tasks. Furthermore, as results from a recent systems simulation suggest, 'old style' PCT thinking, worries about destabilising local health economies and a general lack of skills and analytical abilities have contributed to a somewhat conservative approach to instigating change (Harvey *et al* 2007).

As all the above examples show, while implementation of all the main elements of the policy framework now in place began some time ago, the 'policy journey' has been taken a step at a time and has sometimes involved significant backtracking. As a result the policy framework remains in its infancy, particularly in terms of public health policies. The 2004 review (Wanless 2004) set out a coherent framework for developing a systematic and informed approach to the reduction of risks to health (*see* box, overleaf). The White Paper *Choosing Health,* published in the same year (Department of Health 2004), ignored key elements of that approach, particularly those bearing on the development and monitoring of public health programmes.

Nevertheless, a large number of public health initiatives have been implemented since 2004, including the smoking ban in public places in July 2007, the Five-a-Day campaign to encourage healthier eating, promotion of physical activity, health trainers and many others (Department of Health 2005a). The most recent report from the Department of Health (Department of Health 2007b) identifies a large number of initiatives of various kinds. But many, if not most, of these are small scale and it is too soon to detect their impact on health.

There is no sign as yet of a framework emerging along the lines proposed in the 2004 review (Wanless 2004). Childhood obesity may be the area of public health with the most critical long-term implications. Yet the House of Commons Public Accounts Committee (2007b) concluded that, despite the establishment of a 2004 PSA target involving the Departments of Health, Education and Skills and Culture Media and Sport, little concrete action had been taken. More generally, the Healthcare Commission's 2006 report on the state of the NHS found that 'Although there has been a major policy commitment to improving people's health, progress remains limited' (2006c, p 82).

Organisational change: a costly process

Neither the 2002 nor the 2004 review recommended reorganisation of the NHS. The first review observed that the NHS had been through many reorganisations in the past and that the challenge now was to make the existing structure effective. The authors agreed that greater local freedom was the appropriate way forward, capable of delivering powerful benefits through innovation. They gave strong support to the continuing development of NICE and increased production of new national service frameworks (Wanless 2002).

The 2004 review pointed out that previous NHS reorganisations had not always given careful consideration to their impact on the local delivery of public health objectives. At the time of the review, each of the 303 PCTs had a Director of Public Health post, which meant spreading existing resources very thinly. The authors concluded that change should be evolutionary. 'Given the newness of the structure and that repeated restructuring has tended to weaken the NHS over decades, structural change is not recommended, but where it seems locally that the best way forward is to combine PCTs' forces to tackle public health, that should not be discouraged' (Wanless 2004).

While this review was under way, the government set in train its own review of 'arm's length bodies' (Department of Health 2004a). This extended beyond public health but provided an opportunity to establish an organisational framework that could take public health issues forward in a positive way. There were gaps in responsibilities between existing bodies at the time, and the review recommended assigning responsibility for:
- developing the cost-effectiveness evidence base on public health
- researching the effectiveness of activities, and interpreting findings
- the educational role played formerly by the Health Education Authority
- periodic reassessment of national objectives for all major determinants of health and health inequalities
- regulation of nicotine and tobacco.

Before this review (and, indeed, in the years that followed), both the NHS and the arm's length bodies that support it had been in a state of continual reorganisation. The NHS Plan itself envisaged that the general trend would be towards devolution to the 'front line'. It noted the concurrent establishment of primary care groups or trusts as new purchasing bodies but made no proposals for changing its own regional organisation, the health authorities or the NHS provider trusts.

The Plan proposed that within the department itself the 'increasingly unhelpful split' between public health, the NHS and social services could '...be overcome by combining responsibility for them in a single chief executive post at permanent secretary level with more autonomy and operational control' (para 6.48). It recommended the establishment of a Modernisation Board (and a series of local boards) to advise on implementation, a series of task forces to 'drive implementation' and a Modernisation Agency to support the process of service redesign. The roles of the Commission for Health Improvement, established by the 1998 White Paper, and the Audit Commission were confirmed and no indication was given of an intention to change the roles or organisational structure of other arm's length bodies.

Since 2000, however, all the elements of the structure outlined in the Plan have been revised – in some cases radically and in others more than once (*see* box, overleaf).

The new structure embodies a number of the key features proposed in the 2002 review, specifically the scope for more local action, more independent providers, strong local commissioners and an enhanced role for monitoring of financial and clinical performance through a strengthened regulatory structure.

RECENT ORGANISATIONAL CHANGES IN THE DH, NHS AND RELATED AGENCIES

Department/regions

2001/2 Abolition of health authorities and regional offices and creation of Strategic Health Authorities (SHAs); revision of SHA roles and boundaries 2005/6

2003 Change Programme leading to creation of three business groups and Top Team

2005 High-level McKinsey review leading to a new structure and management board - built round division between departmental Permanent Secretary and NHS Chief Executive plus Chief Medical Officer, '...with greater emphasis on social care, finance and stronger policy and strategy'

2007 New top-level structure introduced prior to capability review

Purchasing

2002 Transfer to PCTs of most health authority functions. Strengthened public health teams in PCTs following 2002 reorganisation

2005 Abolition of original set of primary care trusts (in most areas) and creation of new, larger bodies

2005/6 Introduction of practice based commissioning

2006 PCT Fitness for purpose reviews

Providing

2004 Introduction of foundation trusts. A number of trust mergers but no sustained programme except for ambulance services

Regulators and support organisations

2000 Abolition of Health Education Authority. Replaced by Health Development Agency.

2001 Creation of the NHS Modernisation Agency

2004 Arm's length bodies review; creation of Monitor; abolition of Commission for Health Improvement and creation of Healthcare Commission. NHS University established

2005 Merger of some HDA functions with NICE. Modernisation Agency abolished along with NHS University. Replaced (in part) by NHS Institute for Innovation and Development

2007 Merger of Healthcare Commission, Mental Health Commission and Commission for Social Care Inspection

But because this new structure has taken so long to emerge, its benefits have yet to be realised. Furthermore, the costs of achieving the new structure have been high in more ways than one. Many NHS services and activities require close co-operation both within the health sector and with external bodies, such as local authorities. Organisational changes disrupt not only the formal links underpinning co-operative working but also the informal links based on mutual trust between individual officers and health professionals. These changes, coupled with the twists and turns of health policy, have made day-to-day management more difficult and reduced the capacity to plan for service redesign and other key functions. As the Health Committee noted in relation to workforce planning 'The health service has lost sight of this vision (that is, a clear focus on improving flexibility and productivity) and marginalised workforce planning. The situation has been exacerbated by persistent structural change' (2007, p 104).

Studies carried out in other sectors suggest that these opportunity costs are very high (King's Fund 2006). Within the NHS itself, there is only limited evidence on the impact of structural changes to its organisation. A study of trust mergers on four sites (Fulop *et al* 2002) found that those involved believed the mergers had had a negative effect on the delivery and development of services in general even when they had led to particular benefits, such as the achievement of critical mass. Similarly, a report from the National Audit Office (2003) found that the process of introducing clinical governance into trusts had been disrupted by organisational change.

The Health Committee report on *Changes to Primary Care Trusts* (2006a) reached similar conclusions, based partly on the evidence it received from some PCTs about the likely impact of impending changes to their structure. 'The restructuring of PCTs is likely to have significant effects on their ability to undertake their core functions... After the immediate disruption of reorganisation it is thought to take a further 18 months for the benefits to emerge – a total of three years from the initial reforms' (p 4).

For PCTs, additional problems arose from the fact that the government took several months after the initial announcement of the intended restructure to clarify its position over whether or not PCTs should retain provider functions.

In its response to the committee, the government argued that PCTs had to '...develop and change if they are [to succeed] in implementing the challenging reform programme they face' (p 4). The government also pointed out that it had put in place measures to support

---

ORGANISATION: SUMMARY ASSESSMENT

The structure now in place, with larger purchasing bodies and local clinical engagement through practice based commissioning, has a good chance of being more effective than its predecessor, but has yet to prove itself. Question marks remain, in particular, over the ability of PCTs and PBC to drive changes in service delivery, and the place of public health in the new structure.

Changes to the provider side of the NHS have been less radical. It is too early to assess whether the benefits of foundation trust status outweigh the possible risks to co-operation between trusts.

The new regulatory structure, comprising Monitor, the Audit Commission and the Healthcare Commission, looks far stronger than its predecessor.

The overall structure that emerged by 2007 is still largely untested; and further change is in prospect for the Department itself, in the light of the recent capability review (Capability Review Team 2007). The benefits, if any, of the most recent changes are still to come.

While the original SHAs and PCTs may not have been fit for purpose, the process of organisational change has been costly in terms of disruption, loss of experienced staff and changes in working relationships both within the NHS and with external organisations.

staff during the transition process; but it did not attempt to rebut the claim that the benefits of the changes would take time to materialise and that the changes themselves imposed considerable costs on affected organisations.

Research evidence has not been found about the impact of organisational change on other parts of the health sector, but it may be presumed that they, too, will have suffered disruption threatening their day-to-day efficiency and reducing their capacity to plan and implement improvements.

Service redesign to improve performance

As shown in the previous chapter, the NHS Plan committed the government to a massive programme of capital investment in hospitals and smaller health premises. The case for this programme was largely based on the dilapidated state of the NHS estate, which had suffered from decades of very low levels of investment. But the Plan presented no evidence that the new hospitals would be more cost-effective than the ones they replaced or make a substantial contribution to improved performance in terms of care. In three other ways, however, the Plan identified service redesign as a means to improve performance.

1. Supporting local redesign

The Plan claimed, 'Where [services have been redesigned] the impact has been dramatic. It has resulted in improved services for patients. It has also resulted in improved productivity, made the task of caring for patients easier for staff and in many cases released resources to spend on other services' (Department of Health 2000c, para 6.12). In particular, the Plan promoted the use of 'care pathways' as means of analysing where delays and other problems arise and where changes in working methods and professional roles could improve efficiency and access.

The government had realised as early as 1999 that the process of service reform had to be supported through advisory and learning programmes. In that year, the cancer care collaborative was established to support the relatively stringent waiting time targets being introduced at that time for patients with cancer. Other collaboratives followed and a series of 'action on...' programmes targeted a number of specific areas, such as cataract treatment and orthopaedics.

The Modernisation Agency was established in 2000 to bring these and other initiatives within the ambit of a single body and extend them to the wider NHS. The agency actively encouraged analysis of care pathways along with other methods of improving service delivery (Modernisation Agency 2003).

The range and scope of these and similar programmes has increased steadily. In particular, the 18-week target, set in 2004, has led to an intensive programme of work within both the Department of Health and the NHS Institute for Innovation and Improvement, the successor body to the Modernisation Agency. In addition, the Department promoted some targeted initiatives to improve operational efficiency, such as in pathology and diagnostics where improvements were critical to the achievement of shorter waiting times (see, for example, www.pathologyimprovement.nhs.uk).

2. National service frameworks

The Plan proposed a programme of National Service Frameworks (NSFs), partly to compensate for wide existing variations in service availability and performance. There was some evidence, for example, that cancer care services were not sufficiently specialised (Department of Health 1993, 1995a). This meant that the number of complex procedures carried out in some hospitals was too low to ensure high quality. Better quality care required an organised shift of activities to fewer, better-equipped centres as well as other changes in service delivery, such as well-defined care pathways within and between organisations. This, in turn, required a shift from individual hospitals and GP surgeries to networks of care covering up to two million people.

Following publication of the Cancer Plan (Department of Health 2000d), which was an NSF in all but name, the government published a number of NSFs covering coronary heart disease, mental illness, older people, diabetes, renal disease, long-term conditions, chronic obstructive pulmonary disease and children's services. The 2002 review endorsed this approach, not only to improve service delivery but also to define, in conjunction with NICE, what a comprehensive health service should comprise in practice (Wanless 2001). To achieve this broader goal required a rolling programme of NSF developments that would eventually cover almost all the needs the NHS aimed to meet. The 2004 review recommended that all the NSFs should be kept up-to-date and include costings, resource requirements and research needs (Wanless 2004).

3. Shifting care into the community

Public consultation preceding publication of the NHS Plan had elicited support for the provision of care closer to people's homes. However, many of the measures set out in the Plan involved strengthening the hospital sector, particularly through the rapid growth in consultant numbers, hospital beds and new buildings. The 2002 review argued that the balance of care between acute hospital and other settings was wrong and recommended better integration between NHS and local authority services, backed by financial incentives (Wanless 2002). It went on to recommend a major experiment, drawing on IT resources to determine whether a major shift in the balance of care would improve NHS performance. This experiment was not carried out but in 2006, following extensive public consultation, the government proposed a substantial shift of care from acute hospitals to community settings and set in train a number of measures, including extensive pilots, to achieve this objective (Department of Health 2006j).

A start had already been made on improving care for chronic conditions, using the Quality and Outcomes Framework (QOF) for general practice and specific targeted interventions for those most at risk of needing hospital care. Care for people with chronic illness has been an important feature of the NHS since its inception, but from 2004 onwards the government put in place a series of measures designed both to provide better care of those with long-term conditions and to reduce overall health care costs, particularly in acute hospitals. But these changes were introduced before the necessary analytic work had been completed to identify those most at risk. Early monitoring suggests that so far costs have not been reduced (Gravelle *et al* 2007). However, a substantial programme aimed at forecasting the risk of admission has been under way since 2004 (King's Fund 2007) and the Department of Health has recently established a number of demonstration sites to investigate further the potential of this approach. Further analysis and better targeting may show that substantial savings are achievable.

THE IMPACT OF SERVICE REDESIGN

The technical support targeted directly at improving the process of care delivery has focused on such areas as access times, lengths of stay and increases in day surgery. But there is very little published evidence on what the impact of these measures has been.

A series of studies carried out by the University of Birmingham was generally sceptical about the scale of change actually achieved (Ham *et al* 2003). However, since those reports were completed, the need for change in service delivery has been more widely recognised (particularly since 2004, with the introduction of the 18-week maximum waiting time target) and the number of programmes vastly extended. But there is no means available to measure the impact of all the activity involved: although a large number of case studies are available, none gives a full account of the costs and benefits involved. It is reasonable to assume that some of the gains in waiting times could not have been achieved without the support of the Modernisation Agency and its successor, but there is no way to demonstrate the scale of that effect.

The previous chapter gave evidence of improvements in the services covered by NSFs. As noted above, these were intended to improve standards across the country, but to achieve this goal the way services were provided had to change. The Cancer Plan, for example, has led to the creation of nationwide cancer networks designed to ensure that patients receive specialised care when they need it. Before this, care was often provided by non-specialists with neither the experience nor the facilities to provide high-quality care. Such changes had been resisted for many years and could only have been achieved with strong central leadership. However, it is not possible to attribute the improvements in cancer survival rates to any one specific source of change; better service design, increased funding and staffing levels and new drugs have all contributed (Richards 2006, 2007).

Other changes have also been centrally driven, through targets, standards or incentives, as the following examples show.

Heart disease The Health Commission's review of the NSF found that it had '...given impetus to improving services, most notably the treatment of heart attacks, faster diagnosis of angina and reduced waits for revascularisation' (Healthcare Commission 2005b), although it had less impact on reducing levels of heart disease and providing rehabilitation after treatment.

Stroke The numbers treated in specialist units have increased rapidly (Royal College of Physicians 2007), as recommended in the NSF for older people, but other service areas (including the role of therapists and speed of access to imaging) have lagged behind.

Diabetes and renal disease The Quality and Outcomes Framework for GPs seems to have led to greatly improved diagnosis of these conditions.

There is little systematic evidence on changes in the balance of care. The Department of Health has published data since 2003 that record the number of procedures carried out in primary care settings, but it remains unclear how many of these were transferred from secondary care. The limited available evidence (Sibbald *et al* 2007) does not suggest that significant economic or quality benefits can be confidently expected, although access should be improved.

The previous chapter showed that the government has honoured its commitment to invest in new hospitals and other health premises. However, the initial emphasis on hospital building was essentially backward-looking: the capital stock was old and in need of replacement, but the massive investment from 1997 was instigated without sufficient regard to the context in which it was likely to be used. That context was changed by the government's own policies – introduction of independent sector treatment centres, Payment by Results and the shift to community care – as well as by external factors such as the European Working Times Directive (EWTD). But after its electoral defeat at Wyne Forest over the planned closure of the Kidderminster hospital, the government backed off closure as a route to improved performance.

However, tensions remained between the need to centralise and the desire to preserve and improve access, and these were heightened by financial pressures from 2004 onwards. In many parts of the country, a drive for better quality and lower costs, combined with other factors, such as EWTD, is leading to plans for substantial reconfiguration of services. During the 1990s, reconfiguration had focused on the need for fewer hospital sites, presumed to enjoy lower costs and produce better quality care. But the evidence base for justifying change in terms of cost, quality and access was, and remains, weak. The series of papers issued on the clinical case for change (Department of Health 2007f,l,m,n,w) contained very little evidence to justify their proposed change of direction in terms of potential benefits. The one piece of statistical evidence cited in these papers – relating to improved care for heart patients – was based on clinical judgement rather than research (Hansard 2007a). The recent review of London's health service (Darzi 2007) contains more evidence, but only for a limited number of services; and the case for its main proposal, that a network of 'polyclinics' should be established, has yet to be fully demonstrated. A critical evidence gap therefore remains.

SERVICE DESIGN: SUMMARY ASSESSMENT

The government was right to make service redesign a key policy objective. This issue had been neglected by previous administrations and had to be tackled if service quality, costs and access were all to be improved. It was also right to recognise that achieving change throughout the NHS and across the full range of services required substantial technical support and strong central direction through NSFs and similar initiatives. The Government has not yet committed itself to a continuing programme of NSF development as envisaged in the 2002 review (Wanless 2002), although in some cases guidance on improvement has been published in other ways.

The extent to which hospital reconfiguration is required to raise quality in the medium-term remains uncertain, as do the scale of the potential gains. It is also unclear what access and quality benefits will flow from reducing activity levels in acute hospitals, and at what cost.

Major uncertainties remain about how far hospital services can be transferred to other locations without loss of quality or increased costs. Throughout most of the period under review, the government has failed to acknowledge the need for flexibility in the light of uncertainty over the future balance of care; this failure is particularly apparent in its commitment to the rapid development of new hospitals using PFI.

Support programmes: from workforce to research

The NHS Plan recognised that reforms of both policy and delivery could be achieved only if a number of supporting elements were put in place. In 2000, the NHS was characterised by sharp divisions in professional roles and low uptake of new medical and information technology. Although efforts had been made to monitor performance and improve quality, for example through clinical audit programmes and the national confidential enquiries into perioperative deaths, the concept of clinical governance only started to be introduced in 1999 (Department of Health 1999a). At the start of the 1990s, a new research and development strategy had been announced with the aim of increasing the contribution research spending made to the NHS, but little had been achieved by 2000 (Harrison 2002).

In brief, at the time the NHS Plan was published, the basic elements underpinning productivity and quality improvements in other areas of the economy were not in place within the NHS. For this reason, the 2002 review recommended a number of changes designed to increase the productivity of the following NHS resources: workforce, IT and clinical governance (Wanless 2002).

WORKFORCE

The NHS Plan committed to large increases in the workforce and, while it did not directly address the question of their productivity (House of Commons Health Committee 2007), it did support removal of demarcations between different professions. The 2002 review recognised the critical importance of workforce planning (Wanless 2002). It envisaged the need for changes in the composition and role mix of the workforce in order to compensate for particular skill shortages, and it foresaw enhanced roles for nurses and assistants. It also saw changes in pay and conditions as critical to enhanced efficiency.

As the previous chapter showed, attempts to improve professional performance through changes in staff contracts have had only limited success, at considerable cost. The new GP contract has contributed to higher-quality performance, but at a high price. The new contract for hospital consultants has generated additional costs without apparent benefit to patients and has not yet led to any obvious improvement in productivity. Agenda for Change has allowed for greater flexibility in the workforce, but at a high cost that has yet to be justified.

Many new professional roles have been created, including emergency care practitioners and more specialised nurses, while the extension of prescribing rights has facilitated the development of new forms of service, using pharmacists, nurses and optometrists. Similarly, extension of referrals rights to optometrists has reduced waiting times for eye surgery.

The overall effect of these new contracts on productivity is difficult to assess, especially given how recent most of the changes are. But in many areas, including emergency care, surgical capacity and new community services, changes in the boundaries of professional roles have been critical to service improvement. Improved access to pharmacy care, for example, depends on new contractual arrangements combined with extended roles for community pharmacists. Nevertheless, there is some evidence that it is taking time for these improvements to be realised, partly because they continue to be resisted by other professionals (Pharmacy Practice Research Trust 2007).

Evidence presented to the Health Committee (2007) suggested that changes in professional roles have not always been well implemented, with doubts in some cases about their cost-effectiveness. Nevertheless, it is undoubtedly true that the NHS now has access to a larger range of 'delivery options', provided not just within its own ranks but also by the independent sector. The principle that service change requires changes in professional roles and competences is now widely accepted (Modernisation Agency 2003), and as a result the NHS is now a much more flexible organisation than it was in 2000.

The 2002 review argued that improved workforce planning was critical to the achievement of improved performance (Wanless 2002). As the Health Committee found, the process of workforce planning remains weak and there has been no sustained focus on the need to increase staff productivity. The Department of Health has not yet been able to find effective ways of linking forecasts of service development with the education and training of health professionals; and the recent debacle over medical recruitment is a striking example of this persisting serious weakness.

INFORMATION AND COMMUNICATION TECHNOLOGIES

Both the NHS Plan and the 2002 review envisaged that IT would facilitate major improvements in service delivery. But, as seen in Chapter 2, implementation of the ICT programme has been slow, with substantial benefits yet to be realised. Although the IT programme has contributed to the introduction of Choose and Book (albeit behind schedule) and to improvements in diagnostic performance, its main anticipated benefits have not been achieved.

CLINICAL GOVERNANCE

In 1998 the government published *A First Class Service: Quality within the NHS* (Department of Health 1998a) – the first major move to introduce systematic processes to support the improvement of clinical care. Subsequently, the 1999 Health Act (Secretary of State for Health 1999) imposed a statutory duty on all providers to establish systems of clinical governance. The 2002 review identified increased time spent by NHS staff on clinical governance activities as the main driver for improvements in safety (Wanless 2002). It assumed that by 2010/1, 10 per cent of staff time would be devoted to clinical governance and that the benefits of this would begin to show relatively quickly.

The evidence cited in Chapter 2 shows that expectations in relation to infections and other adverse incidents have not been realised, and it is not yet clear whether the clinical negligence bill has fallen in line with the 2002 review's forecast. The House of Commons Public Accounts Committee (2006) concluded that insufficient progress had been made in reducing risks and that the National Patient Safety Agency, set up in 2001 to co-ordinate incident reporting with a view to promoting patient safety, had yet to demonstrate good value for money. The Healthcare Commission's 2006 review of the state of the NHS found some signs of progress in reducing risks to patients, but with a clear trend yet to emerge. Its report makes it clear that much remains to be done, particularly where hospitals are concerned, over and above the risks posed by MRSA and other infections (Healthcare Commission 2006c). A new drive to reduce clinical errors was introduced in March 2007 (Department of Health 2007a).

In other areas progress has also been below expectations. Clinical audit was introduced in the 1990s but did not develop as originally envisaged, with either individual clinicians or care team. In recognition of this relatively slow development, *Trust Assurance and Safety* (Secretary of State for Health 2007c) proposed a substantial expansion of clinical audit. Other areas, however, have already seen substantial improvements, with a number of national monitoring systems in place for specific diseases (including some cancers, diabetes and various aspects of heart disease treatment), prescribing patterns and quality of care at the institutional level through the work of the Healthcare Commission.

There is only limited evidence of the impact of these activities, partly because they are so new but also because of the inherent difficulty of isolating the impact of one intervention against a background of continuous change. In 2006, the Healthcare Commission set out how it proposed to evaluate its activities, but the proposal itself makes clear how difficult it will be to isolate the effects of its activities from the context in which it operates and to evaluate cost-effectiveness.

The White Paper (Secretary of State for Health 2007c) also proposed a strengthening of continuing professional development and other measures aimed at improving performance in general as well as eliminating poor performance more effectively than in the past. These proposals are too new to have had any impact, but there is little evidence of the effectiveness of measures of this kind, mostly because of a lack of rigorous research (Sutherland and Leatherman 2006). The White Paper impact assessment fails to provide convincing estimates of the benefits the new arrangements – some of which are only in outline – will bring.

Clinical governance at the level of individuals, teams, organisations and systems of care is underpinned by the work of NICE in relation to individual interventions and the treatment of specific conditions. NICE has now established itself as an essential part of the English health care system and, through imitation, in others as well. But that does not constitute proof that it is effective in influencing clinical behaviour on the ground. An early review (Sheldon *et al* 2004) found that '...NICE guidance has been associated with the uptake of some technologies, although this has been variable'. The authors point to many factors that might impede the adoption of NICE guidance, including barriers at the level of individual clinician, organisations and the wider system. A study commissioned by NICE (Abacus 2005) also found considerable variation in response to its guidance.

Subsequent studies commissioned by NICE confirm this broad picture of implementation depending on a broad range of factors at local and national level (NHS National Institute for Health and Clinical Excellence 2005). These studies focus mainly on drugs. A study of its recommendations for services for people with multiple sclerosis found that organisational change and lack of funding had seriously reduced the scope for systematic monitoring across all the relevant services (Royal College of Physicians 2006). It did, nevertheless, establish that the seven main NICE recommendations had generally not been complied with.

Clinical governance now comprises a wide range of policies, some bearing on individual clinicians, some on organisations and some on specific services. In principle, these should form a coherent system for improving the quality of patient care, including the process of care delivery. But, as the evidence in Part 2 will demonstrate, it is hard to provide a full account of improvements in clinical care and process over the past 5–7 years and thus harder still to demonstrate links between the policies and their results. Nevertheless, two conclusions can be reached:

1. The government was right to introduce an explicit focus on the quality of care, although that in itself does not guarantee that services will improve.

2. The evidence is not available to demonstrate how the various elements of clinical governance perform *as a system* and hence whether its design and implementation could be improved.

NEW TECHNOLOGY

The anticipated improvement in quality of care depends in part on innovation in medical technology. The NHS Plan referred only fleetingly to the potential of technology to transform care delivery, focusing on new drugs and the potential of genetics. Subsequently, no target or implementation process was introduced to promote technical innovation across the NHS as a whole. Innovation has, of course, continued in the form of new drugs and new devices (Department of Health 2007 j,x,aa). But no large-scale vision of the potential of new technology has emerged.

By contrast, the 2002 review's vision for the health service in 2022 was one in which patients receive 'the best treatments…. supported by up-to-date and effective use of technology' (Wanless 2002). The interim report reiterated the UK's historical position as a late and slow adopter of medical technology. It concluded that some technologies would reduce unit costs, but that new technology as a whole would continue to put upward pressure on health care spending as it produced improvements in quality. The interim report also presented a preliminary estimate that technology and medical advances had contributed around two percentage points to the annual rate of growth of health spending over the previous 20 years, and suggested that over the next two decades technology spending would need to grow at an even faster rate to catch up – and keep up – with other countries.

The interim report included a discussion about genetics and stem cell technology, highlighting significant uncertainties and differences of opinion about their likely impact over the 20 years to 2022. The 2002 review concluded that their impact on health care spending over this time was unlikely to be great and therefore did not factor in any additional spending specifically to reflect developments in genetics (Wanless 2002). It did note, however, that as stem cell technology develops, it would be important to revisit this assumption in future. Given recent developments in this technology, these views still hold.

In its slow uptake scenario, the 2002 review assumed low rates of technology uptake in health care services, which would contribute around two percentage points a year to growth in health spending (Wanless 2002). The solid progress and fully engaged scenarios predicted higher rates of technology uptake, contributing around three percentage points a year to growth in health spending. The balance of technology spending might differ between these two scenarios, with more spending focused on public health measures, such as screening, in the fully engaged scenario.

In 2003, a Healthcare Industries Task Force was established to promote better working relationships between the NHS and industry with a view to improving the take-up of new technologies (Department of Health 2003c). In 2005, the Health Committee's report *The use of new medical technologies within the NHS* (2005) noted the department's concern about their continued slow take-up and endorsed the recommendations of the task force, which had not been implemented in full.

A further report from the task force (HITF 2007) made more recommendations designed to speed up innovation. In particular, it called for support for changes to the NHS procurement process to promote '...uptake of technologies and innovations which can lead to improvements in health care provision, patient safety and value for money'. In addition, the UK Clinical Research Collaboration, established after publication of *Best Research for Best Health* (Department of Health 2006b), has been tasked with speeding up the transfer of research findings into treatment, particularly through an expansion in clinical trials.

In some areas, such as diagnostics, the extra spending has allowed the NHS to make up some of its 'technological deficit'. In other areas, take-up remains low relative to other countries and in some, such as radiology, there is still considerable ground to make up. In that particular case, the need for more investment seems evident; but, as the task force report acknowledged, evidence of the value of new technologies is generally poor, so it is not possible to estimate the scale of the 'lost' benefits or the costs of achieving them.

In its 2007 report, the task force pointed to progress in some areas, such as evaluation techniques, improved procurement methods and the creation of healthcare technology co-operatives and the National Innovation Centre; but it acknowledged that more needed to be done, particularly to make staff more aware of the potential of new technology to improve care. It looked to improvements in NHS procurement techniques to ensure that patients enjoyed access to new technologies. However, the 2007 report produced neither evidence of the impact of changes already made nor of what might be expected in future.

RESEARCH

Neither the NHS Plan nor the 2002 review gave detailed attention to departmental and other publicly-funded research programmes as a whole. However, as mentioned, the 2002 review called for a major experiment to test the benefits of a shift in care from hospital to community and also envisaged close links between national service frameworks and research programmes (Wanless 2002). The 2004 review emphasised the urgent need for research into the effectiveness of public health interventions. Its absence had hindered the development of a systematic, evidence-based programme (Wanless 2004). Both reviews argued for comprehensive research programmes to be linked to each NSF.

The absence of an effective link between research programmes and NHS service delivery and efficiency was first identified in 1988 (House of Lords 1988). The then government responded with a new research commissioning structure and time-limited research programmes. It recognised the research shortfall relating to service delivery by setting up the NHS Service Delivery and Organisation (SDO) research programme in the 1990s, along with smaller programmes aimed at promoting technical innovations, such as New and Emerging Technologies Programme (NEAT)(Harrison 2002).

In 2005, the Department of Health carried out a review of its own research funding (2006b); this was followed by a wider-ranging review for the Treasury led by Sir David Cooksey (HM Treasury 2006). As a result, a number of new programmes have been announced that bear on operational efficiency, patient safety and public health (Department of Health 2007q,y). Extra funding has been allocated to primary care research and the SDO research programme has been expanded. In 2004 the National Prevention Research Initiative was established to focus on obesity, cancer, coronary heart disease and diabetes. There has also been a new public health initiative within the framework of the UK Clinical Research Collaboration, which will bring together research funding partners to agree a long-term research strategy (ESRC 2007).

These programmes promise greater support for health care delivery and prevention in future, but are still in their infancy and have had little impact so far. An evaluation by the SDO programme of the impact of its own funded research provided substantial evidence of the quality of the work and its favourable reception in this country and abroad. But it was not possible to take the further step of measuring its long-term economic impact on the NHS. What is clear, however, is that the contribution of non-clinical research to NHS performance has been very limited so far, with some nervousness about the level of continuing support it will receive.

SUPPORT PROGRAMMES: SUMMARY ASSESSMENT

The support programmes have made important contributions to improved performance in some areas.

The reform of NHS pay structure has not yet been successful, but potentially important flexibilities within the workforce have been achieved.

Arrangements for clinical governance are well developed, particularly at national level, although their specific impact is hard to detect.

In some key areas, particularly information and medical technology and non-clinical research, it is not yet possible to identify substantial improvements arising from policies introduced in the past five years.

How effective is the policy process?

The experience of the past decade suggests that the 'policy journey' has proved tougher than the government anticipated. In key respects, the Department of Health was not fully prepared for the task of managing an unprecedented process of change. As a recent report has shown (Capability Reviews Team 2007) the Department's analytical capacity has not been great, while its influence has been limited. In addition, political pressure to produce quick results has led to some policies, such as the management of long-term conditions, being introduced with little prior evaluation and others, such as NHS Direct, being implemented nationally before the results of pilot studies were available. In many areas research evidence was weak, reflecting long standing gaps in publicly funded research (Harrison 2002).

Although steps have been taken recently to fill some key gaps, these have come too late to influence performance in the period under review. Relevant international experience was not systematically evaluated and applied in all relevant areas: in the case of Payment by Results (PbR), the early design of the scheme took insufficient account of international experience, which is only now being systematically assessed in the context of the current review (Department of Health 2007s).

While the government was right to aim to reduce the influence of the centre in the day-to-day operation of the NHS and place greater emphasis on monitoring performance through the regulators, it did not fully acknowledge the implications of this change of role. The task of setting the 'rules' or framework within which the NHS should work calls for an ability to estimate the impact of any policy instrument; and this, in turn, requires an understanding of how the system works, how it will respond to such interventions as new incentives, and how the various elements fit together with each other and the available resources. In a complex system like the NHS, it is extremely difficult to take full account of interactions between the various elements. Nevertheless, some avoidable mistakes seem to have been made.

Failure to bring the various elements together was a key factor underlying the deficits that emerged from 2004/05 onwards, when it became clear that, despite the rapid increase in funding, some NHS and primary care trusts were overspending their incomes. Many factors contributed to this situation, including the financial regime itself, failure of workforce planning and poorly designed contracts for GPs and consultants, the costs of which were significantly underestimated by the centre. The number of professionals working in the NHS had grown rapidly, but the cost implications of this were poorly recognised. As a report from the Health Committee (House of Commons Health Committee 2006d) pointed out, financial management was weak at both national and local levels.

Other examples of failure are evident in service configuration. First, the system of PbR, as initially introduced, did not support a shift from hospital to community care, since the tariff could not be unbundled to allow payment for the separate elements of care along the pathway. This failure reflects the initial focus on elective care and support for the choice programme; as the objectives of PbR were broadened, the weaknesses in its initial design became apparent.

Second, the proposed shift of services to community settings has been embarked upon without taking full account of the fact that any substantial shift of this kind threatens to undermine the economics of acute hospitals by leaving some with spare capacity and hence higher costs. The massive investment programme in new hospitals took insufficient account of the potential for such a shift or of the case for larger hospitals based on the need for further specialisation (Darzi 2007). In some cases, trusts are committed by long-term contracts to Private Finance Initiative (PFI) buildings for decades ahead, which presents an additional set of problems. Crucially, there is still is no satisfactory 'failure' regime for trusts that are not financially viable (Palmer 2005).

Additionally, while the government has emphasised the benefits for elective surgery of creating 'focused factories', which separate elective from emergency work (Department of Health 2000b), it has ignored the potential loss of 'system efficiency' that such a policy can create. No attempt has been made, for example, to estimate the impact on the cost of emergency care of providing extra capacity to deal with peaks in demand that were previously met by diverting resources from elective care (Kjekshus and Hagen 2005).

Such weaknesses were clearly identified in the recent capability review (Capability Review Team 2007), which pointed to the following weaknesses in the Department of Health's performance.

TABLE 10: POLICY-MAKING SCORECARD: GOVERNMENT PERFORMANCE AGAINST CABINET OFFICE CRITERIA

Cabinet Office criteria	Government performance
Forward looking Takes long-term view, based on statistical trends and informed predictions of the likely impact of policy	Despite the pledges in the NHS Plan and the National Service Frameworks, the commitment to being forward looking has been rhetorical only. There has been no serious forecasting or planning, for example, of health determinants or other critical assumptions.
Outward looking Takes account of national, European and international factors and communicates policy effectively	Some use has been made of overseas experience but the initial design of Payment by Results, for example, took too little account of the extensive experience of similar schemes in other parts of the world.
Innovative and creative Questions established ways of acting and encourages new ideas	A wide range of new policies have been introduced – sometimes in areas that previous governments had ignored, such as the quality of care.
Evidence based Makes use of best available evidence from a wide range of sources and involves key stakeholders at an early stage	Many policies have been announced without prior evaluation or piloting. For example, community matrons were introduced from 2004 onwards before the analysis had been done to work out how they could be effectively deployed.
Inclusive Takes account of the impact on the needs of all those directly or indirectly affected by the policy	Although the government has deliberately enlisted the support of clinicians for its proposals at national level, it has not systematically engaged professionals as a whole.
Joined up Looks beyond institutional boundaries to the government's strategic objectives	In some areas (for example, the links between health and local authority services over discharge), policies have been joined up. However, more generally, the links between different policy areas have not been taken sufficiently into account.
Evaluation Undertakes systematic evaluation of early outcomes of policy	Very few policies have been evaluated or even properly piloted. In the case of the National Service Frameworks for example, monitoring reports regularly attribute improvements in health to policy and clinical changes and ignore the other factors at work.
Reviews Keeps established policy under review to ensure that it continues to deal with the problems it was designed to tackle, taking account of associated effects elsewhere	A review process has not been established as a regular requirement of National Service Frameworks or in other policy areas.

- There is little evidence of a systematic process for learning from past experience.

- The Department's capacity to formulate whole-system strategy based on effective modelling and analysis of the interactions of different policies remains fragile.

- Policies tend to be developed in organisational 'silos' and cross-boundary integration issues are not routinely considered.

Table 107, p 63, measures the government's performance against its own criteria for good policy-making

---

EFFECTIVENESS OF THE POLICY PROCESS: SUMMARY ASSESSMENT

Overall, the policy process does not score well against the government's own criteria for good policy-making.

In some areas, such as hospital building, progress has been rapid but at the cost of ignoring important risk factors. In others, policies have been introduced without adequate preparation or the implementation process has been drawn out. The various elements sometimes conflict with each other or the connections between them have not been acknowledged.

It is not possible to estimate the impact of these shortfalls on performance, but it is clear that the proper role of the Department of Health has still be to worked out.

OVERALL ASSESSMENT OF THE POLICY FRAMEWORK

The government was right to take the view in 2000 that fundamental reform was required if the NHS was to improve its performance and make effective use of the resources at its disposal. The areas where the most notable improvements have been made, such as waiting times and other aspects of service quality promoted by NSFs, have been centrally- driven.

The government was also right to acknowledge subsequently that its initial approach had to be changed. King's Fund research (Appleby *et al* 2004) suggests that, while the pressure to improve performance exerted by targets and active central management produced positive results, it made some changes requiring a longer-term perspective harder to achieve. Furthermore, targets alone cannot achieve the across-the-board improvements in cost and quality that are needed.

Changes in organisational structure have created an environment in which careful planning across a number of organisations has been hard to achieve. Although the new organisational structure may prove more effective than the one in place in 1997, it is difficult to identify significant improvement resulting from recent changes.

Although it is hard to demonstrate the contribution of service redesign, it is clear that improvements in access and quality of care could only have been achieved by changes in service delivery.

The contribution of support programmes has been limited, but they are clearly critical to improved performance in future.

The central question of which have been the most effective routes to improvement is impossible to answer in a rigorous way. The evidence available for estimating the impact of the wide range of policies the government has pursued is extremely limited. Evidence about the accumulation of present policies must be collected and analysed in the immediate future.

IS HEALTH POLICY MOVING IN THE RIGHT DIRECTION?

It is clear that policy development, organisational change, reform of service delivery, the resource programmes and the policy process have all displayed significant weaknesses. The question now is whether the general approach the government has developed by 2007 is the best way to promote better quality and greater efficiency.

First, it is important to recognise the major improvements that have occurred. The government has succeeded in:

- identifying the main elements of a new way of managing health policy – one less reliant on targets and central direction and more on devolution of purchasing power, greater provider autonomy, a range of incentives, contestability, standards, regulation and information – while retaining central direction in key areas

- establishing a vastly improved national audit and monitoring regime

- offering sustained, if low-key, support for self-care

- beginning to address systematically the needs of people with long-term conditions

- consistently promoting the need for service redesign and supporting the creation of flexibility in professional roles

- promoting a wide range of measures aimed at improving the quality and cost-effectiveness of clinical care

- setting in train measures that allow research and development spending to provide more support for service improvement.

However, the government's public health policies fall far short of those envisaged in the 2004 Review (Wanless 2004). Public health budgets have been cut back and the supporting proposals set out in the review, such as the need for independent and transparent advice on the determinants of health, and systematic evaluation, have not been adopted.

With this major exception, the Department, the NHS and related bodies are now in better shape than in 2002 to deliver both improved quality and increased productivity. But because many key elements of the new framework have only just started to come into effect, or are not fully worked out, it remains unclear how effective they will prove to be. Much will depend on the Department's ability to react appropriately to the recent capability review. Huge challenges remain.

- **Commissioning and choice** It remains to be shown whether the new purchasing structures, coupled with patient choice, can act as an effective spur to improved performance.

- **Competition** How effective can this be in improving performance without prejudice to co-operation and service planning? With cancer networks, for example, ways must be found to reconcile the incentives created for trusts, particularly those with foundation status, with patients' need for access and continuity of care.

- **Targets and standards** The balance between targets, standards and incentives needs to be worked out systematically.

- **Central v local** The balance between central direction and local discretion has yet to be determined.

- **Balance of care** The shift towards local provision, following the White Paper *Our Health, Our Care, Our Say* (Department of Health 2006j), indicates the government's strong commitment to changing the balance of care. But the policy rests on uncertain foundations in terms of quality and economics, and research is vital to test it before widespread implementation. The findings of this research may well significantly influence the design of service provision, which is likely to vary according to the needs of each locality.

In other areas, too, there is a clear need to improve implementation.

- **Financial control** The Department has made a commitment to better policy costing (Secretary of State for Health 2007b) and acknowledged that this has been inadequate in the past.

- **Workforce planning** The Department has acknowledged the need for improvement, and new approaches are being developed.

- **ICT** Development and implementation is acknowledged to be behind schedule.

The conclusion must be that the policies being pursued across the four key areas of policy, organisation, service design and support programmes deserve only conditional approval at this stage. A great deal of work is needed to refine and develop such key policies as PbR and practice-based commissioning, to fully implement some of the initiatives described above and to find the right balance between competition, standards, incentives and patient choice.

It will, therefore, be some time before a clear view can emerge about the effectiveness of the current set of policies. Hence there can still be no guarantee that sufficiently improved performance, in terms of outcomes or productivity, will be achieved at the levels required by the solid progress or fully engaged scenarios, even if the general direction is right.

Finally, there are two significant issues the government has been slow to address.

Demand management

The need for demand management across the NHS as a whole has been given only limited attention. NICE, established in 1999, has been recognised worldwide as a major success, along with the work of the Health Technology Assessment programme. But these developments did not form part of a comprehensive policy on managing the demand for care. In effect, the rapid increases in resources from 2000 allowed issues of scarcity to be put to one side until they re-emerged from 2005 in the form of financial deficits. As a result, important issues have been neglected; for example, the government has continued to press for reduced waiting times for elective care but paid no attention to treatment thresholds. Given the incentives created by PbR, there is a clear risk that providers will expand activity to a point where the benefits at the margin are low. This risk is already emerging with cataract surgery (Johnston *et al* 2005). With the guidance issued in 2006 (Department of Health 2006c) this issue is now 'on the table', but PCTs have been largely left to their own devices to determine how it should be tackled.

This gap is part of a larger failing: throughout this chapter, it has been hard to pin down the contribution that the various elements of government policy have made to the improvements noted above. The government has been unsystematic in its approach to policy evaluation; it has introduced impact assessments but these are prepared in advance of actual implementation and are generally of low quality (because relevant information and research is limited), with little *ex post* monitoring of policy impacts.

The 2002 review recommended a systematic process for weeding out interventions of low value. There are signs that the numbers of some such procedures have declined, but it was not until late 2006 that NICE began a programme of work in this area. The 2004 review recommended that the NSFs should be developed as self-contained planning systems, which would link resources required to results to be obtained, and research findings to reviews. But there has been virtually no progress in this area and, significantly, no systematic programme for developing new NSFs.

Clinical engagement

Change on the scale needed to increase the rate of improvement within the NHS can only be achieved if the need to change is acknowledged and supported by the workforce. The government recognised in principle in 2000 that clinical engagement was required, but the policies pursued seem to have had the opposite effect of alienating many clinicians. The indications are that the government has recognised this problem and has promoted practice-based commissioning in the expectation that it will harness the energies of GPs for developing new services or supporting service redesign.

At national level, the government has given clinicians the lead role in developing NSFs, and a number of papers have been published supporting the clinical case for change. In February 2007 the government held a 'clinical engagement summit' to encourage clinical leaders to support the reform agenda (Department of Health 2007d), while the terms of reference for the latest departmental review of the NHS, to be carried out by Professor Sir Ara Darzi, place particular emphasis on clinical engagement (Darzi 2007).

But there is also evidence that the will to change is not yet universal among clinicians. Research carried out for the Health Foundation (Davies *et al* 2007) suggests that clinicians in general are wary of quality improvement programmes. The process of reform itself has undoubtedly strengthened these feelings: there is ample evidence that the central style of policy-making alienated clinicians, who resented their priorities being determined in this way (Appleby *et al* 2004).

IS THERE AN ALTERNATIVE?

This is an obvious question to ask, not just about the detail but about the broad thrust of current health policy. Critics have called for fundamental changes, including a switch in the basis of funding. The 2002 review following the NHS Plan recommended no significant change at the time and there seems no compelling need to change that judgement, which is now widely supported across the political spectrum (Wanless 2002). A switch of funding base would not only be disruptive in the short-to-medium term, but would not in itself do anything to address areas where progress has been slow or performance poor. The government has accepted the need to review prescription and other charges, which the 2002 review recommended, but has clearly ruled out major change in this area.

Others have proposed a much more rapid and extensive introduction of more competition and private sector involvement. The 2002 review supported the introduction of new suppliers – a policy the government adopted from 2002 onwards (Wanless 2002). What experience so far has shown is that the NHS is short of the skills and information needed to exploit market opportunities, and markets created without the necessary skills are expensive solutions to problems that could be solved in other ways (House of Commons Health Committee 2006b). In addition, some services, such as the major facilities required for emergency care, are natural monopolies within their catchment areas and are therefore immune to competitive pressures from other providers. Hence, the cautious approach the government has taken, allied with permissive legislation that allows new forms of provision to emerge or be commissioned, seems the right way forward, supported by national performance standards applicable to all providers.

Recently the British Medical Association (BMA) has made a number of proposals designed to rectify weaknesses identified in this report (British Medical Association 2007). These include:
- an independent review of the public health function
- more mature commissioning
- greater local autonomy for health professionals and managers
- a focus on outcomes rather than process
- better clinical information systems
- a renewal of clinical governance.

Taken together, however, these recommendations do not adequately address the central issue of how to improve and maintain performance in both cost and quality terms. The BMA is right to seek a better relationship between clinicians and management, since tensions between these groups have been unproductive, but this cannot be entirely attributed to the impact of political interference.

However the NHS is constituted and structured, the need for external accountability for effective use of resources will remain, and that implies a continuing need for a combination of incentives and sanctions to drive performance. Every health care system yet invented has at least the potential for internal conflicts, and there will be a continuing need to anticipate what conflicts might arise, to watch carefully for warning signs and to manage them as they arise. That has not always happened in recent years.

In summary, this would be a dangerous time to embark on further significant change when the new combination of levers to enhance performance has not yet been given the chance to prove itself.

The need now is to ensure that the policy framework the government has evolved in recent years is developed rather than fundamentally reformed. In other words, changes in policy and practice must continue, but structural change avoided wherever possible.

4 Recommendations

This report set out to review changes in health and the NHS in the light of the funding and policy recommendations and modelling assumptions made by the 2002 and 2004 reviews (Wanless 2002, 2004). Previous chapters have examined and assessed the funding of the NHS, the use of the extra resources allocated to the service and the effectiveness with which those resources have been used to generate improvements in productivity, output and health outcomes. The relevant evidence is set out in more detail in Part 2.It has also considered major policy initiatives and developments since the publication of the 2002 review.

It was an ambitious aim, and inevitably the report has been limited by the availability of data and relevant research and by constraints on time and resources. Nevertheless, there is a strong imperative to carry out reviews such as this: the stakes are high, not just in monetary terms, but also in terms of the high value the public place on health – and by implication health care.

It would be difficult to reach an overarching conclusion about the progress of the NHS since 2002 risks without oversimplifying a complex set of indicators. What can be said is that the funding increases recommended by the 2002 review up to 2007/8 have been acted on. In many ways, the NHS has been moving in the direction envisaged in the 2002 review and, as the rest of this report has shown, there have been real and demonstrable achievements. The NHS is generally performing better now than it was in 2002.

However, while it is too early to assess many of the key initiatives from which improvement is sought, the findings of this report suggest that there have also been shortfalls, policy failures and inconsistencies of management, which have left many uncertain about the direction in which the health service is moving and the way the components of the whole system are supposed to work together. Importantly, neither the assumed rate of productivity improvement nor the changes in personal behaviour that the more optimistic scenarios in the 2002 review envisaged have been achieved. These failures will have implications for levels of future NHS funding as the diverging funding paths of the three scenarios by definition depend on significant improvements in these areas.

It is also worth noting that it has been a consistent theme of this report that the government has failed to establish a direct link between financial investment and resources, on the one hand, and the value of results achieved on the other. As a result, it has been challenging for the analysis in this report to provide insights into where substantial gains from individual policies, reorganisation, service redesign or improvements in support programmes may arise.

In the light of the funding and policy framework recommendations of the 2002 and 2004 reviews, and now this current report's assessments, there are 11 recommendations that would help take forward policy on health and social care and address some of the shortfalls in performance identified.

1. Continue to encourage use of recent system reforms to achieve the desired results

The 2002 review set out a framework for how responsibilities could be distributed (Wanless 2002, para 6.5):

- **standards** to be set by departments and agencies of government, essentially as a regulator

- **processes** to be controlled by government and designed to ensure that resources can be used effectively to achieve the standards

- **delivery** arrangements for the provision of care to meet the standards to be locally determined and controlled, working within the processes established. Generally it is at local level that management of resources to achieve outcomes should take place.

The framework set out in the 2002 review is still appropriate. The evidence that has emerged in recent years has reinforced the need to move away from a centralist model that tended to alienate staff, even when pay increased substantially, seemed to be subject to a law of diminishing returns and encouraged distortions and perverse behaviour. Policy needs to continue to encourage local health care organisations to ensure the effective delivery of health services, to manage resources efficiently and to achieve outcomes. It is too early to assess how well the health system as currently configured is capable of achieving these goals. Reforms to the NHS need careful evaluation; in particular the capability of primary care trusts and practice based commissioners to deliver value for money in terms of improved health and health services.

It is recommended that commissioners are encouraged to use available data and the processes now in place more effectively to design and monitor outcome-based policies to which a range of providers will need to respond and that information and knowledge should be provided to local commissioning bodies to enable them to commission services in the most appropriate ways incorporating health and social care best practice.

2. Monitor policy successes and failures

This report has concluded that in a number of key respects policy-making and implementation since 2002 has been weak. These weaknesses have also been identified in reports by the National Audit Office, the Health Committee, the King's Fund and others noted in this review. Furthermore, although the general direction in which government health policy is moving is believed to be right, there remain significant uncertainties about how effective some of its elements will prove to be or how they will work together. In its 2007/8 business plan, the Department of Health acknowledged the need for improvement in its central analytic capacity.

It is recommended that the government strengthens its analytic capacity to monitor how effective policies are. It needs to be prepared to alter direction or change pace if policies are unlikely to deliver the desired impact, even with more time and a supportive financial regime. The government needs to take full account of the impact of further change in its assessments and to consider how best to manage any potentially negative effects. In addressing weaknesses, it must strengthen its capacity to link clinical and service objectives with the resources needed to achieve them.

 ## 3. Assess the performance of health care delivery systems

The way in which the various delivery components will work together in the future is not certain. The Darzi review of the NHS announced by the Prime Minister and Health Secretary is considering, inter alia, establishing a vision for the next decade based less on central direction and more on patient control, choice and local accountability, responsive to patients and local communities (Secretary of State for Health 2007).

The 2002 review argued that the balance of care between the acute hospital and other settings was wrong. It also foresaw a much greater role for primary care with a different skill mix. It envisaged that GPs would focus on patients with more complex needs, become more specialist and provide a wider range of diagnostic and treatment services.

The 2004 review recommended a primary care experiment to assess the benefits of additional resource in information systems, in monitoring risk and in services. A further benefit was foreseen to be the production of evidence about the effectiveness of information to assist personalised risk management and an understanding of disease prevalence in local populations. It was recommended that the experiment should have been directed towards areas of inequality, given that access to services is a crucial issue to be resolved.

This experiment was not taken forward but there are now pilots under way designed to shift substantial volumes of care from acute hospitals to community settings. They need to be researched carefully in relation to clinical outcome, patient satisfaction and cost effectiveness. They should provide opportunities to tackle important issues of productivity and quality, for example: to produce new incentives to transform the care of millions of mostly older people with long-term conditions, supporting them in managing their own health and reducing reliance on expensive secondary care; to show how to tackle large variations in performance; and to produce an out-of-hours service fit for its public in the 21st century when people are likely to become increasingly demanding.

There is a danger in the short term that some PCTs, nervous about destabilising their existing provider network, will fail to reform primary care. Unless PCTs become impartial commissioners on behalf of their populations and enhance their analytical powers, the market-based incentive system is unlikely to be effective in shifting care to the community (Palmer 2006; Harvey *et al* 2007). These incentives need to be developed further; for example, there need to be clear rules to address failures not only of providers unable to generate adequate income as configurations of services change around them, but also of individual services (Palmer 2005, 2006). Practice-based commissioning has the potential to encourage a wider range of health care to be delivered outside hospitals – but significant scaling-up and strengthening of primary care organisations will be needed for both commissioning and service delivery (Harvey et al, 2007

It is relevant that, in a report in respect of independent sector treatment centres, the Health Committee showed that the government persistently overstated their impact and did not put in place satisfactory arrangements for demonstrating their value (House of Commons Health Committee, 2006b; Healthcare Commission, 2007a) As a result in this and other cases, the benefits of new policies, or of additional spending, are unclear and an uncertain basis for national policy-setting.

Similar issues about the need for careful research arise in the delivery of health and social care services to those requiring both; it requires greater clarity at the interface as well as more effective systems that encourage more productive joint local working together.

It is recommended that, given the potentially high costs of reconfiguration, detailed research is carried out into new models of delivery to assess patient impact and cost effectiveness. It is also recommended that the rules about failure of institutions and services are clarified before significant commitments are made by the local organisations given responsibility for implementation. Much of this research should concentrate on local service providers.

It is also recommended that the experiment recommended in the 2004 review is carried out to provide important learning for the future of primary care delivery.

4. Produce regular long-term resource estimates

The 2002 review recommended that future reviews should integrate modelling and analysis of health and social care. In response to this, the 2006 review, commissioned by the King's Fund, *Securing Good Care for Older People* (Wanless 2006), carried out a forecast of resources required for social care for older people. That review was made difficult by the absence of an adequate definition of social care. It found many criticisms of the current system including continued unrest about the interface between health and social care and about the inconsistency of service delivery. It also concluded that policy in this area is not well defined although, using scenario planning to define different possibilities for social care, it was possible to produce a range of possible costs over 20 years.

The 2002 review recommended that a further review should be conducted in, say, five years' time (that is, about 2007) to re-assess the future long-term resource requirements for both health and social care. The government has not done this. This report, while not aiming to fill this gap, has established that, as expected, there have been significant variations in some areas from the original assumptions.

There are good reasons to carry out forecasting on a regular basis given the long-term nature of many of the decisions needing to be taken as well as the need to set short-term resourcing decisions in the context of longer-term plans. Regular reworking of the forecasts (and of the scenarios considered appropriate) would help inform debates about the effectiveness of spending, the comparability of quality of outcomes (domestically and internationally), funding levels and funding sources; these debates would, not least, help to create conditions for better engagement of the public with the difficult policy process of allocating scarce national resources.

The approach – using scenarios to capture particular uncertainties – seems robust. It would involve analysing all the components of the forecasts previously made, using the latest available information and evidence about, for example, demographics, the health status of the population and the consequent likely demands, progress on productivity, progress on public health issues, progress on defining social care policy and the resulting needs and the long-term costs of delivering a comprehensive service. Relevant areas of related research seem likely to include:

- estimates of the contribution of technologies/ medical advances to growth in health spending
- consideration of the impact of developments in genetics
- estimates of the impact of the NHS on the health status of the people it treats.

Twenty years seems a reasonable period for the look forward, and regular updates should have the benefit of developing knowledge and research programmes.

As with the 2002 review, regular forecasts would concentrate mainly on the likely long-term demands. In translating this into a spending path for the whole 20-year period, there would always need to be attention given to the likely resources available in the short term. When resources are relatively constrained, the early years of the 20 year period would be expected to concentrate on delivering productivity improvements and ensuring processes delivered the benefits needed to assist longer-term effectiveness, recognising the likely need in the future for increased rates of resource development.

The forecasting work will need involvement from within government, including the Treasury and the Department of Health, but it would be beneficial if the work was carried out independently to ensure that the processes used for the estimates and forecasts were transparent and seen to be free of any political interference. The work should be commissioned and funded by government but could be tendered to a consortia of relevant organisations or established as a function within the Healthcare Commission or another independent agency.

It is recommended that the Treasury/Department of Health establish a mechanism for commissioning and publishing regular independent estimates of the long-term resources likely to be needed for health and social care services. Five yearly re-forecasts may be appropriate or it may be more helpful to produce a forecast ahead of each Comprehensive Spending Review. All forecasts would be expected to show ranges based on whatever different scenarios were considered appropriate. The forecasting models used in this work should be made publicly available.

5. Measure and manage productivity

A particularly difficult task required in any modelling of long-term resource estimates is the assessment of future productivity. It is important because public perceptions about how productively resources are used will continue to influence general attitudes towards publicly funded health and social care services; the best possible information needs to be identified and publicised by a trusted body.

Of course, it is actual productivity improvements that matter, and recent performance is not in line with the more optimistic scenarios developed in 2002. It is difficult for many of those directing parts of the health system to see how effectively the whole system is operating, and there is evident danger of benefits in one sector being achieved at the expense of higher costs elsewhere. Targets and incentive systems to improve productivity should focus on clinical quality and health outcomes. The reimbursement system, Payment by Results, should play a part in providing a more automatic mechanism to encourage the NHS to seek out more productive ways of meeting patients' health care needs.

It is recommended that incentive systems to improve productivity should focus on clinical quality and health outcomes. The present system of incentives and standards should be progressively developed and refined in the light of experience of their impact. Measurement of the impact by the Healthcare Commission and others will assist. It is recommended that this continuing work into productivity should consider the whole system.

 ## 6. Collect more data to support modelling

The effectiveness of work such as the assessment of productivity would be greatly enhanced if improvements were made in the way the performance of the NHS is monitored. Since 2002 a vast amount of additional data has become available. But as this current review and that of others has shown the data remains limited and some central questions cannot be answered using available data. For example, information on the cost of policies and the relationship between cost and outcome is particularly weak for health services and public health policies. The contribution that extra resources are making to lower levels of heart disease or to improve cancer survival rates remains obscure. Information about primary care is not collated to assist forecasting and assessment.

It is recommended that the Health and Social Care Information Centre work with those commissioned to produce long-term resource forecasts, relevant analysts within the Department of Health and the Treasury and other researchers to define further requirements for and improvements that could be made to health and social care information to assist the modelling of future spending forecasts.

 ## 7. Define 'comprehensive, high-quality' service

In order to forecast resource requirements it is necessary to define the scope and nature of health and social care services to be funded. Forecasts in the 2002 review were required to be based on the provision of comprehensive, high-quality services and, in that review, an attempt was made to define services on the basis of National Service Frameworks (NSFs), NICE judgements and audit of local delivery. Yet none of the NSFs, despite their importance as drivers of improvement, has well-defined costings and none attempts, when reporting their progress, to define the links between the standards they set out, the costs and the clinical results. Until these links are made, the productivity (in terms of all types of health care process and health outcome benefit) will remain unknown.

Prevention strategies should also be more fully developed within the NSFs. Work such as that being carried out within, for example, the Foresight Programme (2007) on obesity or at the London School of Hygiene and Tropical Medicine on heart disease should be supported and pursued, over time, across all main diseases and risk factors.

It is recommended that the updating of existing NSFs and the rolling-out of new NSFs should form the basis of the centrally determined standards for health care. They should be kept up to date and should include costings and resource requirements (including

staffing implications) and should set out research needs. The combination of all the NSFs would help to inform those responsible for management of delivery, so that commissioners could use the range of local levers available to them to achieve national standards.

In social care, the meanings of 'comprehensive' and 'high quality' are not yet defined and it is recommended that a work programme should be established to fill the huge gap this creates in understanding the long-term financial implications of an ageing population. The report commissioned by the King´s Fund – *Securing Good Care for Older People* **(Wanless 2006) recommends the way forward for people aged over 65.**

 ## 8. Model workforce requirements

The Department of Health needs effective ways of linking forecasts of the ways in which the NHS will develop with the scale and mix of the workforce required and with the education and training of health professionals, clinical and managerial. They need to pay particular attention, if they are to capitalise on the systems and processes now in place, to the capacity of the relevant staff to manage the levers for change available.

On remuneration, particularly given the evidence of the last few years, they need to think through how the recently designed remuneration systems can help not only to recruit, retain and motivate staff but also to increase the likelihood that they can encourage delivery of the desired outcomes. The challenge of getting value from the expensive contracts of the last few years will be huge. The costs of all the major new contracts are more obvious than the benefits and the absence of systematic national evaluations is a critical weakness; without such evaluations it is doubtful whether it will ever be known if the benefits outweigh the costs (Buchan and Evans 2007). Equally important will be the capacity of such national evaluations to inform local management about how they can use the levers being made available to them.

The Department has welcomed the challenge posed by the recent Capability Review (2007) to deliver a comprehensive staff development programme and to address specific capability and skills issues. The balance between local plans and control and national forecasting will need assessment as part of their reviews.

It is recommended that the future forecasting of long-term resource requirements in health and social care should pay particular attention to the workforce plans produced by the Department of Health. These will allow an assessment of whether sufficient staff will be available who will be able to deliver the volumes forecast to be needed and who will also be able to capitalise on the systems designed to help them produce the required standards of service and efficiency.

It is recommended that full-scale evaluations of the recently introduced contracts are carried out to assist efforts, nationally and locally, to obtain adequate benefits.

 ## 9. Review the implementation of Connecting for Health

The weaknesses of ICT in the health service have long been evident and the programmes of recent years have represented a determined attempt to improve. The deliverables are critical to many future productivity and service enhancements but, as indicated in chapter

2, there have been serious criticisms made about the current situation and implementation of Connecting for Health, despite some positive developments. Future productivity and quality gains envisaged in the plans for the NHS and reflected in the future forecasts of costs require the effective use of ICT budgets. There is much money still to be spent. There is a need for an audit of the technical aspects of the Connecting for Health programme and the financial costs and benefits before deciding whether or not to continue with the implementation of current plans. Unless there is greater clarity about the costs and benefits of the programme, it will be difficult to make assessments of the long-term costs and investment needs of the NHS.

It is recommended that Connecting for Health is subject to detailed external scrutiny and reporting so that forecasting of long-term costs and benefits can be made with more confidence.

 ## 10. A framework for public health

The 2004 review recommended a conceptual framework to take forward public health in England in a systematic way. It was designed to give suitable long-term confidence to those working in public health and to ensure that their activity was effectively and efficiently targeted.

The review also commented that, in spite of numerous policy initiatives being directed towards public health they have not succeeded in rebalancing health policy away from the short-term imperatives of health care. As a result, it observed, public health practitioners generally seemed to feel undervalued. The situation in 2007 is no better, and a significant opportunity has been lost. The health care system must move to a system that concentrates on keeping people as healthy as possible. This requires the right incentives for commissioners and appropriate contractual arrangements for providers.

The setting of quantified national objectives for changing the prevalence of all the important determinants of health status for the medium and long term was recommended. Such objectives would be designed to help inform future resource planning projections as well as immediate decisions. A great deal of research, analytical thinking and consensus building was envisaged. These national objectives would inform local planning and implementation by networks of local authorities, health organisations and community and voluntary groups. It is such local ownership and action that seems likely to deliver results. This seems to have been recognised in principle, for example, in *Choosing Health* (Department of Health, 2005b) which followed the 2004 review but has not, so far, been facilitated in any broadly successful way in practice.

Another important recommendation was that the government should seek advice about the levels at which the objectives should be set and their impact on health inequalities. It was suggested that an arm's length body should be given responsibility, and it was envisaged that people drawn from a wide range of organisations should give the advice, partly to help mobilise the widespread support needed. This and other aspects of the framework were not taken forward.

Coupled with the severe disruption of the public health workforce as a by-product of wider reorganisation and the ease with which budget allocations for public health can be reallocated when overall budgets are tight, it is perhaps not surprising that progress has fallen well below the most optimistic scenario in the 2002 review. Yet any future forecasting that reassesses long-term health and social care resource requirements is likely to reaffirm the economic sense of well-targeted spending on prevention.

Many organisations have roles to play in delivering improvements in public health, including primary care, which could be used much more effectively if financial incentives were well designed to support good health outcomes and not just activity, for example, by revisions to the Quality and Outcomes Framework (QOF).

Local government has a crucial role but it has been difficult for it to do as much as it could because of capacity problems, the impact of health service reorganisations on local arrangements for co-operation, and the lack of alignment of performance management mechanisms.

It is recommended that the 2004 review recommendations are implemented.

 ## 11. The benefits of measuring health status

Although surveys (such as the Health Survey for England), and to an extent the decennial census, record information on the population's self-assessed health status, no equivalent information is collected routinely on NHS patients. The benefits of measuring individuals´ health status and recording this as part of people´s medical records, are potentially great, from improved measures of productivity and comparative performance benchmarking, through to the sort of information people and purchasers need to inform their decisions about prevention of illness, treatment and commissioning (Appleby and Devlin 2004).

It is recommended that large-scale trials are carried out to explore the potential benefits and costs of routine recording of the health status of people treated and advised by all providers working for the NHS.

Part 2 →
The evidence

Introduction

The five years since the 2002 review has witnessed a considerable increase in health care funding across the United Kingdom. Given this unprecedented investment, the key questions are how well this money has been used and to what extent the desired outcomes, in terms of the health and system effectiveness, have been achieved.

A helpful way of reviewing the evidence is by means of a conventional 'production path' (*see* Figure 5, p 11), starting with a description of financial inputs to the NHS, moving on to how these are converted into resources (such as labour and capital), then to how these are combined to produce outputs, or activity (such as numbers of patients admitted to hospital), and finally to the outcomes (health) these activities help to produce.

A subsequent series of questions concerns how well the NHS has performed in terms of economy, efficiency and effectiveness; that is, its success in converting money into resources, resources into outputs and outputs into outcomes. The most interesting performance indicators are the outcomes – but these are also the most difficult to describe and measure. Nevertheless, the most crucial question of all is: how has the population's health changed as a result of investing more of society's scarce resources in health care?

Although a substantial volume of data has been collated and analysed for Part 2 of this report, it does not claim to offer comprehensive coverage of every aspect of NHS funding, activity or population health. To do so would be prohibitively difficult and, in any case, unnecessary to support the policy analysis and conclusions in Part 1. Where data is inadequate, we have made the appropriate interpretive caveats.

It is also important to point out that virtually all the evidence presented in Part 2 is focused on England; although this bias is unsatisfactory in some respects, it also recognises the inherent problems of comparing four countries with varying health service organisations, definitions of data and trends in reform policy.

Finally, although the base year focus of this review is 2002/3, data from earlier years has been included where this has been considered useful for trend analysis.

5 Funding: what was spent

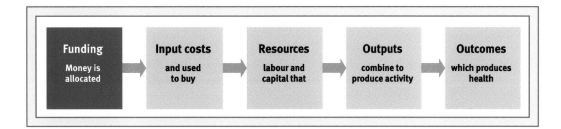

In April 2002, the Chancellor of the Exchequer announced that the NHS would benefit from average annual real-term growth of 7.4 per cent over the five years to 2007/8.

This chapter considers actual spending in the light of this promise and the funding recommendations of the 2002 review. It then goes on to look at funding prospects up to 2022/3.

The primary task of the 2002 review was to 'identify the key factors which will determine the financial and other resources required to ensure that the NHS can provide a publicly funded, comprehensive, high quality service available on the basis of clinical need and not ability to pay'. The 'key factors' identified by the review were a combination of demand drivers, including demographic changes, lifestyle and health-seeking behaviour, and supply factors, such as assumptions about future NHS productivity gains and the design and roll-out of national service frameworks (NSFs) (Wanless 2002).

The review calculated three possible spending paths for the NHS for the two decades to 2022/3, the most attractive of which was the fully engaged scenario. It is worth reiterating that the review was not simply a funding forecasting exercise or a means to address the longstanding problem of under-funding. Although it did show that substantial increases in the share of national wealth devoted to health care would be needed to achieve the high-quality and comprehensive service sought, at the volumes expected to be demanded, this was predicated on substantial changes in service delivery and public engagement with health.

Following publication of the 2002 review, Gordon Brown, then Chancellor of the Exchequer, announced in the 2002 Budget that, over the five years to 2007/8, the NHS across the United Kingdom would benefit from average annual real-term growth of 7.4 per cent. In his Budget speech, delivered on 17 April, he went on to say:

The report by Derek Wanless states that the NHS needs a long-term sustainable financial framework in support of reform and modernisation and it sets out the financial needs for the next two decades – starting with a five year period of high and sustained

growth and, once we have tackled decades of underinvestment, moving to lower rates of growth... in the three five year periods after 2008.
(Brown 2002)

The Chancellor went on to say that 'Reform and investment will bring booked appointments for operations and are reducing maximum waiting times in stages from 18 months to 15 months, then 12 months, then 6 months, then 3 months'. However, he emphasised that reform was a precondition of these new resources (Brown 2002).

This commitment by the government ensured that funding growth should be sufficient to cover the 2002 review's most costly scenario – slow uptake – for health care spending, at least for the five years to 2007/8. After this, the varying assumptions of the three scenarios implied that spending would diverge in line with progress in order to achieve the health and health care goals set out in the review (Wanless 2002).

Funding recommendations of the 2002 review

The 2002 review developed a detailed model to project health expenditure to 2022 for each of the three scenarios. For the majority of NHS expenditure the model initially established baseline unit costs and activity rates across care areas for 2002/3. From here, preparing projections about the future involved adjusting the unit costs and activity rates based on assumptions about future demographics, the costs of future NSFs, changes in age-specific use of care, and other factors (including reduced waiting times and changes in productivity) for each of the three scenarios. The model therefore generated activity, unit cost and total cost projections for each year between the 2002/3 baseline and 2022/3. The costings model was based on data for England only, and an adjustment, based on population, was needed to produce projections for the United Kingdom as a whole. Private sector health spending was assumed to remain at 1.2 per cent of gross domestic product (GDP) over the two decades.

The 2002 review concluded that total real UK NHS spending needed to rise from an estimated £68 billion in 2002/3 to between £154 billion and £184 billion in 2022/3, representing real growth, at a minimum, of around 126 per cent. Table 11, opposite, summarises the 2002 review's funding recommendations, at 2002/3 prices.

The first decade of spending was focused on 'catching up' with best practice in other countries, while spending in the second decade was focused on 'keeping up'. Between 2002/3 and 2007/8, NHS spending in the United Kingdom would need to grow at an annual average rate of between 7.1 and 7.3 per cent, with growth rates easing back in the five years after 2007/8 but still remaining well above historic averages. The review noted that this early growth was likely to be at the upper end of what could sensibly be spent, given resource and capacity constraints, especially in relation to the workforce.

During the second decade, when an increasing amount of 'catch up' spending would have been utilised, real growth in the final five years would reduce further, to 2.4 per cent a year in the fully engaged scenario or 3.5 per cent in the slow uptake scenario, as the emphasis switched to 'keep up'.

Overall, by 2022/3 total health care spending was projected to consume between 10.6 and 12.5 per cent of UK GDP, depending on the scenario used.

TABLE 11: SUMMARY OF HEALTH SPENDING IN THE UK UNDER DIFFERENT SCENARIOS, 2002/3 TO 2022/3

	Actual spending	Projected spending			
	2002/3[1]	2007/8	2012/13	2017/18	2022/3
Total health spending (% of GDP)[2]					
Solid progress	7.7	9.4	10.5	10.9	11.1
Slow uptake	7.7	9.5	11.0	11.9	12.5
Fully engaged	7.7	9.4	10.3	10.6	10.6
Total NHS spending (£ billion)[3]					
Solid progress	68	96	121	141	161
Slow uptake	68	97	127	155	184
Fully engaged	68	96	119	137	154
Average annual real growth in NHS spending (%)[4]					
Solid progress	6.8	7.1	4.7	3.1	2.7
Slow uptake	6.8	7.3	5.6	4.0	3.5
Fully engaged	6.8	7.1	4.4	2.8	2.4

Source: Wanless 2002
[1] Estimates
[2] All figures (apart from NHS spend) include 1.2 per cent for private sector health spending.
[3] 2002/3 prices
[4] Growth figures are annual averages for the five years up to the date shown (four years for 2002/3).

These spending projections represented a significant departure from real long-term changes in NHS funding. Between 1949/50, the first full financial year of the NHS, and 1999/2000, annual real growth in NHS spending had averaged 3.4 per cent (*see* Figure 12, overleaf). By comparison, the 2002 review recommended an accelerated annual growth of around 7.2 per cent between 2002/3 and 2007/8, reducing to around 3 per cent by 2022/3. As Figure 12 also shows, NHS spending growth between 2000/1 and 2002/3 had already begun to increase above the long-term trend and in line with the 2002 review's projections. Continuation of the historic long-term growth rate for the NHS would have meant total spending of around £133 billion by 2022/3 – some £20 billion less than recommended under the fully engaged scenario.

Actual health care spending since 2002

So how did actual health care spending in the United Kingdom compare with these projections? Table 12, overleaf, compares the 2002 review's original spending recommendations with actual spending.

Despite the difference in base-year spending (actual spend in 2002/3 was £66.2 billion compared with the 2002 review's estimated spend of £68 billion), actual (real, GDP-deflated) spending has matched the review's recommendations, with a planned increase of just over £30 billion by 2007/8, of which about 30 per cent has been absorbed by inflation. However, care is needed in making these comparisons: while actual spend is close to the review's recommendations, because GDP is higher than originally forecast,

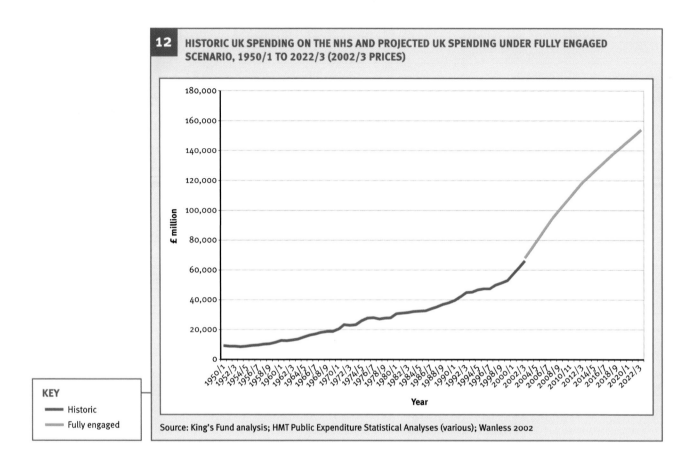

12 HISTORIC UK SPENDING ON THE NHS AND PROJECTED UK SPENDING UNDER FULLY ENGAGED SCENARIO, 1950/1 TO 2022/3 (2002/3 PRICES)

KEY
— Historic
— Fully engaged

Source: King's Fund analysis; HMT Public Expenditure Statistical Analyses (various); Wanless 2002

both increases are now worth less – by around 0.3 percentage points in 2007/8 – as a proportion of GDP. For *total* health care spending, this reduction is offset to some extent by adopting a revised (and slightly higher) estimate of the proportion of GDP devoted to private health care spending: 1.4 per cent compared with the review's figure of 1.2 per cent. This revision (adopted by the Department of Health in 2004) effectively adds

TABLE 12: ACTUAL UK NHS SPENDING COMPARED WITH 2002 WANLESS PROJECTIONS UNDER DIFFERENT SCENARIOS, 2002/3 TO 2007/8

	Spending (£ billion)[1]					
	2002/3	2003/4	2004/5	2005/6	2006/7	2007/8
Projections						
Solid progress[2]	68.0	72.9	78.1	83.6	89.6	96.0
Slow uptake[2]	68.0	73.0	78.4	84.1	90.3	97.0
Fully engaged[2]	68.0	72.9	78.1	83.6	89.6	96.0
Actual	66.2	72.5	78.0	82.9	90.0[3]	96.5[3]

Source: Wanless 2002; HM Treasury 2002a, HM Treasury 2006
[1] 2002/3 prices
[2] Wanless figures for intervening years between 2002/3 and 2007/8 have been interpolated as equal changes between these years.
[3] Figures for 2006/7 and 2007/8 refer to planned spending.

between £2.1 and £2.4 billion to total health care spending each year from 2002/3 to 2007/8 (at 2002/3 prices).

PATIENT CHARGES

While the Exchequer provides the vast bulk of funds for the NHS, significant sums are also raised from patient charges. Charges for prescriptions and dental work currently raise around £1 billion per annum in the English NHS, for example, while other charges, such as for car parking and sight tests, raise a further £200 million or so. These sums are small by comparison with the overall NHS budget, but not insignificant.

The 2002 review noted that out-of-pocket payments could play a role in generating income for the NHS and helping to extend choice for patients, as long as they complied with the basic principle that access to health care should be based on clinical need rather than ability to pay. In particular, the 2002 review suggested that the current exemption system for prescription charges was illogical and should be reviewed by the government; but it was only following the 2006 investigation by the House of Commons Health Committee (2006a) that the government agreed to do this. The remit of this prescription charge review is constrained by an overall commitment that any recommendations should be cost neutral for the NHS, which rules out abolition of the charges. However, it will examine possible revisions to the list of exempt medicines, the implications of a flat-rate charge with no exemptions, and exemptions based solely on ability to pay. The review was due to report in the summer of 2007.

The introduction of additional non-clinical services – such as bedside communications and electronic information services – could enhance patient choice. These are now fairly widespread in the NHS, usually provided by private sector companies under contract to individual hospitals, with charges levied on patients. However, the Health Committee (House of Commons Health Committee 2006c) noted that the cost of bedside telephone calls were very high, partly because of the need to recoup investments to compensate for the relatively poor take-up by hospitals of additional bedside electronic services. The Department of Health's own review of such charges, following complaints from patients and an Ofcom investigation (Ofcom 2006), suggests that the solution is likely to lie in renegotiated agreements at hospital level and greater take-up of the additional services on which the original prices were based (Patient Power Review Group 2007).

Health care spending beyond 2008/9

With actual total health care funding so far broadly following the trajectory suggested by the 2002 review, what are the prospects for future spending?

Figure 13, overleaf, shows the relationship between historic (1990/1 to 2007/8) NHS spending in the UK and the three review scenarios. All figures are set at 2002/3 prices and use the original cash projections for the three scenarios. In order to stay on the fully engaged funding path, real NHS spending would need to increase by around 4.5 per cent per year from 2008/9 to 2012/3, by 3.1 per cent to 2017/8 and by 2.4 to 2022/3. Of course, whether or not such levels remain appropriate to achieve the outcomes needed to catch up and keep up with other developed countries depends on many factors that are subject to significant change.

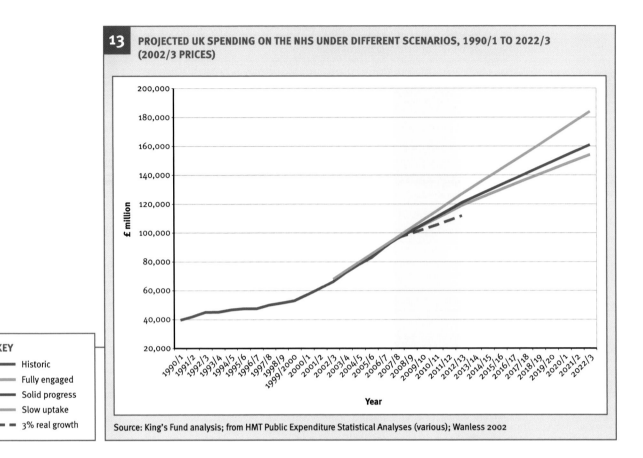

13 PROJECTED UK SPENDING ON THE NHS UNDER DIFFERENT SCENARIOS, 1990/1 TO 2022/3 (2002/3 PRICES)

KEY
— Historic
— Fully engaged
— Solid progress
— Slow uptake
--- 3% real growth

Source: King's Fund analysis; from HMT Public Expenditure Statistical Analyses (various); Wanless 2002

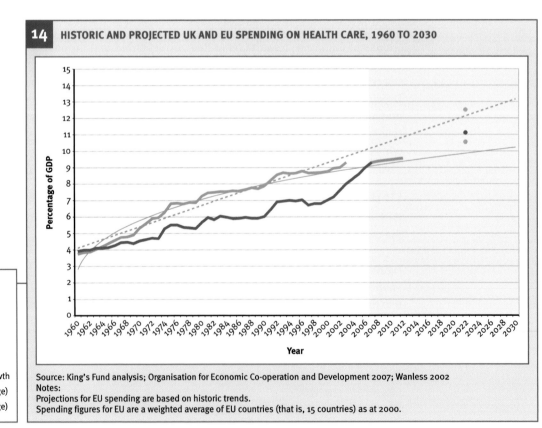

14 HISTORIC AND PROJECTED UK AND EU SPENDING ON HEALTH CARE, 1960 TO 2030

KEY
— EU average
— Actual UK
• Slow uptake
• Solid progress
• Fully engaged
— 3% real NHS growth
--- Linear (EU average)
— Power (EU average)

Source: King's Fund analysis; Organisation for Economic Co-operation and Development 2007; Wanless 2002
Notes:
Projections for EU spending are based on historic trends.
Spending figures for EU are a weighted average of EU countries (that is, 15 countries) as at 2000.

If NHS spending for the next five years were to revert to its long-term average real increase of 3 per cent per annum, all other things being equal, actual NHS spending would by 2012/3 fall short of the fully engaged spending path by around £7.2 billion, the solid progress path by £9.2 billion and the slow uptake path by £15.2 billion.

The recommendations of the 2002 review were based on an assessment of the resources required to achieve defined outcomes, not necessarily to match spending in the EU generally. But matching the proportion of EU GDP spent on health *did* become an objective for the government. By comparison with the UK's European neighbours, a 3 per cent real annual growth for the NHS to 2012/3 would place the UK near the bottom end of estimated average (weighted) EU health care spend as a proportion of GDP (*see* Figure 14, opposite). Note that this is based on total health care spending – both public and private – for the 15 EU countries in 2000.

While the boost in NHS funding in the United Kingdom from the turn of the century represented a significant investment, it is clear from Figure 13 that the United Kingdom had lagged behind the rest of the EU for many decades. The cumulative under-spend (relative to the non-weighted average of EU spending) between 1972 and 1998 was calculated at £220 billion (at 1998 prices) or £267 billion on an income-weighted basis (Wanless 2001).

SUMMARY: FUNDING

- The 2002 review described three future scenarios and made funding projections for each over two decades. It concluded that total real spending on the NHS in the UK needed to rise from an estimated £68 billion in 2002/3 to between £154 billion and £184 billion in 2022/3 (Wanless 2002).
- The 2002 budget confirmed that the NHS would receive an average annual real increase in funding of 7.4 per cent over the five years to 2007/8, compared with the review's recommendation of between 7.1 and 7.3 per cent.
- NHS spending in the United Kingdom between 2002/3 and 2007/8 has broadly increased in line with the review's original cash recommendations. However, higher levels of GDP mean that, as a proportion GDP, NHS spending has been about 0.3 per cent lower than the review suggested.
- Total NHS and private funding in the United Kingdom in 2007/8 now stands at around £113.5 billion (£96.5 billion on the NHS and an estimated £17 billion on private care) which is £2.4 billion higher than assumed by the 2002 review. This takes UK total health spending into the bottom of the range for estimated average EU health care spending in 2007/8.
- In the near-term, future NHS funding will depend on decisions taken in the 2007 Comprehensive Spending Review. Indications are that NHS funding growth will slow to around a 3 per cent a year real increase up to 2010/1. If this were the case, all other things being equal, total health care spend at 2002/3 prices would by 2012/3 fall short of the fully engaged spending path by around £7.2 billion, the solid progress path by £9.2 billion and the slow uptake path by £15.2 billion.

6 Input costs: why they rose

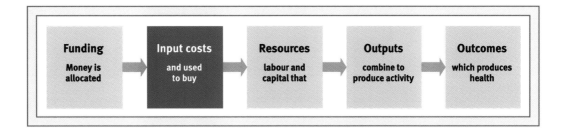

Although NHS funding increased by more than £43 billion (65 per cent) in the five years after 2002, inflation – in the form of higher pay and prices – has reduced the effective funding available to improve the service. This chapter focuses on the additional costs generated by new employment contracts for virtually all the 1.3 million staff in the NHS in the UK. It explains the objectives of the new contracts and considers their impact on productivity and other benefits.

The total cash increase in UK NHS funding between 2002/3 and 2007/8 has been £43.2 billion – an increase of 65 per cent However, inflation – in the form of higher pay and prices – has reduced the effective funding available to develop and expand the volume and quality of health care services. The previous chapter showed that, using a measure of general inflation across the economy as a whole (the GDP deflator), real spending had increased by 46 per cent (equivalent to £30 billion), with around 30 per cent of the additional cash absorbed by inflation. But the GDP deflator does not accurately represent inflation as experienced by the NHS itself.

Historically, given the types and volumes of staff, equipment and consumables purchased by the NHS, NHS-specific inflation has tended to be higher than the GDP deflator (*see* Figure 15, overleaf). Using an NHS-specific measure of inflation to deflate the cash increases reduces the change in volume expenditure between 2002/3 and 2007/8 to around £24.3 billion, with around £18.9 billion (43 per cent) of the £43.2 billion cash increase absorbed in higher pay and prices. Table 13 and Figure 16, overleaf and p 91, summarise these adjustments.

The assumptions about pay and price inflation made by the 2002 review appear to be close to the actual NHS-specific rates of inflation between 2002/3 and 2007/8 (as Figure 16, p 91, shows). It should be noted that (in the absence of official figures) the estimates for actual NHS inflation used for 2005/6 to 2007/8 (based on the Payment by Results tariff uplift calculated by the Department of Health) are almost certainly underestimates.

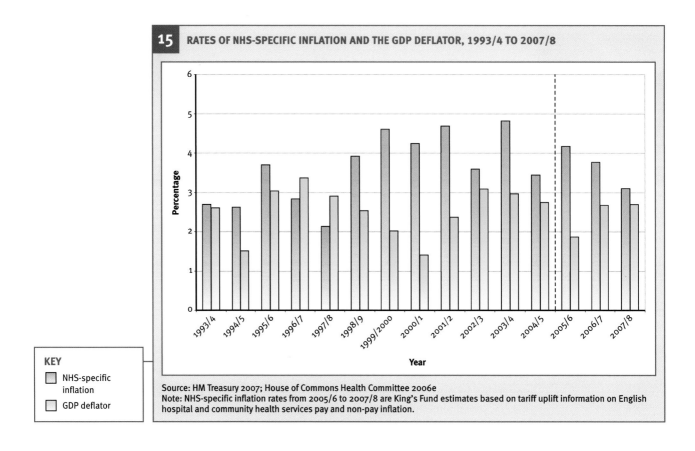

15 RATES OF NHS-SPECIFIC INFLATION AND THE GDP DEFLATOR, 1993/4 TO 2007/8

KEY
- NHS-specific inflation
- GDP deflator

Source: HM Treasury 2007; House of Commons Health Committee 2006e
Note: NHS-specific inflation rates from 2005/6 to 2007/8 are King's Fund estimates based on tariff uplift information on English hospital and community health services pay and non-pay inflation.

One element of the general increase in NHS costs that absorbed a significant proportion of the total cash increase between 2002 and 2007 was pay, reflecting the impact of new contracts for NHS staff.

TABLE 13: UK NHS SPENDING, 2002/3 TO 2007/8

	2002/3	2003/4	2004/5	2005/6	2006/7[1]	2007/8[1]	2002/3–2007/8
Cash (£ million)	66,200	74,700	82,500	89,400	99,400	109,400	43,200
% change		12.8	10.4	8.4	11.2	10.1	65.3
Real[2] (£ million)	66,200	72,543	77,969	82,917	89,993	96,482	30,282
% change		9.6	7.5	6.3	8.5	7.2	45.7
Volume[3] (£ million)	66,200	71,266	76,086	79,146	84,803	90,523	24,323
% change		7.7	6.8	4.0	7.1	6.7	36.7

Source: King's Fund analysis; Wanless 2002; HM Treasury 2002a; HM Treasury 2006
[1] Planned spending
[2] Cash figures adjusted using GDP deflator (HM Treasury 2007)
[3] Cash figures adjusted using NHS-specific inflation rates for 2003/4 and from 2005/6 to 2007/8; inflation rate based on King's Fund estimate, using Payment by Results tariff inflation uplift information on English hospital and community health services pay and non-pay inflation

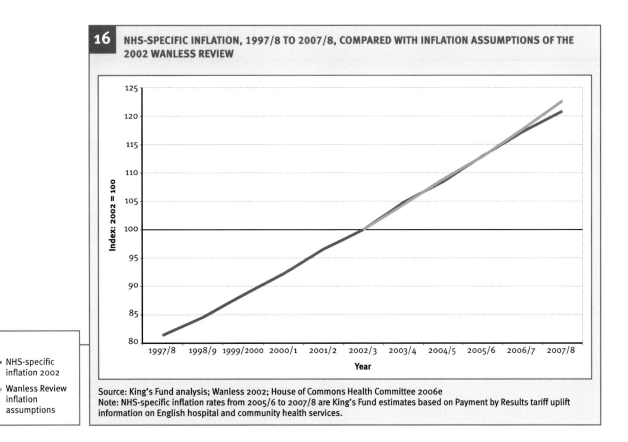

16 NHS-SPECIFIC INFLATION, 1997/8 TO 2007/8, COMPARED WITH INFLATION ASSUMPTIONS OF THE 2002 WANLESS REVIEW

KEY
— NHS-specific inflation 2002
— Wanless Review inflation assumptions

Source: King's Fund analysis; Wanless 2002; House of Commons Health Committee 2006e
Note: NHS-specific inflation rates from 2005/6 to 2007/8 are King's Fund estimates based on Payment by Results tariff uplift information on English hospital and community health services.

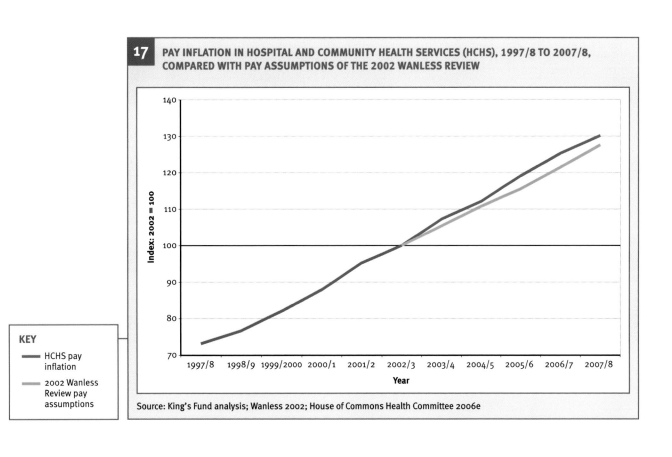

17 PAY INFLATION IN HOSPITAL AND COMMUNITY HEALTH SERVICES (HCHS), 1997/8 TO 2007/8, COMPARED WITH PAY ASSUMPTIONS OF THE 2002 WANLESS REVIEW

KEY
— HCHS pay inflation
— 2002 Wanless Review pay assumptions

Source: King's Fund analysis; Wanless 2002; House of Commons Health Committee 2006e

TABLE 14: NHS-SPECIFIC INFLATION RATES, 1997/8 TO 2007/8

Year	Hospital and community health services (HCHS)				Family health services (FHS)				Other (%)	NHS total (%)
	Pay (%)	Prices (%)	Capital (%)	GMS[1]/ PMS[2] (%)	GDS[3]/ PDS[4] (%)	PhS[5,6] (%)	GOS[6,7] (%)	FHS total (%)		
1997/8	2.5	0.4	4.2	5.1	0.3	2.9	2.9	3.0	3.1	2.1
1998/9	4.9	2.5	3.0	2.3	4.6	2.5	2.5	3.0	2.7	3.9
1999/2000	6.9	1.2	2.8	10.4	1.0	2.0	2.0	4.1	2.4	4.6
2000/1	7.2	-0.4	5.8	3.7	4.0	1.4	1.4	2.7	2.3	4.2
2001/2	8.3	0.1	6.5	1.0	2.8	2.4	2.4	2.1	2.5	4.7
2002/3	5.0	1.1	4.4	5.2	4.0	3.1	3.1	3.9	3.4	3.6
2003/4	7.3	1.4	-3.8	9.7[8]	1.8	3.0	3.0	4.6	2.9	4.8
2004/5	4.5	1.1	3.4		2.5	2.8	2.8		2.8	3.4
2005/6	6.2[9]	1.0[10]				1.9	1.9		1.9	4.2[11]
2006/7	5.2	1.0				2.7	2.7		2.7	3.8
2007/8	3.9	1.0				2.7	2.7		2.7	3.1

Source: House of Commons Health Committee 2006e
Notes:
Shaded cells: No data available and no reasonable basis on which to estimate
[1] GMS = General medical services
[2] PMS = Personal medical services
[3] GDS = General dental services
[4] PDS = Personal dental services
[5] PhS = Pharmaceutical services
[6] PhS and GOS inflation = GDP deflator
[7] GOS = General ophthalmic services
[8] Discontinuity in data series. No data available for 2004/5 onwards
[9] Estimates for HCHS pay from 2005/6 to 2007/8 based on Payment by Results tariff uplift
[10] 2005/6 to 2007/8: King's Fund assumption of 1 per cent per annum price inflation (based on recent years' price changes)
[11] Overall NHS inflation estimated by King's Fund: based on historical non-linear statistical relationship between HCHS pay inflation and overall NHS inflation rate

Pay and the new contracts

Health care is labour intensive, and staff pay accounts for around two-thirds of the total NHS budget. In 2006/7, pay for all hospital and community health services staff cost the NHS in England around £100 million a day; and a 1 per cent pay rise for all NHS staff in England would cost around £360 million a year. Actual pay rises between 2002 and 2007 are difficult to estimate for all sectors of the NHS due to a recent discontinuity in official pay inflation measures for GPs. However, for hospital and community health services staff (making up around 90 per cent of all NHS staff) pay has increased by around 30 per cent between 2002 and 2007 – a real rise of around 15 per cent (*see* Table 14, above). Over this period, average earnings in the economy as a whole rose by a more modest 17 per cent in cash terms.

The overall rate of pay inflation in the NHS has been slightly ahead of the assumptions made by the 2002 review (*see* Figure 17, p 91). The gap between the estimate of actual pay inflation and that assumed by the 2002 review for 2007/8 is of the order of £700 million. However, there is some uncertainty over this figure: estimates of pay inflation from 2005/6 to 2007/8 are based on the inflation uplift used by the Department of Health to update Payment by Results tariffs (which include the additional costs of new contracts for consultants and arising from Agenda for Change); but these inflation uplifts are likely to underestimate the actual rate of pay inflation in the NHS because the impact of the new contracts was underestimated by the Department of Health.

The five years since 2002 have witnessed major overhauls of the employment contracts for virtually all 1.3 million NHS staff in the UK. All these new contracts have generated additional costs for the NHS. The 2002 review identified pay modernisation as important for the creation of workforce capacity: not just to encourage staff to stay in (or return to) the service, but also to promote greater flexibility in the workforce, with more scope for team working and fewer barriers between staff groups, both contributing to an altered skill-mix in the service (Wanless 2002).

The main policy objectives of the new deals for NHS staff are reviewed below, along with their costs and benefits.

AGENDA FOR CHANGE

The most significant contractual change, in terms of numbers and costs, is Agenda for Change. This new deal for NHS staff not covered by the Doctors and Dentists Pay Review Bodies was phased in from December 2004 after more than five years of negotiations between unions and employers. The Department of Health estimates that around 99 per cent of staff are now on new Agenda for Change contracts.

Agenda for Change used a revised system for evaluating jobs according to various factors – skills, effort and knowledge – with a view to setting consistent pay rates across the NHS for jobs of equal assessed value. Pay scales were also overhauled so that just two remained: one for staff covered by nursing and other staff review bodies, and another for everyone else.

AGENDA FOR CHANGE

The key objectives of Agenda for Change were to:
- ensure that the new pay system leads to more patients being treated, more quickly and being given higher quality care
- assist new ways of working which best deliver the range and quality of services required, in as efficient and effective a way as possible, and organised to best meet the needs of patients
- assist the goal of achieving a quality workforce with the right numbers of staff, with the right skills and diversity, and organised in the right way
- improve the recruitment, retention and morale of the NHS workforce
- improve all aspects of equal opportunity and diversity, especially in the areas of career and training opportunities and working patterns that are flexible and responsive to family commitments
- meet equal pay for work of equal value criteria, recognising that pay constitutes any benefits in cash or conditions
- implement the new pay system within the management, financial and service constraints likely to be in place.

Agenda for Change: final Agreement (Department of Health 2004a, p 2)

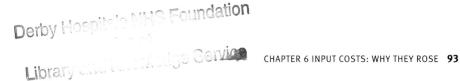

TABLE 15: ESTIMATED COSTS OF IMPLEMENTING AGENDA FOR CHANGE, 2005/6 TO 2008/9

Year	Annual cost (£ million)	Cumulative cost (£ million)
2005/6	950	950
2006/7	440	1,390
2007/8	390	1,780
2008/9	420	2,200

Source: House of Commons Health Committee 2006e

The Department envisaged a wide range of benefits emerging from the new deal, as set out in the box, below. The estimated costs of implementation are shown in Table 15, above.

Although Agenda for Change was introduced fairly recently, there is some evidence about its implementation and its impact. For example, a survey of 2,283 nurses across the United Kingdom, conducted for the Royal College of Nursing in 2006, found that, while the vast majority agreed with the *principles* of job evaluation, only one in four felt the process had been carried out well at local level. Of the sample, 44 per cent felt they were potentially better off as a result of Agenda for Change, 37 per cent believed their circumstances would not change and 12 per cent expected to be worse off (Bell and Pike 2006). However, only one in five thought the new pay system was fairer than before. The survey also looked at nurse morale and found that only 4 out of 10 nurses were not worried they would be made redundant in 2006, compared with 8 out of 10 the year before. There was a similar reduction in agreement with the statement: 'nursing will continue to offer me a secure job for years to come'. Of course, 2006 was a particularly difficult year in terms of the general financial situation in the NHS, with the need to substantially recover after the overspending of previous years. And the proportion of nurses stating that they planned to leave their current employer in the following two years was, at 25 per cent, 5 per cent lower than in 2005.

TABLE 16: RECRUITMENT AND RETENTION OF NURSES AND OTHER HEALTH PROFESSIONALS IN NHS TRUSTS, 2006

Health professionals	Extent of recruitment (rec) and retention (ret) difficulties (%)									
	No problem		Minor problem		Quite a problem		Major problem		Don't know	
	Rec	Ret	Rec	Ret	Rec	Ret	Rec	Ret	Rec	Ret
Nurses	55	50	35	42	7	5	1	1	3	3
Allied health professionals	42	47	36	38	17	11	1	1	4	3
Other scientific, therapeutic and technical staff	48	49	35	41	11	5	1	0	6	5
Ambulance staff	80	67	17	27	0	0	0	0	3	7

Source: Review Body for Nursing and Other Health Professions 2007

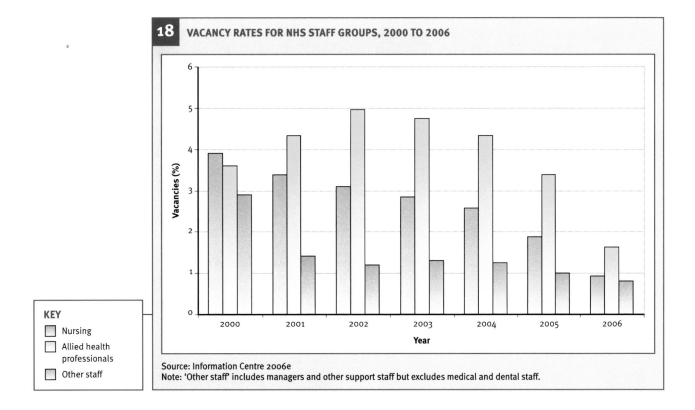

18 VACANCY RATES FOR NHS STAFF GROUPS, 2000 TO 2006

KEY
- Nursing
- Allied health professionals
- Other staff

Source: Information Centre 2006e
Note: 'Other staff' includes managers and other support staff but excludes medical and dental staff.

There are also some limited case study examples of the benefits of Agenda for Change collated by NHS Employers (*see*, for example, www.nhsemployers.org/kb/kb-986.cfm). Many of these benefits arise from the job evaluation process, leading, for example, to consistent grading of staff with similar roles and responsibilities. There is also some tentative evidence from these case studies that Agenda for Change has facilitated a greater acceptance of role flexibility.

The 2007 report of the Review Body for Nursing and other Health Professions provides some data on recruitment, retention and vacancy levels among staff covered by the review (around 800,000 full-time equivalents, all subject to Agenda for Change). The Review Body suggests that recruitment and retention is not a major problem for most employers (*see* Table 16, opposite) and was less difficult in 2006 than in 2005.

Trends in three-month vacancy rates between 2002 and 2006 for nurses, allied health professionals and scientific staff in England were all downward. For qualified nurses, the 2006 vacancy rate was 0.9 per cent compared with 3.1 per cent in 2002, with the rate of reduction accelerating after 2004 (*see* Figure 18, above).

An important question is whether or not nurses' productivity improves as a result of Agenda for Change. Factors driving productivity changes are, of course, complex because productivity depends, among other things, on how nurses' roles relate to other staff groups and to the technologies, systems and processes supporting them. It would be wrong to ascribe any observed short-term changes solely to changes in nurses' pay and contracts. One crude measure of labour productivity occasionally used (admissions per full-time equivalent staff) tentatively suggests that nurse productivity has started to improve. Figure 19, overleaf, shows that from 2003/4, emergency admissions per nurse

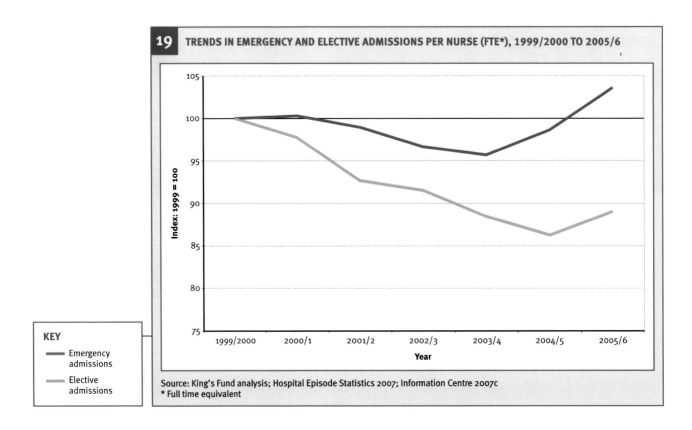

19 TRENDS IN EMERGENCY AND ELECTIVE ADMISSIONS PER NURSE (FTE*), 1999/2000 TO 2005/6

Index: 1999 = 100

Year

Source: King's Fund analysis; Hospital Episode Statistics 2007; Information Centre 2007c
* Full time equivalent

KEY
━━ Emergency admissions
━━ Elective admissions

started to increase, with a similar trend for elective admissions from 2004/5. Much more detailed research into productivity across the whole health service will be needed before firmer conclusions can be drawn.

There is no national evaluation of Agenda for Change. However, a King's Fund study (Buchan and Evans 2007) suggest a mixed picture so far. While the views of key stakeholders, including unions, managers and NHS employers, are generally neutral-to-positive, there is limited hard evidence of benefits, while implementation costs are difficult to assess and, in some respects, such as unsocial hours payments, yet to be resolved.

THE NEW CONSULTANTS' CONTRACT

The NHS Plan promised a consultant-delivered hospital service, underpinned by a new contract that would harness their commitment to the NHS. As has been recognised (Williams and Buchan 2006), there was formerly a collusive arrangement between the NHS and its consultants whereby the former relied heavily on the latter to work for longer than their contracted hours in return for considerable autonomy and freedom to undertake private work alongside NHS commitments. Although of some mutual benefit, this arrangement was seen to reduce consultants' accountability to their employers while also creating a degree of resentment about their long working hours.

After some protracted negotiations, the new contract was formally implemented in October 2003. The 'old' contract, based on a series of fixed commitments and flexible sessions, which also (as its detractors noted) allowed for 'moonlighting' in the private sector, was

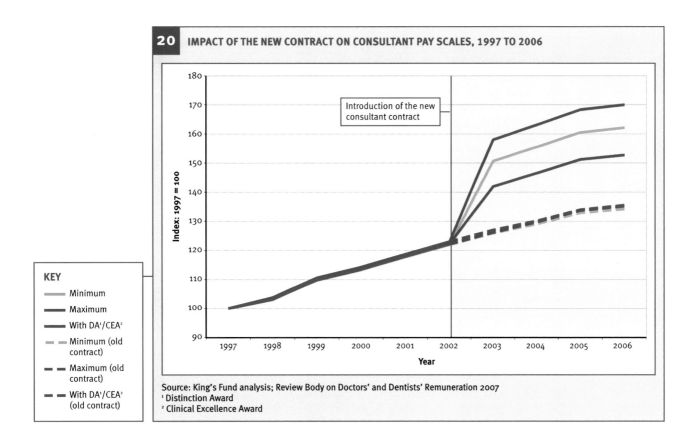

20 IMPACT OF THE NEW CONTRACT ON CONSULTANT PAY SCALES, 1997 TO 2006

KEY
— Minimum
— Maximum
— With DA¹/CEA²
– – Minimum (old contract)
– – Maximum (old contract)
– – With DA¹/CEA² (old contract)

Introduction of the new consultant contract

Index: 1997 = 100

Year

Source: King's Fund analysis; Review Body on Doctors' and Dentists' Remuneration 2007
¹ Distinction Award
² Clinical Excellence Award

replaced by what the then Secretary of State, Alan Milburn, described as a 'something for something' deal (*see* box overleaf).

The costs of the new deal were considerable. Consultant pay scales increased by up to 20 per cent at minimum and 25 per cent at maximum between 2002 and 2003 (*see* Figure 20, above), and earnings per head rose by a third between 2001/2 and 2005/6. The total consultants' pay bill for the English NHS rose by 55 per cent between 2002/3 and 2005/6. Around a quarter of this rise was due to increased numbers of consultants, with the remaining three-quarters due to increases in the per capita costs of employment. In terms of average earnings per head, consultant pay rose from £86,746 in 2002/3 to £109,974 in 2005/6 – a rise of nearly 27 per cent.

The financial costs of the new consultants' contract are well documented, but less evidence about benefits is available at this relatively early stage. Williams and Buchan's early analysis of the new deal suggested that, two years after implementation, there was still little evidence of benefit. The greatest benefit they noted was greater transparency about consultants' work due to job planning. In addition, managers now have some new levers to control, for example, pay progression, and some slack has been removed from the system by imposing some restrictions on external activities (Williams and Buchan 2006).

However, these benefits (some of which have yet to be realised) need to be weighed against the total extra cost of the new contract, which was originally underestimated by the Department of Health and NHS employers. Williams and Buchan also point to some unintended consequences of the new contract, including a potential erosion of professionalism, incentives towards patterns of retirement and a lack of impact on the scale of consultants' private work; the latter finding is ironic, given the original aspirations of the contract (Williams and Buchan 2006).

THE NEW CONSULTANTS' CONTRACT

The new contract applied to all new consultant appointments in England from 31 October 2003. Existing consultants who indicated a commitment to transfer to the new contract between November 2003 and March 2004 were eligible for backdated pay increases. In addition to hospital consultants holding substantive posts, the contract also covers locum consultants, dental consultants, consultant clinical academics, dental clinical academics and senior academic GPs (clinical academics specialising in primary care).

The contractual framework incorporates a new pay structure, including a higher starting salary and extra pay for those with the heaviest on-call duties. Salary increases are no longer automatic (although the majority are expected to progress), with pay progression linked to a number of factors, including satisfactory performance against agreed job plans.

Mandatory job planning is the bedrock of the contract. A job plan is designed to be a prospective agreement that sets out a consultant's duties, responsibilities and objectives for the coming year. The aims are to enable consultants and employers to prioritise work more effectively and agree how consultants can best support the objectives of the service and how employers can support them in this.

There is a new system for organising a consultant's working week. The basic contract for a full-time consultant is 10 four-hour programmed activities (PAs) per week. PAs are separated into four types:
- direct clinical care, including emergency duties and on-call work, operating sessions, ward rounds and outpatient clinics
- supporting professional activities (SPAs), including training, continuing professional development, teaching, audit, job planning and appraisal
- additional NHS responsibilities, such as serving as a Caldicott guardian, clinical governance lead, postgraduate dean, clinical tutor, medical director, clinical director or lead clinician
- external duties, which may include trade union duties and certain work for the General Medical Council as well as 'reasonable quantities of work for the royal colleges in the interests of the wider NHS' (Department of Health 2004g p vi).

Trusts can contract separately for additional PAs where a consultant has regular additional duties that cannot be contained within a standard 10-PA contract. The NHS also has first call on a consultant's time. In order to be eligible for pay progression, consultants must offer their trust one extra PA per week before undertaking paid clinical work outside their NHS contracts. The relationship between private practice and NHS work is clarified by *A Code of Conduct for Private Practice* (Department of Health 2003a). Adherence to this forms part of the eligibility criteria for a new scheme of clinical excellence awards (replacing the distinction awards and discretionary points schemes) and should be assessed at the annual job plan review (Department of Health 2004e).

Emergency work is divided into predictable work, which should be scheduled into the working week as part of a consultant's PAs, and unpredictable work performed while on-call (such as being called to the hospital to operate). Work between 7am and 7pm, Monday to Friday, is paid for at standard rates; work outside these hours and at weekends or on public holidays is during premium time and split into PAs of three hours each. Consultants who participate in on-call rotas are eligible for an availability supplement based on the frequency of their rota commitment and whether or not they typically need to return to hospital immediately or perform complex interventions (category A) or can provide advice by phone (category B).

Source: Williams and Buchan (2006)

The National Audit Office (2007a) reports mixed success for the new contract in realising the Department of Health's expectations. It notes that the contract has contributed to improving the management of consultants' time, preventing an increase in private practice, securing extra work and improving recruitment and retention. However, benefits such as extending patient services and increasing direct clinical care have not yet materialised; while others, such as improved productivity, reduced pay drift and shorter waiting times, are either too difficult to assess or too early to measure. There is little evidence that ways of working have changed as a result of the contract and, although most consultants now have job plans, few trusts have used job planning as a lever for improving participation or productivity.

The report goes on to point out that average consultant pay in 2005/6 was £109,974 (an increase of 27 per cent in three years), and that by the end of March 2006 the Department

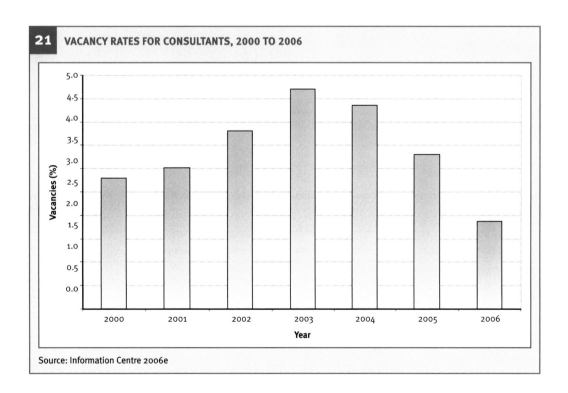

21 **VACANCY RATES FOR CONSULTANTS, 2000 TO 2006**

Source: Information Centre 2006e

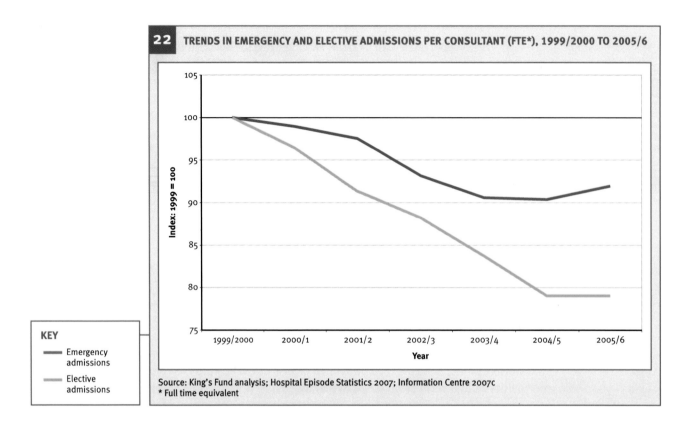

22 TRENDS IN EMERGENCY AND ELECTIVE ADMISSIONS PER CONSULTANT (FTE*), 1999/2000 TO 2005/6

Index: 1999 = 100

Year

KEY
— Emergency admissions
— Elective admissions

Source: King's Fund analysis; Hospital Episode Statistics 2007; Information Centre 2007c
* Full time equivalent

had spent £715 million on the new contract – £150 million more than the original estimate of £565 million. These additional costs arose partly as a result of the contract's higher-than-anticipated baseline workload (in terms of the number of programmed activities and levels of on-call responsibility). They also arose from the fact that many trusts have implemented the contract without sufficient reference to the additional funding for the contract allowed for in primary care trust allocations and their level of income – in part dictated by the tariff for elective and non-elective care. The National Audit Office's conclusion is that '...the contract is not yet delivering the full value for money to the NHS and patients that was expected from it...".

Two further pieces of evidence are worth noting. First, as Figure 21, p 99, shows, the three-month vacancy rate for consultant posts, which rose between 2000 to 2003, has since fallen.

Second, the absence of firm measures of productivity means that, at best, only crude labour productivity measures can be examined. If hospital admissions per full-time equivalent consultant are taken as a measure, productivity for English consultants has been falling since 1999/2000, by more than 20 per cent to 2004/5 for elective admissions and by 10 per cent for emergencies (*see* Figure 22, above). However, these trends appear to have been arrested by 2005/6. Attributing all or part of these changes to the introduction of the new contract is probably unwise, given other simultaneous developments and policy changes, but detailed research on this is vital. Given the amount of money spent on this change, much more needs to be known about what has been gained as a result.

THE NEW GENERAL MEDICAL SERVICES CONTRACT

This contract was developed in response to increasing workload, recruitment and retention difficulties and the belief that the previous payment system for GPs – based on the 'red book' – was no longer fit for purpose. The NHS Plan noted that the red book contract placed more emphasis on *volume* outcomes (such as patient list size and quantity of services provided) than on quality and that the government would work with GPs and their representatives to amend it so as to shift the emphasis towards quality and improved outcomes.

In June 2003, GPs in England voted to accept a new practice-based contract for general medical services (GMS). The contract was implemented in April 2004, with personal medical service (PMS) contracts becoming a permanent alternative for the provision of primary care services. The practice-based contract sets boundaries on workload, with services defined as 'essential', 'additional' and 'enhanced'. All practices are required to provide essential services and, although they are also expected to provide additional services, an opt-out option exists. Additionally, GPs can also opt out of providing out-of-hours (OOH) care, which subsequently became the responsibility of primary care trusts (PCTs).

A key element of the new contract is the Quality and Outcomes Framework (QOF), designed to raise organisational and clinical standards in primary care. The framework consists of a system of financial incentives which reward the delivery of quality care through participation in an annual quality improvement cycle. Achievement is measured against a scorecard of 146 indicators across a range of different domains: clinical, organisational, additional services and patient experience. The QOF then assigns a monetary value for each point scored, up to a current maximum score of 1,000 points.

AIMS OF THE NEW GMS CONTRACT

The Department of Health's 2003 document *Investing in General Practice: the new General Medical Services Contract* explained that the new GMS contract would:
- give practices greater flexibility to determine the range of services they wish to provide, including opting out of additional services and out-of-hours care
- reward practices for delivering clinical and organisational quality and improving the patient experience
- facilitate the modernisation of practice infrastructure (including premises and IT); support the development of best human resource management practice and help GPs achieve a better work/life balance; support the development of practice management; and recognise the particular needs of GPs in different localities, including deprived communities, rural and remote areas
- provide for unprecedented and guaranteed levels of investment through a Gross Investment Guarantee, which replaces the current flawed pay mechanisms. The contract allocates resources on a more equitable basis and allows practice flexibility as to how these are deployed from the global sum
- as a result of these mechanisms, support the delivery of a wider range of higher quality services for patients and empower patients to make best use of them
- simplify the regulatory regime around how the contractual mechanisms will work.

TABLE 17: BREAKDOWN OF PCT SPENDING ON GENERAL MEDICAL SERVICES, 2005/6

Breakdown	Spending (£ million)[1] (% of total)	Variance: under/over spend compared with allocation (£ million) (% of allocation)
General medical services (global sum and MPIG[2])	1,993 (26)	+51 (2.6)
Personal medical services contracts	2,023 (26)	-231 (10.2)
Quality and Outcomes Framework	1,098 (14)	+171 (15.6)
Enhanced services	649 (8)	-26 (3.8)
Primary care organisation admin (discretionary payments)	182 (2)	+88 (93.6)
Premises	413 (5)	-38 (8.4)
Information technology	68 (1)	+4 (6.3)
Out of hours	346 (4)	+242 (130)
Other	45 (5)	-20 (30.7)
Dispensing	873 (11)	-44 (4.8)
Total	**7,691**	**+196 (2.5)**

Source: Adapted from House of Commons Health Committee 2006e
[1] Provisional figures based on unaudited accounts
[2] MPIG = Minimum practice income guarantee

---

23   **AVERAGE NET INCOME AND EXPENSES FOR GPs, 2003/4 TO 2004/5**

£81,566

£100,170   + 23%

£120,064

£129,927   + 8%

2003/4   2004/5

Year

KEY
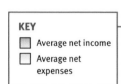
Average net income
Average net expenses

Source: King's Fund analysis; Information Centre 2007e

Funding is held by PCTs, which then allocate it to practices in three main forms:
- a sum to cover the cost of essential and additional primary care services for patients (including, where applicable, out-of-hours services)
- quality payments to reward achievement of standards
- enhanced services payments.

Table 17 (*see* p 101) provides more details on the breakdown of PCT spending on general medical services for 2005/6. QOF payments account for around 14 per cent of all spending, with other GMS payments and spending on personal medical services absorbing just over half of total spend.

The impact of underestimating the cost of one aspect of the new GMS contract – the buy-out of out-of-hours duties – is evident from Table 17: PCT spending on out-of-hours provision exceeded the 2005/6 allocation by 130 per cent.

As a consequence of these contractual changes, GPs have seen significant increases in their net incomes. Analysis by the Information Centre for Health and Social Care found that the average net income from NHS and private work for GPMS GPs (all those working under General Medical Services or Personal Medical Services contracts) increased by 22.8 per cent between 2003/4 and 2004/5 to stand at £100,170 (*see* Figure 23, opposite).

Although average expenses for GPMS GPs rose by 8.2 per cent between 2003/4 and 2004/5, gross earnings outpaced this increase in expenses, generating a 5 per cent decrease in the expenses ratio.

Much of the early evidence on the impact of the new GMS contract on hours worked is anecdotal. However, a survey of all GPs in Scotland (NHS Education for Scotland 2006) found that the average hours worked, excluding out-of-hours, was 38.5 hours a week in 2006; salaried GPs reported an average of 41.5 hours per week, which is three fewer than they worked in 2002.

Most GPs have scored well against the Quality and Outcomes Framework, achieving well over 90 per cent of possible points. The Information Centre found that the average number of QOF points achieved by practices in England in 2004/5 was 958.7 – 91.3 per cent of the total available. The Centre also found that the then maximum score of 1,050 points was achieved by 222 practices (2.6 per cent) and that the median score was 999.1. However, with no baseline measurement available, it is impossible to know whether the QOF is recording real improvements or simply describing current practice.

Concerns remain that the costs of the new GMS contract were significantly under-estimated and mismanaged by the Department of Health. The House of Commons Public Accounts Committee (2007a) commented recently that preparations for the new out-of-hours service were 'a shambles'; that it costs around £70 million a year higher than was envisaged; and that doctors have done particularly well out of the deal. Furthermore, in their Seventeenth Report of Session 2006/7 (2007b), they went on to point out that the costs associated with the new GP contract exceeded Department of Health forecasts by £250 million in 2004/5.

Broader criticisms were raised by the Health Committee's report into NHS workforce planning (2007). This noted that:

- NHS Plan staffing targets had been exceeded
- large pay increases were granted without securing increases in productivity
- attempts to create a more flexible workforce had had mixed results.

The Committee observed that 'The planning system remains poorly integrated [with] an appalling lack of coordination between workforce and financial planning', and concluded that workforce planning must be a priority for the NHS.

SUMMARY: INPUT COSTS

- Of the £43.2 billion cash increase in UK NHS spending between 2002/3 and 2007/8, an estimated £18.9 billion (43 per cent) was absorbed by higher input costs.
- Estimates of combined pay and non-pay NHS inflation between 2002/3 and 2007/8 closely matched the 2002 review's inflation assumptions. However, actual pay inflation exceeded the review's assumptions while actual non-pay inflation was slightly lower.
- The main source of higher costs has been pay increases arising from three new contracts introduced in the last four years – Agenda for Change (covering all non-medical staff) and new contracts for hospital doctors and general practitioners.
- The cumulative additional cost of Agenda for Change from 2005/6 to 2007/8 has been around £1.8 billion. Consultant pay rates under their new contract increased by around 25 per cent and the new GP contract boosted average net income by 23 per cent.
- There is some tentative evidence that these new contracts may have reduced three-month vacancy rates for the staff groups involved. There are also some indications that consultant and nurse productivity, which had been falling since 1999, may be starting to improve.
- However, there is a dearth of robust evidence to demonstrate significant productivity or other benefits arising from the new contracts and pay deals.

7 Resources: investment in staff, buildings and equipment

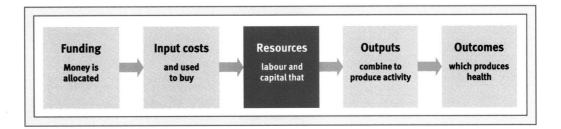

The previous chapter examined the significant impact on NHS input costs of the three new pay deals for NHS staff, which have helped to reduce the effective funding available to improve the service.

This chapter evaluates progress towards government commitments to invest in increased human and other resources, including doctors, nurses and therapists, hospitals and GP premises, hospital beds and equipment and IT systems.

The 2002 review made an implicit commitment to successful delivery of the NHS Plan (Department of Health 2000c), which set out the government's 10-year strategy for reforming the NHS in England. Importantly, the March 2000 budget settlement supported its implementation by channelling money into the NHS to fund extra investment in staff and facilities.

The 2002 review predicated its modelled resource requirements on the belief that the Plan's 10 core principles would remain valid in 20 years' time. It incorporated the commitments of the NHS Plan and, in some instances, recommended additional investment. For example, the review's projected increases in the NHS capital building programme were substantially in excess of those set out in the Plan (Wanless 2002).

Given that the NHS Plan is so integral to the resource requirements of the 2002 review, what progress has been made since its publication in terms of commitments to increase staff and other health care resources? The headline investment in NHS facilities and staff outlined in the Plan were:

- 7,500 more consultants
- 2,000 more GPs
- 20,000 extra nurses
- 6,500 extra therapists
- 7,000 extra beds in hospitals and intermediate care
- more than 100 new hospitals and 500 new 'one-stop' primary care centres
- more than 3,000 GP premises modernised
- 250 new scanners
- modern IT systems in every hospital and GP surgery.

The commitments to staffing, beds, premises and equipment were to be realised by 2004, with modernisation of IT systems also to be achieved in the first five years of the Plan. The major target for the second five years was the delivery of the new hospitals. These resource areas are examined in turn below.

Changes in staffing levels

The NHS Plan committed to achieving, by 2004, the following additional staff:

- 7,500 consultants
- 2,000 GPs
- 20,000 nurses
- 6,500 therapists (or 'allied health professionals').

All these targets referred to headcounts, not full-time equivalents (FTEs). But what actually happened?

Between 1999 and 2006, the number of professionally qualified clinical staff – hospital doctors, nurses and GPs – in the NHS rose by 25 per cent to 674,621, to represent half the total NHS workforce. Although 2006 saw a small decline in the number of professionally qualified clinical staff, the full-time equivalent number actually rose to 571,374.

TABLE 18: NUMBER OF DOCTORS, NURSES, ALLIED HEALTH PROFESSIONALS AND NON-MEDICAL STAFF IN THE NHS (HEADCOUNT), 1996 TO 2006

Year	All doctors excluding retainers	Consultants including Directors of Public Health	GPs excluding retainers and registrars	All qualified nurses including practice nurses	Qualified allied health professionals	All non-medical staff
1996	86,584	20,402	27,811	319,151	48,611	541,726
1997	89,619	21,474	28,046	318,856	49,893	538,972
1998	91,837	22,324	28,251	323,457	51,479	541,831
1999	93,981	23,321	28,467	329,637	53,105	556,584
2000	96,319	24,401	28,593	335,952	54,788	564,905
2001	99,169	25,782	28,802	350,381	57,001	591,370
2002	103,350	27,070	29,202	367,520	59,415	620,747
2003	108,993	28,750	30,358	386,359	62,189	649,555
2004	117,036	30,650	31,523	397,515	65,515	670,381
2005	122,345	31,993	32,738	404,161	67,841	686,231
2006	125,612	32,874	33,091	398,335	67,483	663,519

Source: Information Centre 2007c
Note: More accurate validation in 2006 has resulted in 9,858 duplicate records being identified and removed from the non-medical census. Although this represents less than 1 per cent of total records, it should be taken into consideration when making historical comparisons. These 9,858 duplicate records, broken down by main staff group, are: 3,370 qualified nurses; 1,818 qualified scientific, therapeutic and technical staff; 2,719 support staff to doctors and nurses; 368 support staff to scientific, therapeutic and technical staff; 1,562 NHS infrastructure support staff; and 21 in other areas. The impact of duplicates on FTE has been minimal, with the removal of 507.

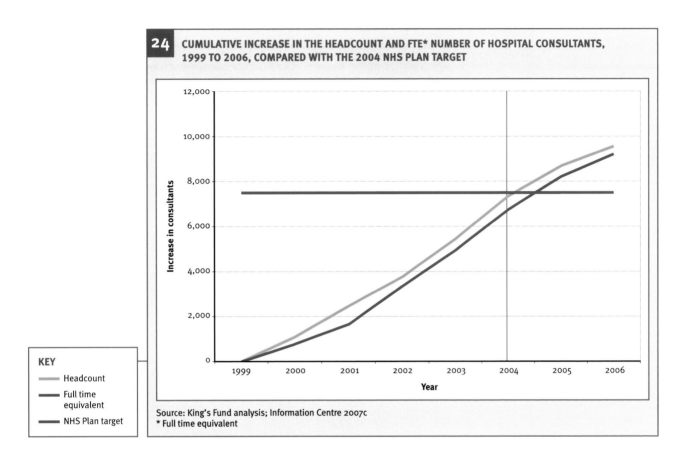

24 CUMULATIVE INCREASE IN THE HEADCOUNT AND FTE* NUMBER OF HOSPITAL CONSULTANTS, 1999 TO 2006, COMPARED WITH THE 2004 NHS PLAN TARGET

KEY
— Headcount
— Full time equivalent
— NHS Plan target

Source: King's Fund analysis; Information Centre 2007c
* Full time equivalent

Hospital consultants

The number of hospital consultants (including Directors of Public Health) increased by 7,329 between 1999 and 2004, just below the government target of 7,500. However, by 2005, a year later than planned, the NHS Plan commitment had been more than met, with an increase of 8,672, representing a rise of 37 per cent; in full-time equivalent terms, this equates to a rise of 8,203 consultants, an increase of 38 per cent (*see* Figure 24, above). By 2006 there were 32,874 consultants in the NHS, equating to 30,619 full-time equivalent staff.

General practitioners

The targeted increase of 2,000 GPs has been exceeded. Between 1999 and 2004 an extra 3,056 GPs – 1,750 full-time equivalents – were recruited to the NHS. By 2005, the headcount had gone up by 4,271 – equal to 2,690 full-time equivalent posts. Interestingly, between 2005 and 2006 there was a further 1 per cent increase in GP numbers but a 6 per cent rise in full-time equivalent staff; this is the first time since the Plan that the annual growth in full-time equivalent GPs has exceeded the headcount growth (*see* Figure 25, overleaf).

The government also pledged to boost medical school places by 1,000, and this target was rapidly met. Medical school places increased by 59 per cent between 1999/2000 and 2005/6, from 3,972 to 6,298. However, around 60 per cent of the increase in medical staffing between 2000 and 2006 was made up of doctors who qualified outside the United Kingdom; given the duration of medical training, the increase in medical school places in the United Kingdom could not be expected to impact on staffing levels until 2006 at the earliest.

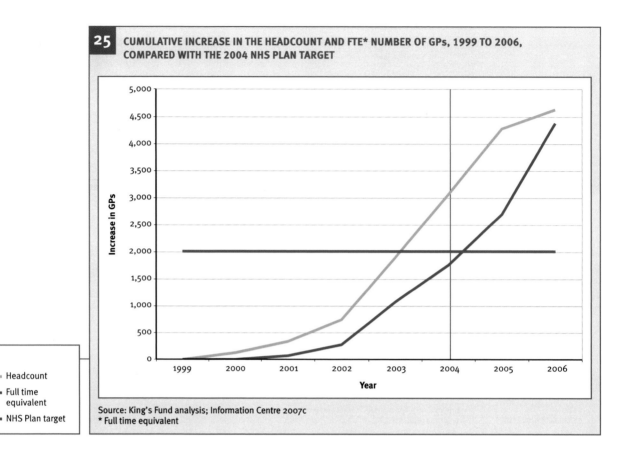

25 CUMULATIVE INCREASE IN THE HEADCOUNT AND FTE* NUMBER OF GPs, 1999 TO 2006, COMPARED WITH THE 2004 NHS PLAN TARGET

KEY
— Headcount
— Full time equivalent
— NHS Plan target

Source: King's Fund analysis; Information Centre 2007c
* Full time equivalent

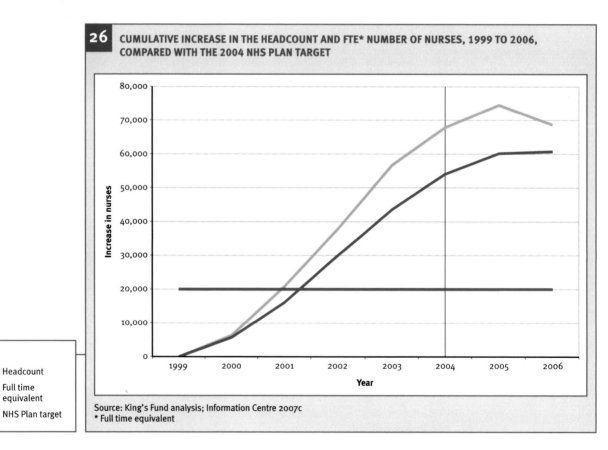

26 CUMULATIVE INCREASE IN THE HEADCOUNT AND FTE* NUMBER OF NURSES, 1999 TO 2006, COMPARED WITH THE 2004 NHS PLAN TARGET

KEY
— Headcount
— Full time equivalent
— NHS Plan target

Source: King's Fund analysis; Information Centre 2007c
* Full time equivalent

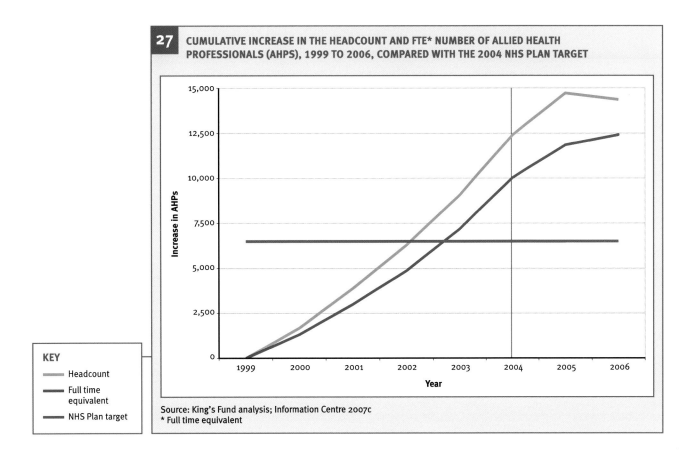

27 CUMULATIVE INCREASE IN THE HEADCOUNT AND FTE* NUMBER OF ALLIED HEALTH PROFESSIONALS (AHPS), 1999 TO 2006, COMPARED WITH THE 2004 NHS PLAN TARGET

KEY
—— Headcount
—— Full time equivalent
—— NHS Plan target

Source: King's Fund analysis; Information Centre 2007c
* Full time equivalent

Nurses and therapy staff

Target increases for nursing and therapy staff have also been exceeded. Between 1999 and 2004 the number of nurses increased by 67,878 to 397,515 (compared with a target increase of 20,000) and the number of qualified allied health professionals (AHPs) rose by 11,039 to 58,959 (compared with a target of 6,500). Over this period, the full-time equivalent figures for nurses and AHPs also exceeded the NHS Plan targets, with increases of 21 per cent and 23 per cent respectively. Between 2005 and 2006, while head counts for both these groups fell, full-time equivalent numbers rose (see Figures 26 and 27, opposite and above).

Non-clinical staff

Non-medical NHS staff, including managers, porters and administrative staff, have traditionally accounted for about half of all personnel in the NHS. Since 1996 the numbers of non-medical staff have increased by around 22 per cent, compared with 31 per cent for medical staff; as a proportion of total NHS staff, non-medical numbers are now at their lowest for a decade. In full-time equivalent terms, the number of non-medical staff in the NHS increased by 26 per cent between 1996 and 2006, compared with 32 per cent for medical staff (see Figure 28, overleaf). In part, this reduction may reflect increased outsourcing of some NHS jobs, but national figures are not available to prove this.

Full-time equivalent managers and senior managers account for almost 7 per cent of all non-medical staff and just over 3 per cent of total NHS staff. Since 1996, their full-time equivalent numbers have increased by around 70 per cent (see Figure 29, p 111). Between 2005 and 2006 both the head count and full-time equivalents fell for the first time in a decade.

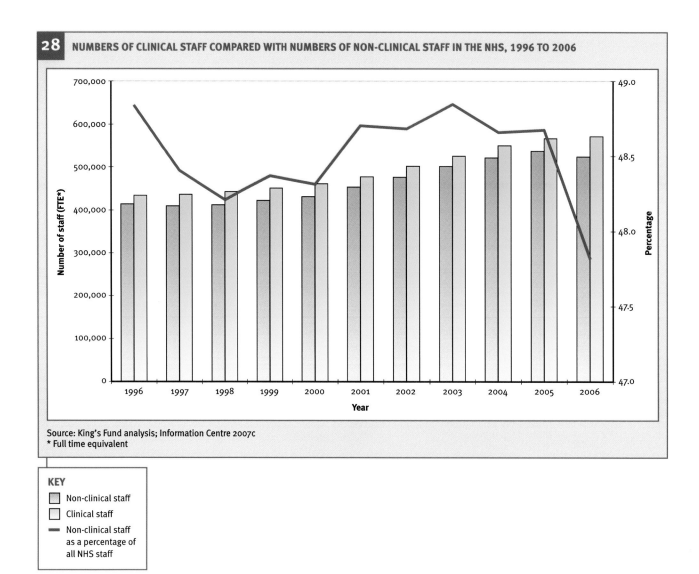

Source: King's Fund analysis; Information Centre 2007c
* Full time equivalent

KEY

▢ Non-clinical staff
▢ Clinical staff
— Non-clinical staff
   as a percentage of
   all NHS staff

Although the opportunity cost of any increase in non-medical staff can be viewed as a potential loss of medically qualified staff, the more important issue is whether the NHS has the right number of managerial and other support staff to enable the service to carry out its primary tasks efficiently and effectively.

Taking a long-term view on workforce capacity building

The NHS Plan heralded a period of rapid growth in the NHS workforce, so that by 2005 the government had exceeded all its (headcount) staffing targets. The Plan also emphasised the need to sustain this expansion in future by increasing the number of training places. How does this expansion of human capital within the NHS compare with the workforce projections outlined in the 2002 review?

The staffing commitments of the NHS Plan were central to delivering the review's vision for increased health activity over the next two decades. The review predicted that the health care workforce might need to increase by almost 300,000 by 2022 under all three

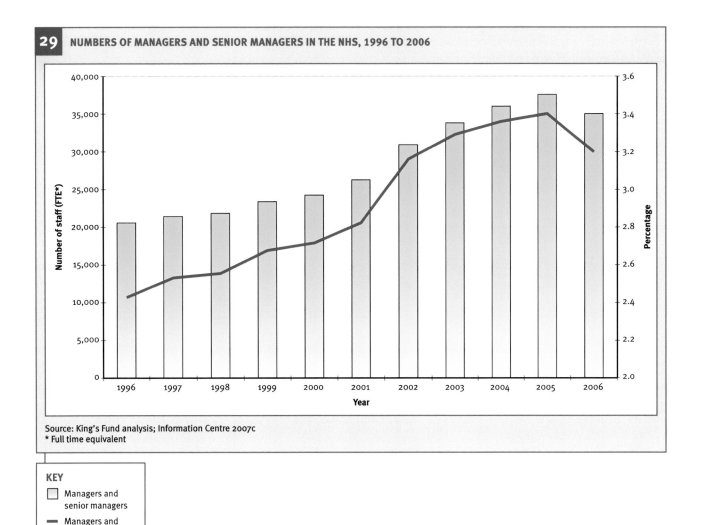

29 NUMBERS OF MANAGERS AND SENIOR MANAGERS IN THE NHS, 1996 TO 2006

Source: King's Fund analysis; Information Centre 2007c
* Full time equivalent

KEY

☐ Managers and
senior managers

— Managers and
senior managers
as a percentage of
all NHS staff

scenarios, with workforce demand growing fastest during the second half of this period. The review noted that the planned increase in nurses was almost sufficient to match future demand, but that the planned increase in doctors would eventually fall short of demand (Wanless 2002).

Table 19, on p 113, and Figure 30, overleaf, apply the 2002 review's projected growth rates for the demand and supply of doctors to derive a time series of the projected demand and supply of doctors in England up to 2020. Given that the government exceeded all its NHS staffing targets by 2005, it is unsurprising that in that year the actual supply of doctors exceeded the review's demand projections. This situation of 'excess' supply suggests the workforce is unlikely to act as a capacity constraint on the pace of investment under each of the 2002 review's scenarios. For example, in the fully engaged scenario it was originally estimated that there would be an excess supply of 1,781 full-time equivalent doctors in 2005, whereas in fact the excess amounted to 15,583 full-time equivalents. However, all other things being equal, it is likely that the increasing demands predicted by the review will absorb this excess supply, by 2008 at the earliest.

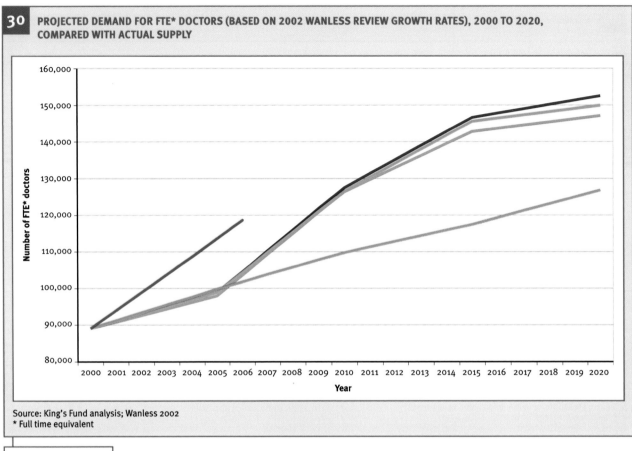

30 PROJECTED DEMAND FOR FTE* DOCTORS (BASED ON 2002 WANLESS REVIEW GROWTH RATES), 2000 TO 2020, COMPARED WITH ACTUAL SUPPLY

Source: King's Fund analysis; Wanless 2002
* Full time equivalent

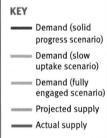

KEY
— Demand (solid progress scenario)
— Demand (slow uptake scenario)
— Demand (fully engaged scenario)
— Projected supply
— Actual supply

The 2002 review's demand projections indicate that the need for more doctors will remain in the longer term, but that the growth rates seen between 2000 and 2006 will need to slow down.

In summary, while short-term growth in the NHS workforce has overshot both the NHS Plan targets and the 2002 review's estimates, the latter's longer-term projections suggest that even more staff will be needed in future.

INTERNATIONAL COMPARISONS

The recent rapid increase in the numbers of clinical staff in the NHS has narrowed the gap between the United Kingdom and its European neighbours. Between 1999 and 2004 the number of physicians per 1,000 of the population rose by 21 per cent in the United Kingdom, a growth rate bettered only by Ireland (at 22 per cent). Nevertheless, despite this rapid growth, the UK ratio of 2.3 physicians per 1,000 population in 2004 remained the lowest of the EU-15 countries, as shown by Table 20, opposite.

TABLE 19: PROJECTED DEMAND AND SUPPLY OF FTE* DOCTORS UNDER 2002 WANLESS SCENARIOS, 2005 TO 2020, COMPARED WITH ACTUAL SUPPLY

	Number of doctors (FTE*)			
	2005	2010	2015	2020
Projected demand				
Solid progress	98,866	127,537	146,667	152,534
Slow uptake	98,866	126,548	145,530	149,896
Fully engaged	97,975	126,388	142,818	147,103
Projected supply	99,756	109,732	117,413	126,806
Actual supply	113,558			

Source: King's Fund analysis; Wanless 2002
Note: 'Doctors' comprises consultants, junior doctors and GPs
* FTE = full time equivalent

TABLE 20: NUMBER OF PHYSICIANS PER 1,000 OF THE POPULATION IN SELECTED OECD COUNTRIES, 1999 TO 2004

Country	1999	2000	2001	2002	2003	2004	% change 1999–2004
Austria	3.0	3.1	3.2	3.3	3.4	3.5	17
Belgium	3.8	3.9	3.9	3.9	4.0	4.0	5
Denmark	2.8	2.8	2.8	2.9	3.0	na	7*
Finland	2.3	2.3	2.3	2.4	2.4	2.4	4
France	3.3	3.3	3.3	3.3	3.4	3.4	3
Germany	3.2	3.3	3.3	3.3	3.4	3.4	6
Greece	4.2	4.3	4.4	4.6	4.7	4.9	17
Ireland	2.3	2.2	2.4	2.4	2.6	2.8	22
Italy	4.2	4.1	4.3	4.4	4.1	4.2	0
Luxembourg	2.5	2.5	2.5	2.6	2.7	2.8	12
Netherlands	3.1	3.2	3.3	3.4	3.5	3.6	16
Portugal	3.1	3.2	3.2	3.3	3.3	3.4	10
Spain	2.9	3.2	3.1	2.9	3.2	3.4	17
Sweden	3.0	3.1	3.2	3.3	3.3	na	10*
United Kingdom	1.9	1.9	2.0	2.1	2.2	2.3	21

Source: Organisation for Economic Co-operation and Development 2007
* Change from 1999 to 2003

TABLE 21: NUMBER OF NURSES PER 1,000 OF THE POPULATION IN SELECTED OECD COUNTRIES, 1999 TO 2004

Country	1999	2000	2001	2002	2003	2004	% change 1999–2004
Austria	9.0	9.2	9.2	9.3	9.4	9.3	3
Belgium	5.3	5.4	5.5	5.6	5.8	6.0	13
Denmark	6.7	6.9	7.0	7.1	7.0	na	4*
Finland	5.7	6.1	6.6	6.9	7.3	7.6	33
France	6.5	6.7	6.9	7.1	7.3	7.5	15
Germany	9.3	9.4	9.6	9.6	9.7	9.7	4
Greece	3.1	3.2	3.4	3.8	na	na	–
Ireland	13.6	14.0	14.8	15.3	14.8	15.0	10
Italy	5.2	5.2	5.4	5.4	5.4	na	4*
Luxembourg	na	na	na	na	12.3	12.7	–
Netherlands	12.7	13.4	13.3	13.6	13.9	14.2	12
Portugal	3.7	3.7	3.8	4.0	4.2	4.4	19
Spain	6.5	6.4	6.6	7.2	7.5	7.4	14
Sweden	9.7	9.8	9.9	10.2	10.3	na	6*
United Kingdom	8.3	8.4	8.5	8.9	9.1	9.2	11

Source: Organisation for Economic Co-operation and Development 2007
* Change from 1999 to 2003

The UK has more nurses per 1,000 population than Spain, Italy or France and, since 1999, has also rapidly closed the gap with Germany (*see* Table 21, above).

THE COST OF INCREASED STAFF NUMBERS

The previous chapter looked in some detail at the extra costs of NHS staff pay increases and the impact of the new staff contracts. However, given the unprecedented rise in the *volume* of staff over the last few years, it is also worth examining this in terms of its cost implications to the NHS.

A recent analysis (Department of Health 2007e) suggested that around 80 per cent of the additional funds for the (English) NHS between 2001 and 2004 were accounted for by increased *employment* (rather than increased pay or other expenditure). This analysis of the costs of extra staff formed part of a wider study into the causes of NHS deficits up to 2004/5. The Department's study first identified the cumulative increase in spending by primary care trusts (PCTs) and strategic health authorities (SHAs) between 2001/2 and 2004/5 *over and above what it would have been if it had followed the trend in spending from 1999/2000 and 2000/1*. It then calculated a similar cumulative figure for the growth in the NHS wage bill (for all staff, excluding agency and practice staff), again over and above the trend increase in employment. The results of these calculations suggested that, of the additional funds above trend of £13 billion, £9 billion were accounted for by the increased volume of staff, with extra pay for these staff adding a further £1.2 billion.

Overall, then, it would appear that nearly 70 per cent of the increase in funding (above trend) was absorbed by increased volumes of staff, and under 10 per cent by inflation in unit costs (leaving around 20 per cent spent on non-staff goods and services, including inflation on these items).

While this analysis asks a valid question – where did the extra money *above trend increases* go? – by definition it fails to consider the destination of the *absolute* increase in funding and, by implication, fails to show the true proportion of that increase that was accounted for by increases in the total wage bill.

A more straightforward analysis, using the same data sets as the Department used, suggests that the cash increase in PCT/SHA spend on hospital and community health services between 2001/2 and 2004/5 was £18.1 billion, and that the increase in the total wage bill accounted for 56 per cent (£10.2 billion) of this overall increase.

TABLE 22: ANALYSIS OF THE INCREASE IN THE TOTAL NHS WAGE BILL, 2000 TO 2004

	2000	2001	2002	2003	2004	Change 2000–2004	Total
Total PCT/SHA spend (£ thousand)	42,100,000	45,800,000	50,300,000	55,000,000	60,200,000	18,100,000	
Actual staff numbers[1]	801,493	837,196	882,114	928,059	968,435	166,942	
Actual wage bill[1] (£ thousand)	19,585,100	21,950,710	24,324,745	26,966,745	29,743,414	10,158,314	
Estimated unit cost[1,2] (£ thousand)	24.4	26.2	27.6	29.1	30.7	–	
Additional cost of existing staff[3] (£ thousand)	–	1,429,502	1,086,978	1,187,519	1,327,045	–	5,031,044
Additional cost of new staff							
due to higher unit costs[4] (£ thousand)	–	63,678	109,338	187,524	276,409	–	636,949
due to increased volume[5] (£ thousand)	–	872,430	1,177,719	1,266,957	1,173,215	–	4,490,321
Total change in wage bill (£ thousand)		2,365,610	2,374,035	2,642,000	2,776,669		10,158,314
due to higher unit costs (£ thousand)	–	1,493,180	1,196,316	1,375,043	1,603,454	–	5,667,993
due to increased volume (£ thousand)	–	872,430	1,177,719	1,266,957	1,173,215	–	4,490,321

Source: King's Fund analysis of data from Department of Health 2007e
[1] Based on data from Department of Health 2007e, Annex A
[2] Unit costs = wage bill/staff numbers
[3] Annual additional costs = staff as at 2000 x change in unit costs
[4] Annual cost = cumulative additional staff each year x change in unit costs each year
[5] Annual cost = annual change in staff numbers x previous year's unit cost

A large proportion of the increase in the wage bill between 2001 and 2004 – around £5.7 billion – was accounted for by increased unit costs (such as higher pay and movement of staff up pay scales) and around £4.5 billion by the costs of employing extra staff. Table 22, p 115, sets out the data and calculations.

This alternative analysis is supported by evidence from trusts' financial returns for 2005/6 presented by the Department of Health to the House of Commons Health Committee (2006d): this showed that around 47 per cent of the (total) cash increase for the NHS in 2005/6 was absorbed by pay inflation and only 9 per cent by increases in the volume of staff.

New hospitals and premises

The NHS Plan promised a significant expansion in NHS infrastructure up to 2010, including:

By 2004
- 500 new one-stop primary care centres
- modernisation of more than 3,000 GP premises
- clearance of at least a quarter of the maintenance backlog

By 2010
- more than 100 new hospitals, replacing old and out-of-date buildings.

The 2002 review's vision for a modern NHS estate in 2022/3 incorporated the physical infrastructure commitments contained in the plan, but outlined more ambitious aspirations for the replacement and upgrading of health service facilities. These included:
- replacement of one-third of hospital and community health service (HCHS) estates by 2022/3, starting with those with most maintenance backlog
- 75 per cent of beds in new hospitals in single en-suite rooms, with a maximum of four beds in other rooms
- upgrading or replacement of the entire primary care estate by 2010/1.

HOSPITALS

The NHS Plan promised more than 100 new hospital schemes in total between 2000 and 2010. In fact, though, the government had launched its hospital building programme in July 1997, and many new hospitals were due to become operational soon after the Plan's publication; indeed the Plan stated, 'We have given the go ahead to 38 major developments. Over half of these will be open to the public by 2003/4 (Department of Health 2000c, p 44).

Clearly there has been significant progress towards the Plan's target. In February 2007, the Department published a series of maps showing the location of new hospitals and primary care facilities. Since 1997, 84 new hospitals have become operational, with a further 25 under construction.

Analysis by the Construction Products Association (CPA) (2006) reported that the government's new hospital programme included 142 major and medium-sized schemes extending beyond 2010. By late 2006, 65 new hospitals had become operational since 2000. The CPA analysis indicates that many of the larger hospital schemes initially included in the new-build programme have been cancelled or subject to pre-construction delays, with the result that hospitals delivered to date have included more medium-sized projects than anticipated.

Information on the layout of new hospital wards is difficult to establish. The government's intention to shift from large public wards to more private and personal accommodation was demonstrated in 2006, when the Department of Health gave the go-ahead to six new NHS hospital private finance initiative (PFI) developments, with up to half of the beds earmarked for single rooms (Department of Health 2006g). However, this falls short of the 2002 review's recommendation that 75 per cent of beds in new hospitals should be in single en-suite rooms (Wanless 2002).

In addition to the new hospital building programme, since July 2006 the government has been inviting primary care trusts to bid for up to £750 million of capital funding over the next five years to develop a new generation of modern NHS community hospitals. Funding was to be made available from early 2007 for trusts to build new community clinics and hospitals, convert old acute hospitals into community hospitals and renovate existing community hospitals to include chemotherapy and mobile cancer scan facilities. In December 2006, the Department announced that £44.5 million had already been made available for four new community hospitals.

The government seems on track to deliver on its promise of building at least 100 new hospitals by 2010. However, the evidence suggests it will fall short of the review's targets for single rooms and maximum room occupancy. Indeed, the government is still struggling to fulfill its commitment to single-sex *wards*. Clearly, an important reason for lack of progress on these fronts is cost.

GP PREMISES AND ONE-STOP SHOPS

Estimates from the Construction Products Association (2005) suggest that the NHS Plan commitment to build 500 one-stop primary care centres and modernise 3,000 GP premises has been met, albeit after the 2004 deadline. In December 2004, the CPA reported that 510 one-stop centres had been completed or were under construction, and that 2,848 GP premises had been (or were in the process of being) modernised. The Department of Health has announced that over 625 new one-stop primary care centres have been created since 2001, with plans for a further 125 by the end of 2008. Since 2001, around 3,000 (or almost one-third) of GP surgeries have been substantially refurbished or replaced.

The 2002 review assumed that the entire primary care estate (consisting of around 10,500 premises) would be upgraded or replaced by 2010/1. The government has now met its pledge to substantially refurbish or replace up to 3,000 GP premises by 2004, and it did so at an estimated rate of around 63 premises per month (based on the CPA analysis). At this rate it would take the government almost another 10 years to refurbish or upgrade the remaining 7,500 or so GP premises. The fact that the government has no additional targets for the continual upgrading of the primary care estate suggests that the review's expectations will not be met by 2010/1.

EXISTING NHS ESTATE

The NHS Plan recognised that historic under-investment in NHS facilities had led to a growing backlog of repairs and set a target to reduce the NHS maintenance backlog by 25 per cent, from an estimated £3.1 billion in 1999 to £2.3 billion by 2004. In fact, though, the overall maintenance backlog has *grown*, and in 2005/6 stood at £3.7 billion – an increase of nearly a fifth since 1999/2000 (CPA 2006).

It would seem very unlikely, therefore, that one-third of the entire hospital and community health services estate will be replaced by 2022/3, as envisaged by the 2002 review.

HOSPITAL BEDS

The number of NHS hospital beds in England has been declining for many years, as part of a global phenomenon. The decline in beds in the United Kingdom (as in most other countries) was partly a reaction to changing technologies that reduced the need for long hospital stays (such as the rapid expansion of day case surgery) and partly driven by policy initiatives, such as the commitment to more community-based mental health and

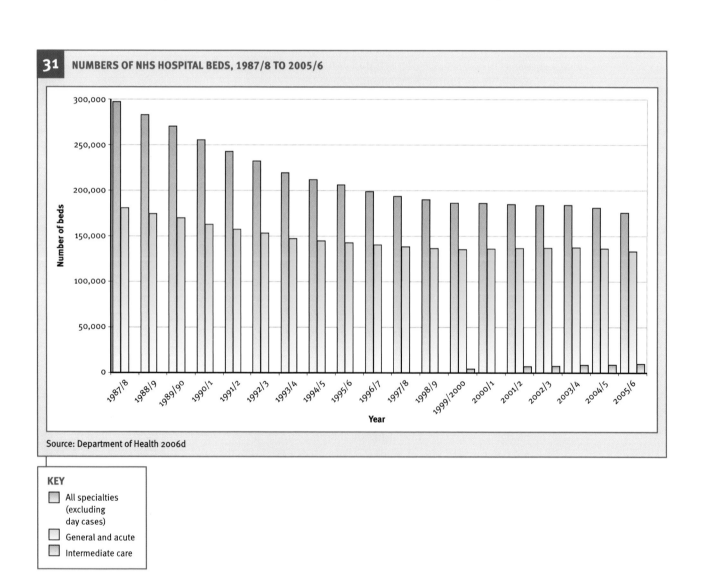

31 NUMBERS OF NHS HOSPITAL BEDS, 1987/8 TO 2005/6

Source: Department of Health 2006d

KEY
■ All specialties (excluding day cases)
□ General and acute
▨ Intermediate care

TABLE 23: NUMBER OF NHS HOSPITAL BEDS BY SPECIALTY, 1999/2000 TO 2005/6

Year	All specialties[1]	Specialty				
		General and acute[2]		Mental illness	Learning disability	Maternity
		Acute	Geriatric			
1999/2000	186,290	107,218	27,862	34,173	6,834	10,203
2000/1	186,091	107,956	27,838	34,214	6,316	9,767
2001/2	184,871	108,535	28,047	32,783	5,694	9,812
2002/3	183,826	108,706	27,973	32,753	5,038	9,356
2003/4	184,019	109,793	27,454	32,252	5,212	9,309
2004/5	180,966	109,544	26,641	31,286	4,415	9,081
2005/6	175,646	108,113	24,920	29,802	3,927	8,883

Source: Department of Health 2006d
[1] Excluding day case only
[2] General and acute = acute + geriatric

learning disability services. However, concern that the decline in hospital beds might have gone too far led to the establishment of the National Beds Inquiry in 1998. The Inquiry concluded that the health service did not have the right number of the right sort of hospital beds in the right places and that *more,* rather than fewer, beds were needed to meet the needs of NHS patients in the 21st century (Department of Health 2000b). The NHS Plan subsequently promised to deliver extra beds.

The commitment was to increase bed numbers by 7,000 by 2004, with 2,100 extra general and acute beds and 5,000 intermediate care beds. Did the government fulfil this commitment – and what happened to bed numbers overall? The long-term trend, as shown by Figure 31, opposite, and Table 23, above, has been for a long-term steady decline in total bed numbers since 1987/8. This decline slowed from 1998/9, however, and between 2002/3 and 2004/5 numbers fell by around 2,900. In 2005/6 bed numbers fell more steeply, by 5,300 in one year.

As Table 24 and Figure 32, overleaf, show, by 2005/6 (a year later than planned), the number of intermediate care beds had increased by more than 5,500.

By 2003/4 (a year earlier than planned) the government had increased the number of general and acute beds in England by nearly 2,200 – around 100 more than planned. However, since achieving the commitment outlined in the NHS Plan, the number of general and acute beds has fallen by over 4,200 (*see* Figure 33, p 121), including a fall of more than 3,000 in 2005/6. There are now fewer general and acute beds in the NHS than when the Plan was published.

The classification 'general and acute beds' comprises acute and geriatric beds (*see* Table 23, above). Further analysis of the rise and fall in the number of general and acute beds since the NHS Plan was published shows that the number of geriatric beds (which made up 21 per cent of general and acute beds in 1999/2000) has been declining since then. By

TABLE 24: NUMBER OF NHS INTERMEDIATE CARE BEDS, 1999/2000 TO 2005/6

Year	Intermediate care beds
1999/2000	4,242
2000/1	na
2001/2	7,021
2002/3	7,493
2003/4	8,697
2004/5	8,928
2005/6	9,771

Source: Department of Health 2006d
Note: The figure for intermediate care beds is a second quarter figure.

2003/4, when the government achieved its target of having an extra 2,100 general and acute beds in the NHS, the rise was entirely accounted for by additional acute beds, which masked a reduction of around 400 geriatric beds. The overall reduction of around 2,050 general and acute beds between 1999/2000 and 2005/6 is made up entirely of reductions in geriatric beds, with a modest rise in numbers of acute care beds (*see* Figure 34, opposite).

The 2002 review also assumed, in the solid progress and fully engaged scenarios, that over 20 years there would be a 5 per cent reduction in births requiring special or intensive care due to reductions in teenage pregnancies and reduced levels of smoking during pregnancy.

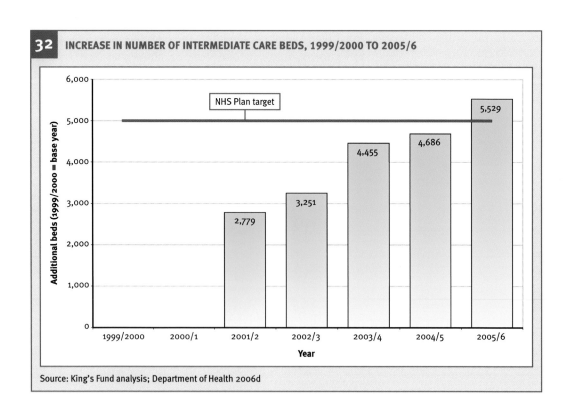

32 INCREASE IN NUMBER OF INTERMEDIATE CARE BEDS, 1999/2000 TO 2005/6

Source: King's Fund analysis; Department of Health 2006d

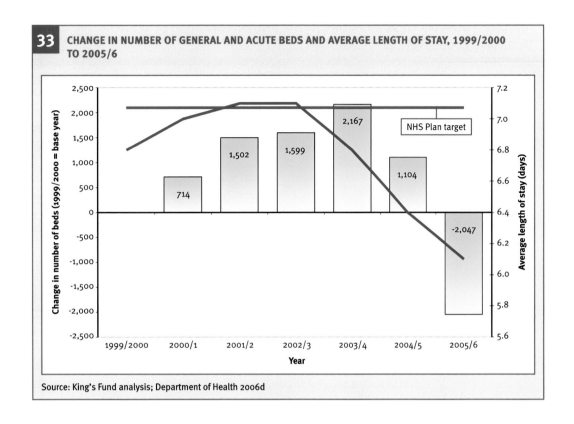

33 CHANGE IN NUMBER OF GENERAL AND ACUTE BEDS AND AVERAGE LENGTH OF STAY, 1999/2000 TO 2005/6

NHS Plan target

Source: King's Fund analysis; Department of Health 2006d

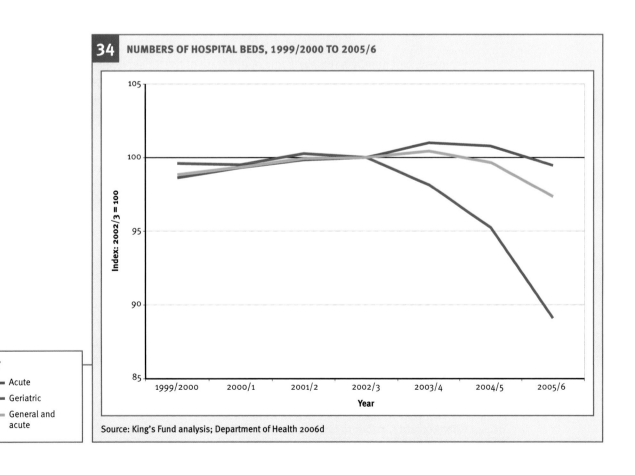

34 NUMBERS OF HOSPITAL BEDS, 1999/2000 TO 2005/6

KEY
— Acute
— Geriatric
— General and acute

Source: King's Fund analysis; Department of Health 2006d

TABLE 25: NUMBER OF ADMISSIONS IN THE UNITED KINGDOM, BY COUNTRY, IN MATCHED UNITS, FROM 2005 AND 2006 SURVEYS

Country	2005		2006		% change 2005–6	
	Total admissions	Number of cots	Total admissions	Number of cots	Total admissions	Number of cots
England	35,258	1,865	35,538	1,887	0.8	1.2
Scotland	3,830	208	4,151	213	8.4	2.4
Wales	1,423	90	1,416	83	-0.5	-7.8
Northern Ireland	1,191	77	1,205	69	1.2	-10.4

Source: Redshaw and Hamilton 2006

Information on the number of babies requiring special or intensive care is not routinely collected, although surveys by the National Perinatal Epidemiology Unit (Redshaw and Hamilton 2006) provide some evidence about trends in admissions. This work showed that admissions to neonatal units in the UK have continued to rise, with admissions to the units studied totalling 74,510 infants in 2005. Based on matched units, there was a 1.5 per cent increase in admissions to UK neonatal units between 2005 and 2006; over the same period, the number of cots in matched units has risen by 0.5 per cent (*see* Table 25, above).

It is far too early to judge whether or not the 2002 review's assumption of a 5 per cent reduction in the births requiring special or intensive care will come to fruition.

For many, bed numbers remain iconic of the state of health services, with more being unambiguously better than fewer. But the way this particular resource is *used* is more significant than its availability. Although the implication of increasing bed numbers is that more patients can be treated, it also tends to lengthen average hospital stays. As Figure 33, p 121, shows, there does seem to be a link between bed numbers and lengths of stay.

Internationally, the United Kingdom still has fewer beds per 1,000 population than some of the larger EU 15 countries, such as Germany or France. However, since 1999 the reduction in the number of hospital beds per 1,000 population in the United Kingdom has been less steep than in Germany and France. Table 26, opposite, shows the international trend for reducing hospital bed numbers as a result of changes in technology and pressure to increase productivity.

Delayed discharges
The 2002 review noted that around 4,200 patients in English hospitals – equivalent to 10 full hospitals – experienced delays in discharge. Around a quarter of these patients were waiting for access to a care or nursing home place, while a further 30 per cent were waiting for an assessment of their discharge needs or eligibility for public funding.

The 2002 review suggested a solution to this problem, pioneered in Sweden, of introducing a charge or fine to encourage local authorities to speed up discharge arrangements, either to nursing homes or (with support if necessary) to patients' own

TABLE 26: NUMBER OF HOSPITAL BEDS IN ALL SECTORS[1] PER 1,000 POPULATION IN SELECTED OECD COUNTRIES, 1999 TO 2004

Country	Beds per 1,000 population						% change 1999–2004
	1999	2000	2001	2002	2003	2004	
Italy	4.9	4.7	4.6	4.4	4.2	na	-14.3[2]
Austria	8.8	8.6	8.5	8.4	8.3	7.7	-12.5
Ireland	4.7	4.7	4.5	4.4	4.3	4.2	-10.6
France	8.3	8.1	7.9	7.8	7.7	7.5	-9.6
Luxembourg	7.4	6.9	6.9	6.8	6.8	6.7	-9.5
Spain	3.7	3.7	3.6	3.5	3.4	na	-8.0[2]
Denmark	4.3	4.3	4.2	4.1	4.0	na	-7.0[2]
Germany	9.2	9.1	9.0	8.9	8.7	8.6	-6.5
Netherlands	5.1	5.2	5.0	4.9	4.8	na	-5.9[2]
Belgium	7.2	7.1	7.0	6.9	6.8	6.8	-5.6
United Kingdom	4.3	4.3	4.2	4.2	4.1	4.1	-4.7
Portugal	3.8	3.8	3.7	3.6	3.6	3.7	-2.6
Greece	4.7	4.7	4.8	4.7	na	na	0.0[3]
Sweden	na	na	na	na	na	na	na
Finland	na	na	na	na	na	na	na

Source: Organisation for Economic Co-operation and Development 2007
[1] Public, not-for-profit and private hospitals
[2] Change from 1999 to 2003
[3] Change from 1999 to 2002

homes. Such a system was introduced in 2004, together with an annual transfer of £100 million from the NHS budget to local authorities to encourage joint working between the sectors. As figure 35, overleaf, shows, delays in transfers of care have declined by nearly a third since 2004. But, as the longer-term trend also shows, this decline has been relatively shallow by comparison with reductions in delays between 2001 and 2003.

It is unreasonable to expect no delays in discharging some patients; and while fining has had a positive impact (not least in focusing management and professional efforts on tackling the problem), it may be that further effort needs to be directed at delays arising from health rather than social care management.

Information and communication technology

The 2002 review identified better use of information and communications technologies (ICT) as key to potential productivity and health gains. It also called for stringent standards, set by the centre, to ensure that systems would be fully compatible across the NHS, ICT budgets ring-fenced and achievements audited.

The development of ICTs in the NHS has had a long – and not always successful – history. The first serious national policy initiative was set out in the NHS Information Management and Technology (IM&T) strategy, published in 1992 (Department of Health 1992a). A

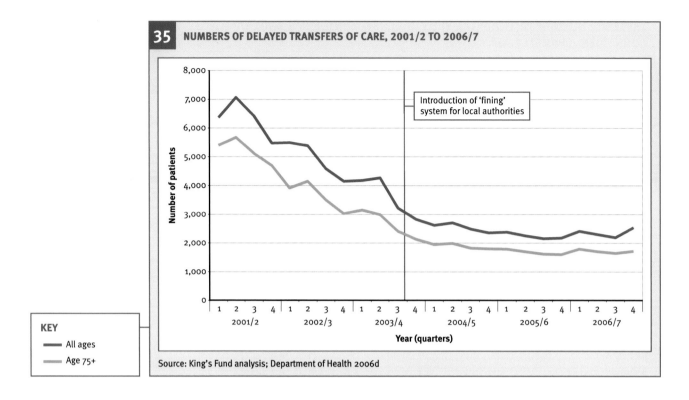

35 NUMBERS OF DELAYED TRANSFERS OF CARE, 2001/2 TO 2006/7

Introduction of 'fining' system for local authorities

KEY
— All ages
— Age 75+

Source: King's Fund analysis; Department of Health 2006d

decade on, the National Programme for IT in the NHS (NPfIT) was responsible for implementing an integrated ICT infrastructure for all NHS organisations in England, to be completed by 2014. NPfIT originally had four key deliverables:

■ an integrated care records service
■ electronic prescribing;
■ electronic appointment booking
■ an underpinning IT infrastructure with sufficient connectivity and broadband capacity to support the critical national applications and local systems.

Connecting for Health, the agency responsible for NPfIT, has since assumed responsibility for other services including Picture Archiving and Communications Systems (PACS), the Quality Management and Analysis System (QMAS) and NHSmail.

The box opposite summarises progress to date on the four key deliverables of NPfIT.

The 2002 review maintained that there was a strong case for a rapid pace of investment, but only if steps were taken to ensure that this would deliver cost-effective solutions (Wanless 2002). The review's ICT resource projections incorporated a substantial increase in investment. In the fully engaged and solid progress scenarios, spending was projected to double to £2.2 billion by 2003/4, peaking at around £2.7 billion in 2007/8. The slow uptake scenario saw the same level of cumulative ICT spending, phased in more slowly.

Actual ICT spending in England is estimated to have increased from £1 billion in 2002/3 to £2.3 billion in 2005/6 (NHS Connecting for Health 2007b). In 2006/7, the planned increase in ICT spending is set to rise by 25 per cent to just under £2.9 billion (*see* Table 27, below), a level that exceeds the 2002 review's peak in spending of £2.7 billion in 2007/8 under the fully engaged and solid progress scenarios.

NPFIT PROGRESS TO APRIL 2007

Integrated care records service

The NHS Care Records Service (NCRS) aims to provide an electronic health care record for every patient in England. The NHS Plan noted that this could become a reality by 2004, when 75 per cent of hospitals and 50 per cent of primary and community trusts would have implemented electronic patient record systems. However, controversy has seriously undermined this aspect of the NPfIT, partly due to the absence of any published plans for the design and implementation of NCRS. It is also unclear what information will be held on individual electronic health care records. Doctors and patient groups remain anxious about who will have access to electronic patient records and the associated risk to patient confidentiality. The government has now agreed to allow patients to 'opt out' of having their records held by NCRS, although the details of the opt-out procedures have not been settled. Consequently, real progress is only just beginning. In the spring of 2007, a number of early adopters began creating 'summary care records' as a prelude to the national roll-out. These records are expected to include significant elements of a patient's care, including major diagnoses, procedures, current and regular prescriptions, allergies, adverse reactions, drug interactions and recent investigation results. However, this will be a challenge. National roll-out is expected to begin early in 2008, but it will be several years before coverage is complete. A date has not yet been specified for the system to be fully operational.

Electronic prescribing

The Electronic Prescription Service (EPS) allows prescriptions to be sent electronically from prescribers to pharmacies. Implementation began in early 2005 (NHS Connecting for Health 2005a), slightly after the 2004 start time envisaged by the NHS Plan. As of April 2007, nearly 16.5 million prescription messages have been issued electronically, with the service being used for around 8 per cent of daily prescription messages. The system is being actively used by 1,700 GP practices in England (around 20 per cent), although only for a minority of their prescribing (NHS Connecting for Health 2007a). Every GP surgery, along with community pharmacies and other dispensers, was expected to have access to the service by 2007, although this target will almost certainly be missed due to slower-than-expected uptake. In time, prescribers operating from other locations, such as walk-in centres and dental practices, will be included in the scheme, and there are also plans to include hospitals issuing prescriptions for dispensing in the community.

Electronic appointment booking ('choose and book')

The 'choose and book' system allows patients at the point of referral to book online appointments from a GP surgery, at a date and time of their choosing. From January 2006, the system also enabled them to choose a provider from a limited list of around four organisations, which will expand over time. The NHS Plan promised to achieve electronic booking of appointments by 2005. Choose and book began (albeit on a limited scale) within this time frame, with the first booking made in July 2004 (NHS Connecting for Health 2005b). Subsequent take-up appears to have been slow. The system currently relies on relatively outdated technology, which has led to dissatisfaction among GPs (Medix 2006). The Department of Health has not achieved its target for 90 per cent of all patient referrals to use choose and book by March 2007.

According to NHS Connecting for Health, as of April 2007 more than 3 million bookings have been made using the system, accounting for around a third of NHS referral activity, from GP surgery to first outpatient appointment (NHS Connecting for Health 2007a). This includes some appointments made by telephone, using choose and book. Around a quarter of GP referrals through the choose and book system are made in the surgery at the point of referral.

New National Network (N3) project
The NHS Plan aimed to have all GP practices connected to NHSnet by March 2002, achieving 95 per cent connection prior to the deadline. Since then, NHSnet has been superseded by a new national network for the NHS known as N3. This aims to link all NHS organisations, providing secure networking services and the broadband capacity to meet all the current and future IT needs of the NHS. Connections to the N3 network started in April 2004, with full implementation expected to take three years. Progress as of April 2007 appears on schedule, with 18,989 connections to N3 and 98 per cent of GP practices connected to the network (NHS Connecting for Health 2007a).

Given the well-documented delays that have beset the NPfIT, and the absence of published plans for the design and implementation of the NHS Care Records Service, it is perhaps not surprising that actual ICT spending has not followed the 2002 review's solid progress or fully engaged spending trajectories. The National Audit Office (2006) concluded that the NPfIT had made substantial progress but continued to face significant challenges, with key parts of the programme falling behind schedule. More recently the House of Commons Public Accounts Committee (2007a) stated that 'The Department is unlikely to complete the Programme anywhere near its original schedule... At the present rate of progress it is unlikely that significant clinical benefits will be delivered by the end of the contract period'.

TABLE 27: SPENDING ON ICT IN THE NHS, 2002/3 TO 2006/7

	Spending (£ million)				
	2002/3	2003/4	2004/5	2005/6	2006/7*
Local revenue	832.0	914.2	1,046.3	1,159.8	1,240.3
Central revenue	186.3	280.8	475.5	523.0	580.0
Total revenue	**1,018.3**	**1,195.0**	**1,521.7**	**1,685.8**	**1,820.3**
Local capital	–	234.3	205.6	238.5	336.4
Central capital	–	23.6	364.4	386.8	725.7
Total capital	**–**	**257.9**	**570.0**	**625.4**	**1,062.1**
Total capital plus revenue	**1,018.3**	**1,452.9**	**2,091.7**	**2,311.1**	**2,882.4**

Source: NHS Connecting for Health 2007b
* Planned spending

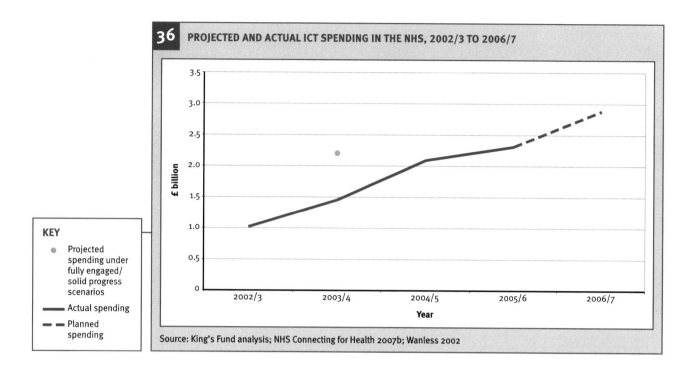

36 PROJECTED AND ACTUAL ICT SPENDING IN THE NHS, 2002/3 TO 2006/7

KEY

● Projected spending under fully engaged/ solid progress scenarios

—— Actual spending

– – Planned spending

Source: King's Fund analysis; NHS Connecting for Health 2007b; Wanless 2002

In 2003/4 actual spending on ICT in the NHS was around £0.7 billion lower than the £2.2 billion envisaged in the solid progress and fully engaged scenarios (*see* Figure 36, above). The 2002 review noted that its ICT investment path would raise spending to more than 3 per cent of total NHS spending. However, since then the government has stated its intention is to increase ICT expenditure to 4 per cent of total NHS spending (Hansard 2004). Should the planned expenditure on ICT in 2006/7 be realised, spend as a percentage of total NHS spending will have increased from 1.7 per cent in 2002/3 to 3.4 per cent in 2006/7.

The relative contribution to total ICT spending from central government (as opposed to the local NHS) has been increasing since 2002/3 (*see* Figure 37, overleaf). In that year, only 18 per cent of total NHS ICT spend came from central government, but by 2006/7 the contribution by central government is expected to have risen to 45 per cent. Much of this change is being driven by large increases in capital spending, predominantly funded by central government (*see* Figure 38, p 129).

Spending on the NPfIT is projected to be £12.4 billion (at 2005/6 prices) over the 10 years to 2013/4 (NAO 2006). Up to the end of March 2006, actual expenditure on the contracts let in 2003 and 2004 was lower than planned: £654 million (estimated outturn) compared with expected expenditure of £1,448 million, reflecting the slow delivery of some systems. Our analysis suggests that the ICT resources set out in the 2002 review should be sufficient to cover the National Audit Office (NAO)'s estimated cost of £12.4 billion for the 10-year programme.

The extent to which the NHS will benefit from these substantial investments remains unclear. A detailed review of NPfIT is beyond the scope of this report, but three factors seem likely to have an impact on the 2002 review's productivity assumptions.

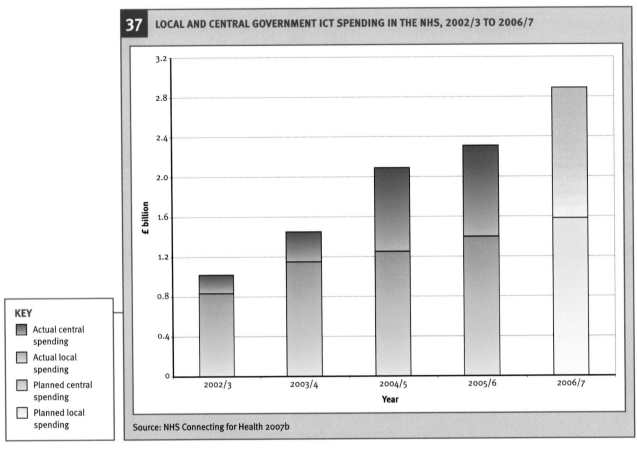

37 LOCAL AND CENTRAL GOVERNMENT ICT SPENDING IN THE NHS, 2002/3 TO 2006/7

KEY

■ Actual central spending

■ Actual local spending

■ Planned central spending

□ Planned local spending

Source: NHS Connecting for Health 2007b

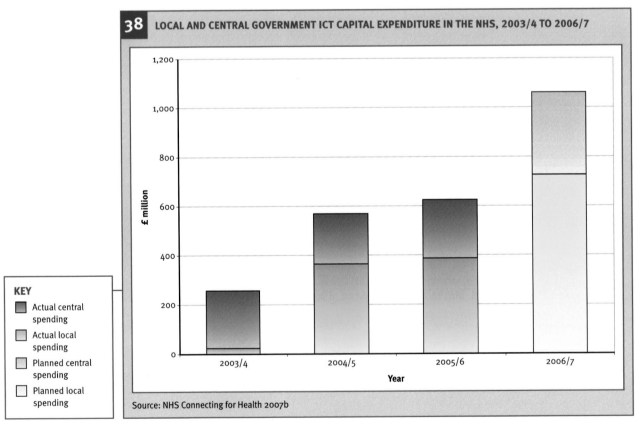

38 LOCAL AND CENTRAL GOVERNMENT ICT CAPITAL EXPENDITURE IN THE NHS, 2003/4 TO 2006/7

KEY

■ Actual central spending

■ Actual local spending

■ Planned central spending

□ Planned local spending

Source: NHS Connecting for Health 2007b

The first is the failure to develop an ICT strategy whose benefits are likely to outweigh costs. The NAO (2006) noted that '...it was not demonstrated that the financial value of the benefits exceeds the cost of the Programme'. This is a serious criticism, implying either the absence of an original business case for investment or investment made in spite of a business case that did not justify the spending. In similar vein, a report by the British Computer Society (2006) concluded that '... the central costs incurred by NHS [Connecting for Health] are such that, so far, the value for money from services deployed is poor'. Surprisingly, systematic reviews of ICTs show that evidence for key technologies, such as NCRS and PACS, is lacking (Delpierre C et al 2004; Poissant L et al 2005). It is difficult to understand why Connecting for Health is being allowed to pursue a high-cost, high-risk strategy that cannot be supported by a business case.

Second, while the 2002 review assumed that investments would be audited and evaluated, apart from the NAO report the necessary work is not being undertaken and it does not seem possible to obtain reliable data on NHS resources being committed to NPfIT. Connecting for Health has so far made negligible investments of less than £0.5 million in evaluation (a fraction of the projected £12.4 billion costs). There seems a real risk that the costs and benefits of NPfIT will never be accurately assessed.

The third factor, which may turn out to be the most important, is that the NPfIT contracts risk creating monopolies in various areas of the programme. The House of Commons Public Accounts Committee (2007a) has noted that 'The use of only two major software suppliers may have the effect of inhibiting innovation, progress and competition'. Connecting for Health chose to award a small number of large contracts to consortia charged with designing and implementing the technologies. But they could instead have set out to create a competitive market for IT goods and services. Is it possible that a robust business case could be created, even now, with a focus on strategies for encouraging a healthy market?

It is clear that there are considerable challenges ahead in modernising NHS IT systems, and continuing debate over the feasibility of some current NPfIT plans. The continuing uncertainty and delays have the potential to undermine the productivity gains envisaged by the 2002 review.

New scanners

The NHS Plan committed the service to investing in 250 new scanners by 2004. This total comprised 50 new magnetic resonance imaging (MRI) scanners, to increase the number of diagnostic procedures by 190,000, and 200 new computerised tomography (CT) scanners (150 replacements and 50 extras), to increase procedures by 240,000.

By April 2006, new and replacement equipment delivered through central programmes included 146 new MRI scanners, 135 linear accelerators, 224 CT scanners and more than 730 items of breast-screening equipment. Of equipment now in use in the NHS, about 71 per cent of MRI scanners, 77 per cent of CT scanners and 75 per cent of linear accelerators were purchased since January 2000.

There is no published data recording when this new and replacement equipment came into use, but progress against the NHS Plan is reflected in the numbers of procedures

SUMMARY: RESOURCES

- The NHS Plan of 2000 set out a 'shopping list' of staff and other resources. In most cases these have either been met or are on target to be met.
- Increases in numbers of NHS staff were targeted for 2004. By 2005 the government had more than achieved these goals for all relevant staffing groups in terms of both numbers and full-time equivalents. Consultant numbers were 16% above target, GPs 166 per cent above, nurses 272 per cent above and AHPs 102 per cent above.
- However, the 2002 review projections up to 2022/3 suggest that even more staff will be required in the relatively near future (Wanless 2002).
- Non-clinical staff numbers have increased substantially, but at a lower rate than for medical staff, and the ratio of non-medical to medical staff is at its lowest for more than 10 years.
- Although the government seems on track to deliver the NHS Plan targets of building 100 new hospitals and modernising over 3,000 GP premises, it seems highly unlikely that the 2002 review's more ambitious aspirations to replace one-third of the hospital and community health estate by 2022/3 and upgrade the entire primary care estate by 2010/1 will be met.
- Backlog maintenance has increased by a fifth between 2000 and 2005 rather than declined by a quarter, as envisaged by the Plan.
- As a result of investment in scanning equipment since the Plan, around three-quarters of MRI scanners, CT scanners and linear accelerators now in use in the NHS are new. Moreover, NHS Plan targets for increased numbers of procedures have been substantially exceeded.
- The National Programme for IT in the NHS (NPfIT) is responsible for implementing an integrated care records service, an electronic prescribing system, an electronic appointment booking system and the underpinning IT infrastructure by 2014. The 2002 review identified better use of ICTs as key to potential productivity and health gains and recommended a doubling of ICT spend by 2003/4, peaking at around £2.7 billion in 2007/8, in the solid progress and fully engaged scenarios (Wanless 2002).
- Actual ICT spending in England is estimated to have increased from £1 billion in 2002/3 to £2.3 billion in 2005/6. Actual spending on ICT in the NHS in 2003/4 was around £0.7 billion lower than envisaged in the solid progress and fully engaged scenarios. Our analysis suggests that the ICT resources set out in the 2002 review would be sufficient to cover the £12.4 billion estimated cost of the 10-year programme.
- The extent to which the NHS will benefit from these substantial investments remains unclear. Three factors likely to have an impact on the 2002 review's productivity assumptions are: failure to develop an ICT strategy whose benefits are likely to outweigh costs; failure to audit and evaluate investments; and the risk of monopolies in parts of the programme. These factors, together with delays to the programme, have the potential to seriously undermine the productivity gains envisaged by the 2002 review.

undertaken. Between 1999/2000 and 2004/5, the number of MRI examinations performed in England rose by 359,000, compared with the 190,000 projected in the NHS Plan, while CT examinations increased by 782,000, compared with 240,000 envisaged by the Plan.

The latest data, for 2005/6 indicates that since 1999/2000 the number of MRI and CT examinations performed in England has risen by 91 and 82 per cent, respectively. It is clear from this that the planned investment in new NHS scanning facilities has been achieved.

8 Outputs: the services delivered

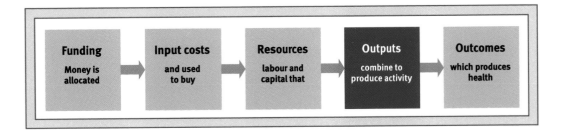

The last chapter looked at investment in human and other resources in line with pledges made in the NHS Plan.

This chapter considers how those resources have been translated into activity, in terms of hospital services, mental health care, primary care, prescribing and other activities, including NHS Direct, walk-in centres and ambulance services.

The NHS produces a considerable range of outputs, whose variety means they cannot easily be added together. In addition, over time the measured units of activity (such as an operation or an outpatient attendance) change in terms of what they deliver in health terms. All of this makes it difficult to calculate trends in total output for the NHS. This is the essential problem in measuring productivity, which has been the object of much conceptual thinking in recent years.

Recent output measure developments by the Department of Health list around 1,700 specific categories of NHS activity, covering primary, secondary, community and other NHS services (see Table 28, overleaf). Using data from the hospital episode statistics (HES), the National Reference Costs (NRC) database and other sources, as appropriate, the table estimates the overall cost of each activity type. (Note that the spend figures in column 4 are estimates drawn from a variety of sources and will not add up to the actual total spend on the NHS in 2005/6. The table is designed to illustrate the relative shares of the total budget spend on different services/activities.)

Hospital services: elective, emergency, outpatient and maternity

Hospital activity includes a large range of services and patient classifications. Figure 38, below, describes the various ways patients treated in NHS hospitals are categorised, based partly on the source of admission and partly on care received. As Table 28, overleaf, indicates, elective, non-elective, outpatient and accident and emergency services account cumulatively for around a third of all NHS spending.

133

TABLE 28: NUMBER OF NHS ACTIVITY CATEGORIES AND ESTIMATED SHARES OF TOTAL NHS SPENDING, 2005/6

Activity	Number of activity categories[1]	Approximate share of total NHS spending	
		(£ billion)[2]	(%)
Elective patients	>500	6.26	9.3
Non-elective patients	>500	8.74	13.0
Outpatients	~300	5.79	8.6
Accident and emergency	9	1.27	1.9
Mental health services	30	5.15	7.6
Primary care prescribing	~200	7.82	11.6
Primary (GMS) care	5	7.70	11.4
NHS Direct calls answered	1	0.10	0.1
NHS Direct online 'hits'	1		
Walk-in centre visits	1	0.005	0.01
Ambulance journeys	1	0.96	1.4
General ophthalmic services	1	0.40	0.6
General dental services	1	1.91	2.8
Others (critical care, audiology services, pathology, radiology, chemotherapy, renal dialysis, community services, bone marrow transplants and rehabilitation)	>100	3.38	5.0
Central budgets[3]		18.00	26.6
Total		**67.49**	**100.0**

Source: Adapted from Department of Health 2004e
[1] Categories for elective, non-elective, outpatients and accident and emergency are measured in health care resource groups. Other categories are a mix of visits, calls and so on.
[2] King's Fund estimates based on National Reference costs (2005/6) (Department of Health 2006e).
[3] This refers to centrally funded organisations (such as the Department of Health itself) and services. There are no routine activity measures to cover this disparate set of budgets.

ELECTIVE ADMISSIONS

The NHS in England carries out around 6 million elective interventions in hospitals each year. The next few pages set out changes in the total volume of elective activity between 1988 and 2005, broken down in various ways. Table 29, opposite, shows the total number of elective admissions by treatment type (inpatient and day case), while Figure 40, *see* p 136, demonstrates cumulative trends in inpatient and day case admissions.

Hospital activity is classified in a number of ways, partly depending on the broad nature of the care provided (for example, did the patient stay in hospital overnight?) and partly based on the source of admission (for example, were they admitted from a waiting list?). The diagram below describes the different categorisations used by the NHS.

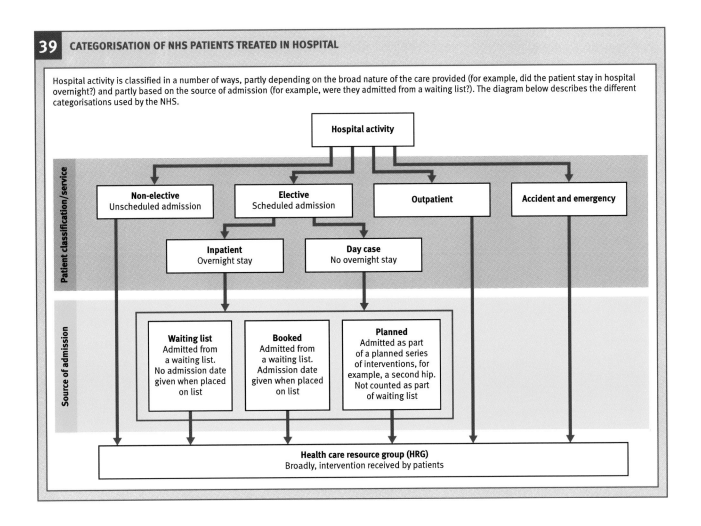

Overall, between 1998 and 2005 elective admissions rose by just over 605,000 (an increase of 11 per cent). While this is equivalent to an average annual increase of around 1.5 per cent, in fact admissions fell in 2000 and 2001, and the bulk of the increase over the whole period took place in just two years – 2002 and 2005. After 2002, elective admissions rose by just under 7 per cent.

TABLE 29: TRENDS IN ELECTIVE ADMISSIONS FOR INPATIENTS AND DAY CASES, 1998 TO 2005

Case type	1998/9	1999/2000	2000/1	2001/2	2002/3	2003/4	2004/5	2005/6	1998–2005 (% change)
Inpatient	2,070,237	1,994,650	1,955,277	1,907,591	1,974,267	1,986,993	1,941,497	1,979,341	
% total	37.7	35.8	35.1	34.8	34.7	34.6	33.5	32.5	-4.4
Day case	3,414,648	3,576,402	3,612,104	3,575,144	3,707,303	3,752,688	3,844,851	4,110,850	20.4
% total	62.3	64.2	64.9	65.2	65.3	65.4	66.5	67.5	
Total	5,484,885	5,571,052	5,567,381	5,482,735	5,681,570	5,739,681	5,786,348	6,090,191	11.0

Source: King's Fund analysis; Hospital Episode Statistics 2007

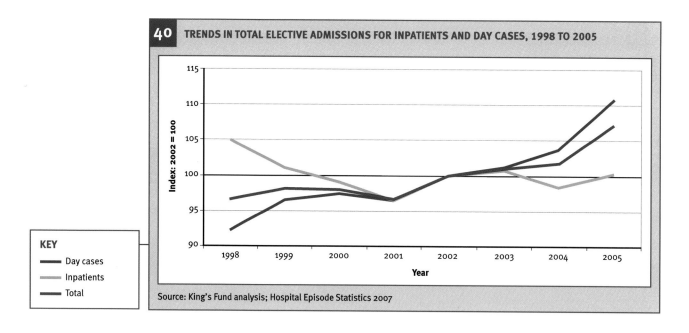

40 TRENDS IN TOTAL ELECTIVE ADMISSIONS FOR INPATIENTS AND DAY CASES, 1998 TO 2005

Source: King's Fund analysis; Hospital Episode Statistics 2007

Within the overall trend, there has been a noticeable change in case type, with inpatient numbers declining by around 90,000 (-4.4 per cent) between 1998 and 2005 and day case numbers increasing by nearly 700,000 (+20.4 per cent). However, this has translated into only a small percentage increase in the day case rate – from 62.3 per cent to 67.5 per cent.

While there has been an overall increase in total elective admissions, the picture at the level of Health Resource Groups (HRGs) is more mixed. As Table 30, opposite, illustrates, nearly a fifth of the *net* increase in total admissions was accounted for by just one HRG

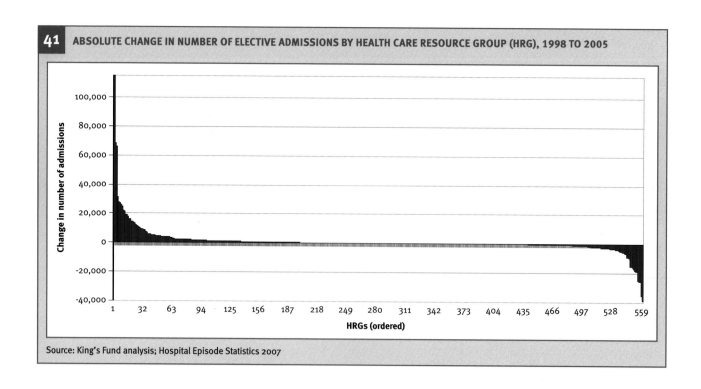

41 ABSOLUTE CHANGE IN NUMBER OF ELECTIVE ADMISSIONS BY HEALTH CARE RESOURCE GROUP (HRG), 1998 TO 2005

Source: King's Fund analysis; Hospital Episode Statistics 2007

TABLE 30: TOP 10 INCREASES AND DECREASES IN TOTAL ELECTIVE ADMISSIONS BY HEALTH CARE RESOURCE GROUP (HRG), 1998 TO 2005

HRG code	Name	Change 1998–2005	% change 1998–2005	Change as % total change
Top 10 increases				
B02	Phakoemulsification cataract extraction with lens implant	114,917	73.5	19.0
F35	Large intestine: endoscopy/internal procedures	68,770	34.7	11.4
S01	Haematology disorder with minor procedure	65,928	66.3	10.9
S22	Planned procedures not carried out	36,686	29.4	6.1
E14	Cardiac catheterisation w/o complications	31,409	44.5	5.2
L48	Renal replacement therapy w/o complications	27,649	172.1	4.6
H04	Primary knee replacement	27,190	97.7	4.5
D98	Chemotherapy with a respiratory system diagnosis	25,819	132.5	4.3
H10	Arthroscopies	24,963	27.8	4.1
L20	Bladder: minor endoscopy procedure with complications	24,304	96.2	4.0
Top 10 decreases				
Q11	Varicose vein procedures	-18,056	-34.7	-3.0
S24	Holiday relief care	-18,353	-38.4	-3.0
C01	Ear procedures: category 1	-18,832	-28.7	-3.1
F06	Oesophagus: diagnostic procedures	-18,885	-7.8	-3.1
M10	Surgical termination of pregnancy	-25,308	-36.8	-4.2
M01	Lower genital tract: minor procedures	-25,633	-53.9	-4.2
C24	Mouth/throat procedures: category 3	-25,730	-20.0	-4.3
B03	Other cataract extraction with lens implant	-28,834	-89.7	-4.8
M06	Upper genital tract: internal procedures	-35,450	-19.6	-5.9
F16	Stomach/duodenum: diagnostic procedures	-38,972	-27.9	-6.4
Gross increase in all HRGs		1,127,116	20.5	
Gross decrease in all HRGs		-521,810	-9.5	
All HRGs		605,306	11.0	100.0

Source: King's Fund analysis; Hospital Episode Statistics 2007

(cataract extraction with lens implant, now the commonest elective procedure), while just three operations accounted for more than 40 per cent of the net increase. Within the overall increase in elective admissions is a decrease of 521,000 admissions for certain HRGs, half of these accounted for by the 'top 10 decreases' listed in the table.

Figure 41, opposite shows the extent to which changes in elective admissions are concentrated among a relatively small number of HRGs, with 32 per cent of the net increase accounted for by just 3.5 per cent of all HRGs.

TABLE 31: TOP 10 INCREASES AND DECREASES IN INPATIENT ELECTIVE ADMISSIONS BY HEALTH CARE RESOURCE GROUP (HRG), 1998 TO 2005

HRG code	Name	Change 1998–2005	% change 1998–2005	Change as % total change
Top 10 increases				
H04	Primary knee replacement	27,182	97.7	29.9
E15	Percutaneous transluminal coronary angioplasty (PTCA)	15,249	143.0	16.8
H02	Primary hip replacement	13,400	39.1	14.7
M03	Lower genital tract: major procedures	10,140	47.7	11.2
J02	Major breast surgery, including plastic procedures, aged >49 or with complications	8,988	44.2	9.9
H10	Arthroscopies	8,950	28.9	9.8
G14	Biliary tract: major procedures, aged <70 w/o complications	5,699	23.5	6.3
F98	Chemotherapy with a digestive system diagnosis	4,961	34.0	5.5
S22	Planned procedures not carried out	4,431	7.6	4.9
E16	Other percutaneous cardiac procedures	4,340	99.4	4.8
Top 10 decreases				
F74	Inguinal umbilical/femoral hernia repair, aged <70 w/o complications	-8,414	-28.4	-9.3
C22	Nose procedures: category 3	-10,762	-32.5	-11.8
C14	Mouth/throat procedures: category 2	-11,195	-40.3	-12.3
B03	Other cataract extraction with lens implant	-12,200	-97.9	-13.4
M06	Upper genital tract: internal procedures	-12,678	-29.6	-13.9
Q11	Varicose vein procedures	-13,675	-50.8	-15.0
M07	Upper genital tract: major procedures	-16,534	-24.6	-18.2
S24	Holiday relief care	-19,175	-40.5	-21.1
B02	Phakoemulsification cataract extraction with lens implant	-25,398	-68.8	-27.9
C24	Mouth/throat procedures: category 3	-27,835	-28.5	-30.6
Gross increase in all HRGs		249,134	12.0	
Gross decrease in all HRGs		-340,030	-16.4	
All HRGs		-90,896	-4.4	100.0

Source: King's Fund analysis; Hospital Episode Statistics 2007

Inpatient HRGs

For elective inpatients there has been a 4.4 per cent net *decrease* in admissions, but this includes notable increases, as Table 31, above, shows. Almost 30 per cent of the net increase in inpatients is accounted for by one intervention – primary knee replacement. Together with increases in primary hip replacements, percutaneous coronary angioplasty (PTCA) and major treatments for the lower genital tract, this accounts for more than two-thirds of the net change in inpatient admissions.

TABLE 32: TOP 10 INCREASES AND DECREASES IN DAY CASE ADMISSIONS BY HEALTH CARE RESOURCE GROUP (HRG), 1998 TO 2005

HRG code	Name	Change 1998–2005	% change 1998–2005	Change as % total change
Top 10 increases				
B02	Phakoemulsification cataract extraction with lens implant	140,315	117.6	20.2
F35	Large intestine: endoscopy/internal procedures	68,624	36.7	9.9
S01	Haematology disorder with minor procedure	65,509	75.6	9.4
E14	Cardiac catheterisation w/o complications	35,198	72.0	5.1
L48	Renal replacement therapy w/o complications	33,088	500.3	4.8
S22	Planned procedures not carried out	32,255	48.5	4.6
D98	Chemotherapy with a respiratory system diagnosis	27,033	244.3	3.9
L20	Bladder: minor endoscopy procedure with complications	22,972	118.1	3.3
A07	Intermediate pain procedures	22,116	27.8	3.2
U01	Invalid primary diagnosis	19,941	65.4	2.9
Top 10 decreases				
M02	Lower genital tract: internal procedures	-13,389	-28.1	-1.9
J09	Malignant breast disorder, aged >69 or with complications	-14,694	-74.5	-2.1
L41	Vasectomy procedures	-14,873	-43.4	-2.1
C01	Ear procedures: category 1	-15,857	-27.6	-2.3
B03	Other cataract extraction with lens implant	-16,634	-84.6	-2.4
F06	Oesophagus: diagnostic procedures	-17,784	-7.6	-2.6
M06	Upper genital tract: internal procedures	-22,772	-16.5	-3.3
M10	Surgical termination of pregnancy	-22,843	-35.6	-3.3
M01	Lower genital tract: minor procedures	-24,931	-57.8	-3.6
F16	Stomach/duodenum: diagnostic procedures	-37,960	-27.8	-5.5
Gross increase in all HRGs		998,188	29.2	
Gross decrease in all HRGs		-301,986	-8.8	
All HRGs		696,202	20.4	100.0

Source: King's Fund analysis; Hospital Episode Statistics 2007

There have been notable reductions in inpatient admissions for mouth and throat procedures, cataract extractions, major treatments for the upper genital tract, and holiday relief care.

Day case HRGs

Drilling down into the net changes in day case admissions, it is evident that more than 20 per cent of this increase (around 115,000) is accounted for by just one operation – cataract extractions with lens implant. This increase is slightly offset by a decrease in inpatient

TABLE 33: TRENDS IN ELECTIVE AND NON-ELECTIVE ADMISSIONS, 1998 TO 2005

Admissions	1998/9	1999/2000	2000/1	2001/2	2002/3	2003/4	2004/5	2005/6	1998–2005 (% change)
Elective	5,484,885	5,571,052	5,567,381	5,482,735	5,681,570	5,739,681	5,786,348	6,090,191	
% total	54.5	54.2	53.6	52.6	52.6	51.3	49.7	49.6	11.0
Non-elective	4,587,628	4,704,763	4,820,434	4,941,706	5,112,779	5,450,772	5,835,137	6,196,392	
% total	45.5	45.8	46.4	47.4	47.4	48.7	50.3	50.4	35.1
Total	10,072,513	10,275,815	10,387,815	10,424,441	10,794,349	11,190,453	11,621,485	12,286,583	22.0

Source: King's Fund analysis; Hospital Episode Statistics 2007

admissions for such procedures, which fell by around 25,000 (*see* Table 31, p 138). Three further HRGs – haematological disorders with minor procedures, large intestine: endoscopy/intermediate procedures and cardiac cathererisation – together account for a further 25 per cent of this net increase.

Within the net increase in all day case admissions, there are also large percentage reductions in day case admissions for some HRGs, as Table 32, p 139, shows.

However, only three of the top 10 total increasing elective HRGs show evidence of a significant switch from inpatient to day case care: cataract extraction, cardiac catheterisation and renal replacement therapy.

NON-ELECTIVE ACTIVITY

As can be seen from Table 33, above, elective admissions accounted for just under half of

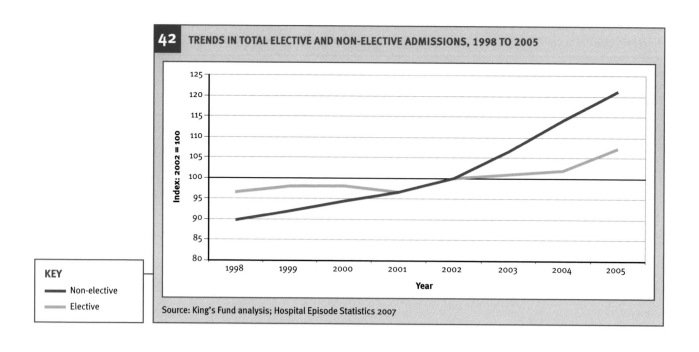

42 TRENDS IN TOTAL ELECTIVE AND NON-ELECTIVE ADMISSIONS, 1998 TO 2005

KEY
— Non-elective
— Elective

Source: King's Fund analysis; Hospital Episode Statistics 2007

TABLE 34: TOP 10 INCREASES AND DECREASES IN NON-ELECTIVE ADMISSIONS BY HEALTH CARE RESOURCE GROUP (HRG), 1998 TO 2005

HRG code	Name	Change 1998–2005	% change 1998–2005	Change as % total change
Top 10 increases				
E36	Chest pain, aged ‹70 w/o complications	72,729	87.7	4.5
L09	Kidney/urinary tract infections, aged ›69 or with complications	55,632	160.9	3.5
F46	General abdominal disorder, aged ›69 or with complications	42,651	78.8	2.7
F47	General abdominal disorder, aged ‹70 w/o complications	41,017	44.6	2.5
D99	Complicated elderly with a respiratory system diagnosis	40,600	79.9	2.5
E35	Chest pain, aged ›69 or with complications	37,174	98.6	2.3
D20	Chronic obstructive pulmonary disorder/bronchitis	35,222	33.4	2.2
E31	Syncope/collapse, aged ›69 or with complications	34,919	92.6	2.2
D13	Lobar atypical/viral pneumonia, aged ›69 or with complications	34,194	105.0	2.1
S25	Other admissions	32,566	50.4	2.0
Top 10 decreases				
U08	Poorly coded dominant procedure	-4,841	-98.0	-0.3
T03	Schizophreniform psychoses w/o section	-4,982	-18.1	-0.3
E19	Heart failure/shock, aged ‹70 w/o complications	-5,433	-31.3	-0.3
P01	Asthma/recurrent wheeze	-5,555	-20.9	-0.3
E34	Angina, aged ‹70 w/o complications	-6,587	-9.9	-0.4
E12	Acute myocardial infarction w/o complications	-6,953	-8.5	-0.4
S23	Rehabilitation	-7,522	-88.5	-0.5
U01	Invalid primary diagnosis	-9,851	-9.0	-0.6
T07	Depression without section	-13,666	-33.4	-0.8
M05	Upper genital tract: minor procedures	-21,784	-46.3	-1.4
Gross increase in all HRGs		1,758,063	37.4	
Gross decrease in all HRGs		-149,299	-3.2	
All HRGs		1,608,764	35.1	100.0

Source: King's Fund analysis; Hospital Episode Statistics 2007

all admissions to hospitals by 2005. Non-elective, or emergency, admissions make up the remainder and have increased proportionately by around five percentage points. Figure 42, opposite, shows cumulative trends in numbers of elective and non-elective admissions between 1998 and 2005.

It is clear that the biggest source of activity growth for hospitals has been emergency admissions, which have risen by more than 35 per cent – about 1.6 million – since 1998. This growth in emergency admissions started to accelerate from 2003/4 onwards. With no

TABLE 35: TRENDS IN ELECTIVE ADMISSIONS BY SOURCE OF ADMISSION, 1998 TO 2005

Source of admission	1998/9	1999/2000	2000/1	2001/2	2002/3	2003/4	2004/5	2005/6	(% change) 1998–2005
Waiting list	2,925,708	2,800,739	2,616,070	2,357,224	2,346,259	2,253,214	2,111,166	2,177,190	-25.6
Booked	1,689,940	1,666,190	1,694,434	1,817,653	1,973,735	2,035,935	2,139,454	2,257,707	33.6
Planned	869,237	1,104,123	1,256,877	1,307,858	1,361,576	1,450,532	1,535,728	1,655,294	90.4
Total	5,484,885	5,571,052	5,567,381	5,482,735	5,681,570	5,739,681	5,786,348	6,090,191	11.0

Source: King's Fund analysis; Hospital Episode Statistics 2007

obvious epidemiological explanation for this trend, the likelihood is that it was caused by changes in clinical behaviour and trusts' admission policies – the latter possibly driven by such imperatives as the need to meet maximum four-hour waits in accident and emergency (A&E) departments.

About a quarter of this net increase in emergency admissions is accounted for by just 10 HRGs (*see* Table 34, p 141).

METHOD OF ELECTIVE ADMISSION

Another way of disaggregating elective activity – and one that touches on the government's dominant health policy of reducing waiting lists and times – is to examine the sources of patient admissions. Table 35, above, shows the total number of elective admissions to English hospitals broken down by source of admission: waiting list, booked and planned (*see* Figure 37, above, for definitions). Figure 43, below, illustrates cumulative trends in elective admissions by source of admission.

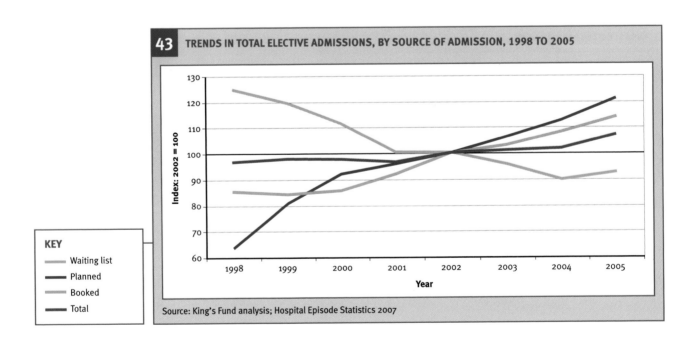

43 TRENDS IN TOTAL ELECTIVE ADMISSIONS, BY SOURCE OF ADMISSION, 1998 TO 2005

KEY
— Waiting list
— Planned
— Booked
— Total

Source: King's Fund analysis; Hospital Episode Statistics 2007

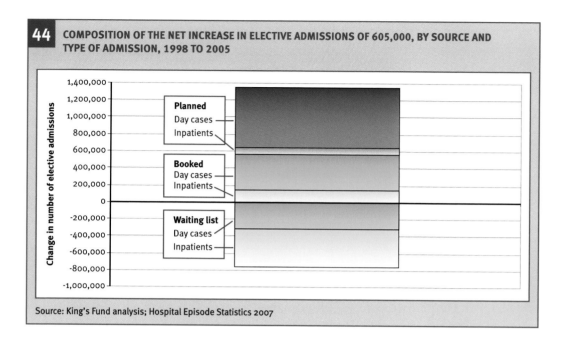

44 COMPOSITION OF THE NET INCREASE IN ELECTIVE ADMISSIONS OF 605,000, BY SOURCE AND TYPE OF ADMISSION, 1998 TO 2005

Source: King's Fund analysis; Hospital Episode Statistics 2007

It is clear that the virtually all of the net increase in elective admissions between 1998 and 2005 was due to a rise of 786,000 (+90 per cent) in planned admissions, which are not counted as part of the waiting list. Conversely, admissions from the waiting list fell by 749,000 (-26 per cent), offset to some extent by a rise of 568,000 (+34 per cent) in booked admissions, which *are* counted as part of the waiting list (*see* Figures 44–46, pp 143–4).

Planned cases are not counted as part of the waiting list. There is no obvious single factor explaining this growth, it may be due to reclassification of some procedures or genuine growth in others (see p 145).

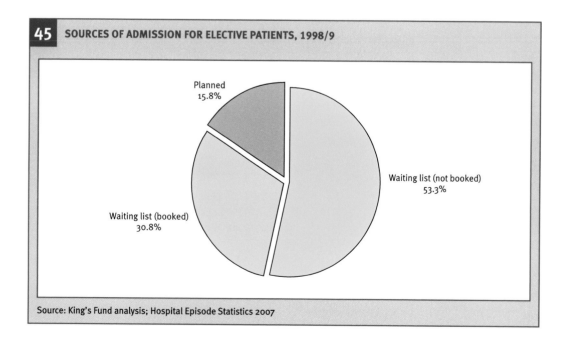

45 SOURCES OF ADMISSION FOR ELECTIVE PATIENTS, 1998/9

Source: King's Fund analysis; Hospital Episode Statistics 2007

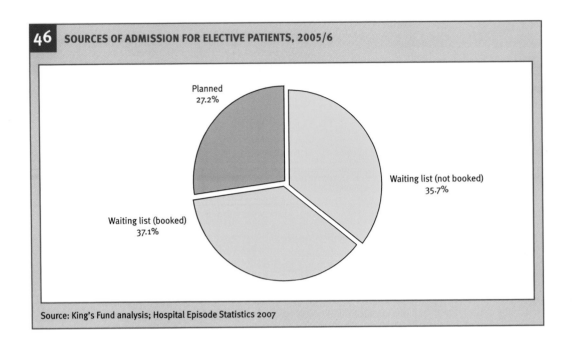

46 SOURCES OF ADMISSION FOR ELECTIVE PATIENTS, 2005/6

Planned
27.2%

Waiting list (not booked)
35.7%

Waiting list (booked)
37.1%

Source: King's Fund analysis; Hospital Episode Statistics 2007

Inpatients and day cases

The overall decrease in inpatient admissions is largely due to a decrease in patients admitted from waiting lists, offset partly by increased booked and planned admissions (*see* Figure 47, below).

The net increase in day case admissions since 1998 is almost wholly attributable to increases in booked admissions and a steep rise in the number of planned day cases, offset by a decline in patients admitted from the waiting list (*see* Figure 48, opposite).

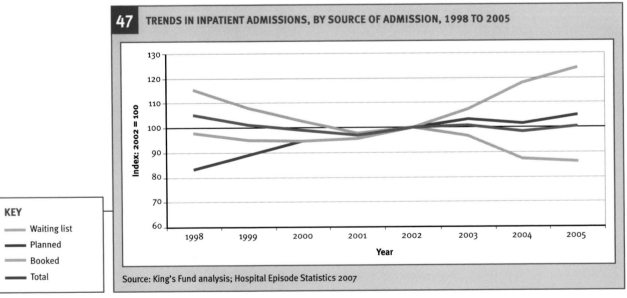

47 TRENDS IN INPATIENT ADMISSIONS, BY SOURCE OF ADMISSION, 1998 TO 2005

KEY
— Waiting list
— Planned
— Booked
— Total

Source: King's Fund analysis; Hospital Episode Statistics 2007

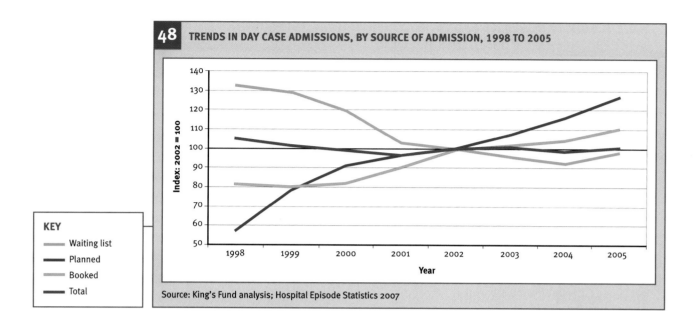

48 TRENDS IN DAY CASE ADMISSIONS, BY SOURCE OF ADMISSION, 1998 TO 2005

KEY
— Waiting list
— Planned
— Booked
— Total

Source: King's Fund analysis; Hospital Episode Statistics 2007

Waiting list and booked admissions HRGs

Within the net decrease in waiting list and booked admissions, analysis at HRG level reveals a more complex picture. Table 36, overleaf, shows, for example, that there were significant increases in booked cases and admissions from the waiting list for a number of HRGs. Again, cataract extraction with lens implant topped the list, with a 50 per cent rise in admissions, accounting for more than 43 per cent of the total net change.

There were also some notable reductions in admissions, with diagnostic or endoscopic HRGs accounting for a quarter of the gross reduction.

Planned cases HRGs

As is clear from the analysis above, there has been a considerable increase in numbers of planned cases since 1998. A more detailed examination of the change in planned cases at the level of HRGs is shown in table 37, *see* p 147.

Comparing the increases in admissions for planned cases with changes in all other elective admissions suggests that for most of the top 10 planned cases HRGs, the increases in admissions are simply part of an overall growth in admissions (*see* Figure 49, p 148). However, for two diagnostic HRGs (for the stomach/duodenum and the oesophagus) and possibly a third (minor endoscopic bladder procedures), large decreases in other elective admissions have been offset by increases in planned cases, which suggests a switch in patient classification. Furthermore, about a third of the large increase in total elective cataract admissions is accounted for by the increase in planned admissions.

TABLE 36: TOP 10 INCREASES AND DECREASES IN WAITING LIST PLUS BOOKED ADMISSIONS BY HEALTH CARE RESOURCE GROUP (HRG), 1998 TO 2005

HRG code	Name	Change 1998–2005	% change 1998–2005	Change as % total change
Top 10 increases				
B02	Phakoemulsification cataract extraction with lens implant	78,386	50.7	-43.4
E14	Cardiac catheterisation w/o complications	29,513	43.6	-16.3
H04	Primary knee replacement	25,726	93.6	-14.2
H10	Arthroscopies	24,563	27.8	-13.6
S22	Planned procedures not carried out	19,302	16.4	-10.7
E15	Percutaneous transluminal coronary angioplasty (PTCA)	16,402	161.4	-9.1
H13	Hand procedures: category 1	13,275	28.5	-7.3
H02	Primary hip replacement	12,650	37.4	-7.0
M03	Lower genital tract: major procedures	11,206	52.7	-6.2
L30	Prostate/bladder Nk: minor endoscopy procedure (male and female)	11,057	117.1	-6.1
Top 10 decreases				
J37	Minor skin procedures: category 1 w/o complications	-18,721	-10.4	10.4
C01	Ear procedures: category 1	-19,016	-29.5	10.5
L21	Bladder: minor endoscopy procedure w/o complications	-19,440	-15.1	10.8
M01	Lower genital tract: minor procedures	-21,358	-57.0	11.8
C24	Mouth/throat procedures: category 3	-26,531	-21.1	14.7
M10	Surgical termination of pregnancy	-27,777	-42.0	15.4
B03	Other cataract extraction with lens implant	-28,809	-91.2	15.9
M06	Upper genital tract: internal procedures	-39,919	-22.5	22.1
F16	Stomach/duodenum: diagnostic procedures	-61,357	-47.3	33.9
F06	Oesophagus: diagnostic procedures	-77,938	-35.4	43.1
Gross increase in all HRGs		500,950	10.9	
Gross decrease in all HRGs		-681,701	-14.8	
All HRGs		-180,751	-3.9	100.0

Source: King's Fund analysis; Hospital Episode Statistics 2007

TABLE 37: TOP 10 INCREASES AND DECREASES IN PLANNED ADMISSIONS BY HEALTH CARE RESOURCE GROUP, 1998 TO 2005

HRG code	Name	Change 1998–2005	% change 1998–2005	Change as % total change
Top 10 increases				
F35	Large intestine: endoscopy/internal procedures	75,397	288.3	9.6
S01	Haematology disorder with minor procedure	62,920	168.8	8.0
F06	Oesophagus: diagnostic procedures	59,053	256.7	7.5
B02	Phakoemulsification cataract extraction with lens implant	36,531	2,352.3	4.6
L21	Bladder: minor endoscopy procedure w/o complications	29,763	46.4	3.8
F98	Chemotherapy with a digestive system diagnosis	29,483	45.1	3.8
L48	Renal replacement therapy w/o complications	26,609	193.8	3.4
A07	Intermediate pain procedures	24,326	207.4	3.1
D98	Chemotherapy with a respiratory system diagnosis	23,912	224.7	3.0
F16	Stomach/duodenum: diagnostic procedures	22,385	226.5	2.8
Top 10 decreases				
S02	Malignant disorder of lymphatic/haematology systems with complications	-2,266	-42.8	-0.3
M16	Non-surgical treatment of gynae malignant, aged >69 or with complications	-2,284	-54.3	-0.3
S23	Rehabilitation	-2,471	-82.8	-0.3
L07	Non OR kidney/urinary tract neoplasms, aged >69 or with complications	-2,493	-61.2	-0.3
S21	Convalescence/other relief care	-2,509	-83.5	-0.3
P07	Neoplasms	-2,636	-25.7	-0.3
C36	Mouth, head, neck/ear diagnosis: category 4, aged >69 or with complications	-3,392	-89.0	-0.4
M01	Lower genital tract: minor procedures	-4,275	-42.3	-0.5
S24	Holiday relief care	-7,835	-27.2	-1.0
J09	Malignant breast disorder, aged >69 or with complications	-14,077	-76.8	-1.8
Gross increase in all HRGs		851,652	98.0	
Gross decrease in all HRGs		-65,595	-7.5	
All HRGs		786,057	90.4	100.0

Source: King's Fund analysis; Hospital Episode Statistics 2007

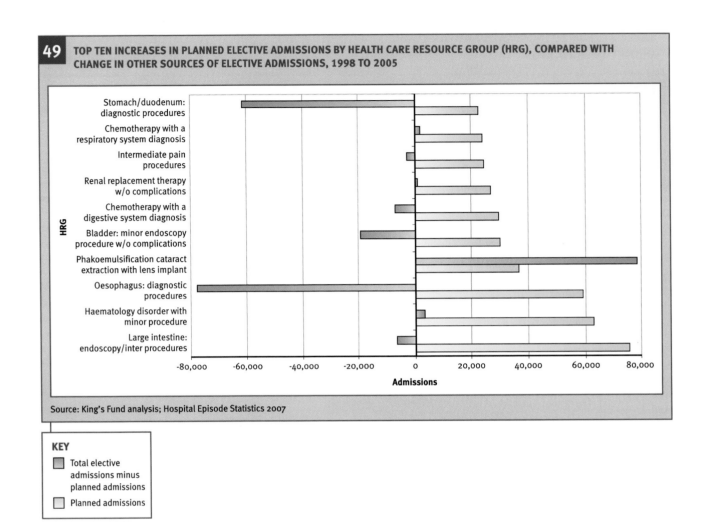

49 TOP TEN INCREASES IN PLANNED ELECTIVE ADMISSIONS BY HEALTH CARE RESOURCE GROUP (HRG), COMPARED WITH CHANGE IN OTHER SOURCES OF ELECTIVE ADMISSIONS, 1998 TO 2005

Source: King's Fund analysis; Hospital Episode Statistics 2007

KEY

Total elective admissions minus planned admissions

Planned admissions

TABLE 38: TRENDS IN HOSPITAL ADMISSIONS FOR PEOPLE AGED UNDER 65 PER 1,000 POPULATION, 2000/1 TO 2005/6

Year	People aged 0–64	
	Coronary heart disease and stroke	All other conditions
2000/1	137,656	5,855,950
2001/2	135,720	5,781,833
2002/3	137,239	5,873,209
2003/4	137,628	6,061,800
2004/5	136,272	6,183,105
2005/6	136,035	6,542,747
% change 2003–6	-0.9	11.4
% change 2001–6	-1.2	11.7

Source: Hospital Episode Statistics 2007

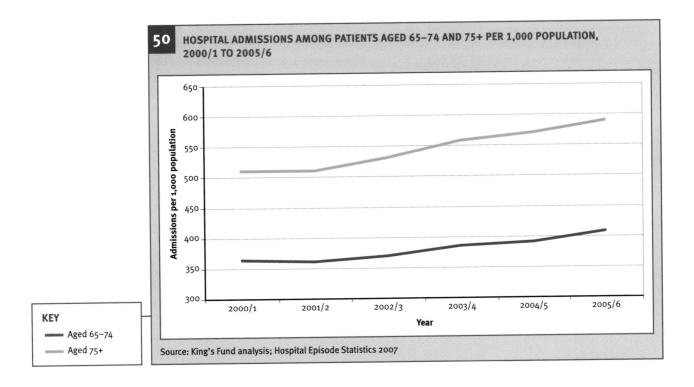

50 HOSPITAL ADMISSIONS AMONG PATIENTS AGED 65–74 AND 75+ PER 1,000 POPULATION, 2000/1 TO 2005/6

KEY
— Aged 65–74
— Aged 75+

Source: King's Fund analysis; Hospital Episode Statistics 2007

2002 REVIEW ASSUMPTIONS ABOUT HOSPITAL UTILISATION

Under the solid progress scenario, the 2002 review projected that over the two decades from 2002/3 there would be a 10 per cent reduction in hospital admissions related to coronary heart disease (CHD) and stroke for 15–64 year olds, with a 5 per cent reduction in those related to all other disease areas. These reductions are higher in the fully engaged scenario, which assumed a 25 per cent reduction in care related to CHD and stroke and an overall 15 per cent reduction for all other disease areas (Wanless 2002).

Table 38, opposite, shows that between 2002/3 and 2005/6 hospital admissions relating to CHD and stroke for people under 64 declined by 1 per cent – too slow a reduction to meet the 2002 review's assumption. The rising trend in admissions for all other conditions will need to be reversed over the next 15 years if the review's assumptions are to be met.

The 2002 review's solid progress scenario also assumed that by 2022 hospital utilisation by the over-75s would match current use by those aged 65–74. As figure 50, above, shows, however, recent (albeit short-term) trends suggest a divergence rather than convergence in utilisation by these age groups.

SUMMARY: ELECTIVE AND EMERGENCY ACTIVITY

- The net increase in total elective activity between 1998 and 2005 arose from an increase in day cases that outweighed a decrease in inpatient activity.
- Day case admissions have increased from 62.3 per cent to 67.5 per cent of all elective admissions.
- The increase in day case activity is almost wholly due to increases in admissions for just a handful of interventions – most notably cataract procedures.
- For three of the top ten increasing elective HRGs, there is indicative evidence of a substitution of day cases for inpatients.
- The net increase in elective admissions is largely attributable to increases in just a handful of operations – such as cataract procedures.
- The largest source of the overall growth in hospital activity has been increases in emergency admissions, with a net increase of around 1.6 million (+35 per cent) between 1998 and 2005, compared with a net increase in elective admissions of 605,000 (11 per cent).
- Thus the proportion of hospital activity accounted for by emergency admissions has risen by 4.9 per cent. However, changes in emergency admissions were less concentrated at the level of HRGs than changes in elective activity.
- Virtually all of the net increase in elective admissions between 1998 and 2005 was due to a near-doubling in planned admissions.
- Admissions from the waiting list fell by more than a quarter between 1998 and 2005, although booked admissions rose by more than a third.

TABLE 39: REFERRAL AND ATTENDANCE RATES FOR OUTPATIENT APPOINTMENTS, 1994 TO 2006

Year	GP referrals to first outpatient appointment	Other referrals for first outpatient appointment	Total referrals	First attendances	Subsequent attendances	Total attendances
1994	7,996,019	1,680,927	9,676,946	10,362,877	28,942,923	39,305,800
1995	8,547,633	2,322,463	10,870,096	10,989,334	29,128,357	40,117,691
1996	8,692,158	2,877,519	11,569,677	11,294,069	29,578,700	40,872,769
1997	8,991,722	3,328,204	12,319,926	11,529,432	30,105,837	41,635,269
1998	9,139,785	3,361,251	12,501,036	11,777,780	30,376,617	42,154,397
1999	9,141,425	3,460,904	12,602,329	12,136,405	30,904,294	43,040,699
2000	9,362,770	3,717,471	13,080,241	12,466,233	31,103,107	43,569,340
2001	9,470,342	4,016,558	13,486,900	12,612,615	31,062,363	43,674,978
2002	9,655,874	4,299,402	13,955,276	12,878,799	30,886,026	43,764,825
2003	9,802,237	4,643,662	14,445,899	13,430,530	31,689,082	45,119,612
2004	9,776,914	4,960,972	14,737,886	13,370,173	31,397,428	44,767,601
2005	9,807,847	5,254,313	15,062,160	13,727,249	31,499,332	45,226,581
2006 Q1[1]	2,385,625	1,371,059	3,756,684	3,358,369	7,774,085	11,132,454
2006 Q2[2]	2,338,430	1,360,046	3,698,476	3,403,297	7,735,627	11,138,924

Source: House of Commons Health Committee 2006e
[1] Q1 = First quarter

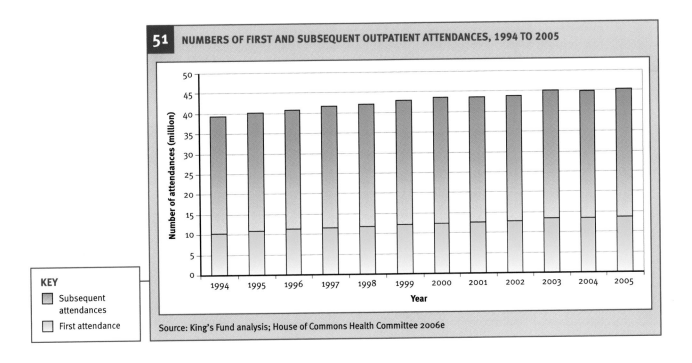

51 NUMBERS OF FIRST AND SUBSEQUENT OUTPATIENT ATTENDANCES, 1994 TO 2005

KEY

■ Subsequent attendances

□ First attendance

Source: King's Fund analysis; House of Commons Health Committee 2006e

OUTPATIENT ACTIVITY

Outpatient care accounts for about 9 per cent of total NHS spending and more than 45 million attendances every year. In 2005/6, more than one in four people in England had a first attendance at an outpatient department. Since the mid-1990s total outpatient attendances have risen by 6 million (15 per cent), although growth has been more modest since 2002 (see Table 39, opposite, and Figure 51, above).

Outpatient demand comes from two main sources: GP referrals and referrals by consultants and other doctors. As Figure 52, below, shows, since 2000 there has been

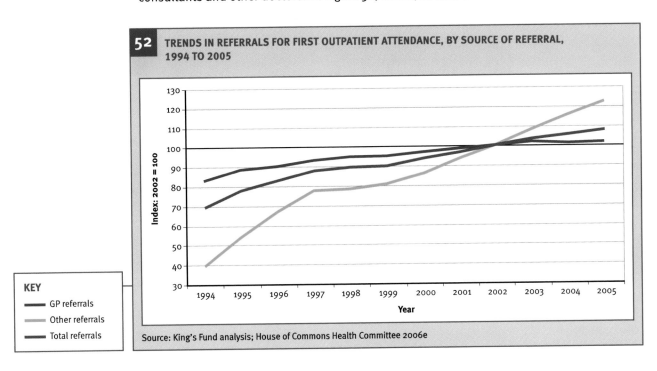

52 TRENDS IN REFERRALS FOR FIRST OUTPATIENT ATTENDANCE, BY SOURCE OF REFERRAL, 1994 TO 2005

KEY

— GP referrals

— Other referrals

— Total referrals

Source: King's Fund analysis; House of Commons Health Committee 2006e

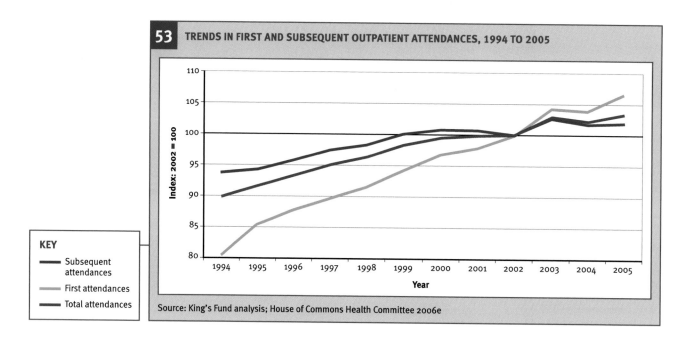

53 TRENDS IN FIRST AND SUBSEQUENT OUTPATIENT ATTENDANCES, 1994 TO 2005

KEY
— Subsequent attendances
— First attendances
— Total attendances

Source: King's Fund analysis; House of Commons Health Committee 2006e

little change in GP referrals, while consultant-to-consultant and other referrals rose by more than a fifth between 2002 and 2005, continuing a long running trend.

Referrals translate into attendances and, as Table 39, *see* p 150, shows, first attendances have risen more or less in line with the absolute rise in referrals. As Figure 53, above, shows, however, total attendances rose by around 3.3 per cent between 2002/3 and 2005/6, an increase wholly achieved in the first year.

MATERNITY ACTIVITY

About 593,400 NHS hospital deliveries took place in England in 2005/6, 8 per cent more

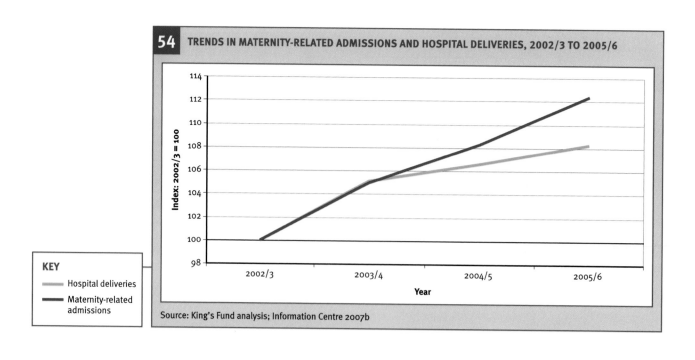

54 TRENDS IN MATERNITY-RELATED ADMISSIONS AND HOSPITAL DELIVERIES, 2002/3 TO 2005/6

KEY
— Hospital deliveries
— Maternity-related admissions

Source: King's Fund analysis; Information Centre 2007b

TABLE 40: ACCIDENT AND EMERGENCY ATTENDANCES, 1987/8 TO 2006/7[1]

Year	New attendances	Follow-up attendances	Total attendances
1987/8	10,879,543	3,024,124	13,903,667
1988/9	10,983,736	2,837,081	13,820,817
1989/90	11,207,099	2,728,203	13,935,302
1990/1	11,204,059	2,512,913	13,716,972
1991/2	11,035,326	2,270,155	13,305,481
1992/3	10,993,202	2,077,009	13,070,211
1993/4	11,364,703	1,923,987	13,288,690
1994/5	11,942,599	1,869,123	13,811,722
1995/6	12,461,909	1,772,381	14,234,290
1996/7	12,483,633	1,642,544	14,126,177
1997/8	12,793,720	1,570,426	14,364,146
1998/9	12,811,064	1,469,324	14,280,388
1999/2000	13,167,495	1,461,530	14,629,025
2000/1	12,953,432	1,339,875	14,293,307
2001/2	12,852,702	1,191,316	14,044,018
2002/3	12,945,413	1,100,162	14,045,575
2003/4	15,312,738	1,204,107	16,516,845
2004/5	16,711,750	1,125,430	17,837,180
2005/6	17,775,225	983,939	18,759,164
2006/7[1]	18,185,755	929,955	19,110,901

Sources: House of Commons Health Committee 2006e
[1] 2006/7 is an estimate based on the first six months of 2006/7 scaled up and reflecting the quarterly pattern of activity in 2005/6.

than in 2002/3 (The Information Centre 2007). As can be seen from Figure 54, opposite, between 2002/3 and 2005/6, the total number of maternity-related admissions (first finished consultant episodes for delivery and non-delivery episodes) rose from 924,000 to 1,038,000, an increase of 12 per cent (Information Centre 2007b).

Between 2002/3 and 2005/6 the number of first attendances at maternity outpatients fell by 11 per cent, from 522,000 to 465,000 (Department of Health 2006e); this reduction probably reflects a shift towards the provision of antenatal care away from hospitals to an increasingly diverse range of community settings.

ACCIDENT AND EMERGENCY ACTIVITY

Accident and emergency services account for some 2 per cent of NHS expenditure, with about 20 million attendances a year; roughly one person in three visits an A&E department at least once in a year.

As Table 40, above, and Figures 55 and 56, overleaf, show, A&E activity had been relatively stable from the late 1980s to 2002/3, with some upward trend in first attendances but a compensating downward trend in follow-up visits. However, between 2002/3 and 2005/6, new attendances rose by more than 37 per cent, or 4.8 million attendances.

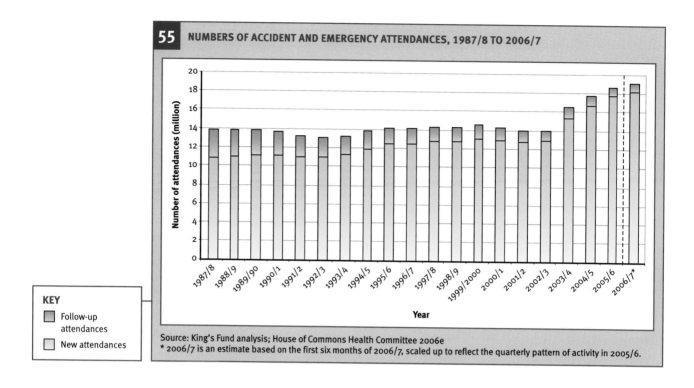

55 NUMBERS OF ACCIDENT AND EMERGENCY ATTENDANCES, 1987/8 TO 2006/7

KEY
- Follow-up attendances
- New attendances

Source: King's Fund analysis; House of Commons Health Committee 2006e
* 2006/7 is an estimate based on the first six months of 2006/7, scaled up to reflect the quarterly pattern of activity in 2005/6.

Assuming little change in the health of the population, this dramatic rise is probably due to changes in the service itself, such as reduced waiting times to meet the four-hour maximum wait target. However, changes in other services, such as GPs' out-of-hours cover, are also likely to have encouraged more visits to A&E.

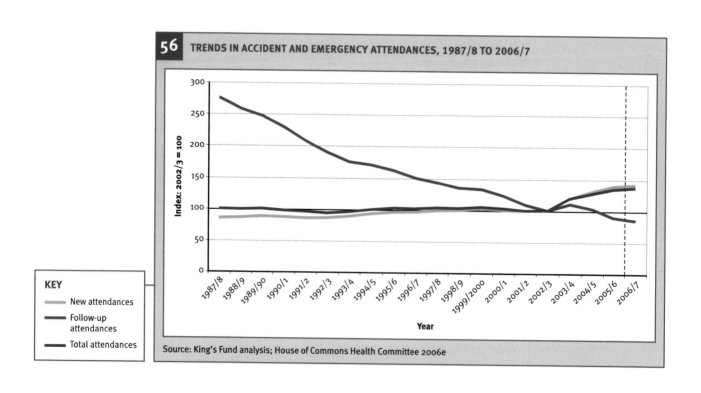

56 TRENDS IN ACCIDENT AND EMERGENCY ATTENDANCES, 1987/8 TO 2006/7

KEY
- New attendances
- Follow-up attendances
- Total attendances

Source: King's Fund analysis; House of Commons Health Committee 2006e

Mental health

NHS activity related to patients with mental health problems is diverse, covering inpatient stays in hospital, prescribing, community-based and primary care services. Hospital Episode Statistics (HES) show that both the number of finished consultant episodes (FCEs) and the number of admissions to hospital with a primary diagnosis related to mental illness declined between 1998/9 and 2005/6, by 10 per cent and 16 per cent respectively

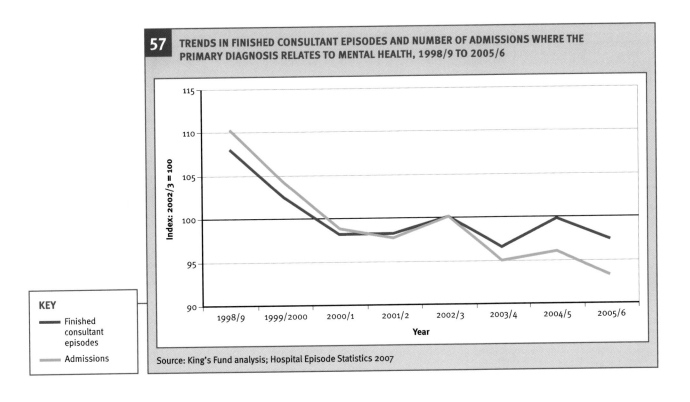

57 TRENDS IN FINISHED CONSULTANT EPISODES AND NUMBER OF ADMISSIONS WHERE THE PRIMARY DIAGNOSIS RELATES TO MENTAL HEALTH, 1998/9 TO 2005/6

KEY

— Finished consultant episodes

— Admissions

Source: King's Fund analysis; Hospital Episode Statistics 2007

TABLE 41: NUMBERS OF FINISHED CONSULTANT EPISODES WHERE THE PRIMARY DIAGNOSIS CONCERNS MENTAL ILLNESS, 1998/9 TO 2005/6

Diagnosis	Year							
	1998/9	1999/2000	2000/1	2001/2	2002/3	2003/4	2004/5	2005/6
Dementia	31,816	29,637	27,759	27,489	28,116	27,457	27,368	25,781
Other organic mental disorder, including symptomatic mental disorders	5,049	4,856	4,789	5,235	5,276	5,289	5,664	5,982
Mental and behavioural disorders due to psychoactive substances	42,427	42,327	40,607	41,248	42,236	46,192	52,624	57,814
Schizophrenia, schizotypal and delusional disorders	38,517	36,806	36,109	37,086	37,736	36,174	39,699	36,414
Mood (affective) disorders	57,376	54,515	52,192	52,569	52,203	47,884	47,916	43,332
Neurotic, behavioural and personality disorders	33,404	30,418	28,926	29,352	30,016	27,761	29,291	27,663
Mental retardation	22,665	19,379	18,781	16,944	17,340	14,625	12,629	11,398
Other mental and behavioural disorders	11,785	12,840	11,580	11,131	12,250	11,614	9,394	10,540
Total	243,039	230,778	220,743	221,054	225,173	216,996	224,585	218,924

Source: King's Fund analysis; Hospital Episode Statistics 2007
Note: The data in this table is ungrossed; it has not been adjusted to account for shortfalls in the number of records received from NHS trusts, or for missing/invalid clinical data (ie, diagnosis and operation codes).

(*see* Figure 57, p 155). Despite this overall downward trend, it is notable that FCEs with a primary diagnosis classified as 'mental and behavioural disorders due to psychoactive substances' have increased significantly since 2002/3, by 37 per cent (*see* Table 41, above).

The number of FCEs for a primary diagnosis related to mental illness has also declined as a proportion of total FCEs, from 2 per cent in 1998/9 to 1.5 per cent in 2005/6; and the proportion of admissions for mental illness has declined by the same amount. These downward trends are partly due to a policy shift towards treating more people with mental health problems in outpatient and/or community settings. Crisis resolution/home treatment teams and other community-based services designed to manage acute episodes of mental illness without admission to hospital were set up between 2001 and

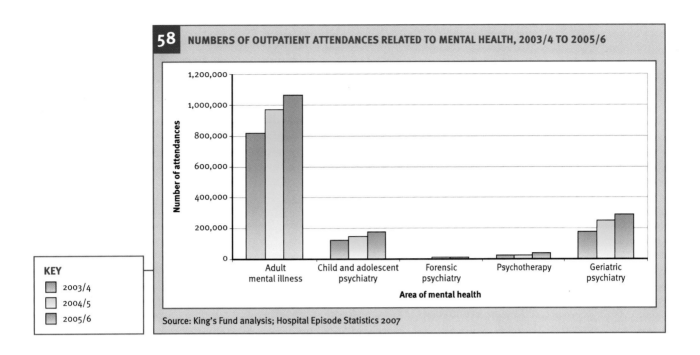

58 NUMBERS OF OUTPATIENT ATTENDANCES RELATED TO MENTAL HEALTH, 2003/4 TO 2005/6

KEY
- 2003/4
- 2004/5
- 2005/6

Source: King's Fund analysis; Hospital Episode Statistics 2007

TABLE 42: NUMBERS OF PATIENTS (WHO HAD PRIOR INPATIENT OR OUTPATIENT CARE) CONTACTED, BY PROFESSION OF CONTACT, 2003/4 AND 2004/5

Profession of contact	Year	Total patients	Total contacts
Clinical psychologist	2003/4	99,610	476,820
	2004/5	126,050	618,520
Community psychiatric nurse	2003/4	332,270	2,780,580
	2004/5	367,680	2,869,080
Consultant psychotherapist	2003/4	11,550	87,460
	2004/5	11,280	83,860
NHS Direct Mental Health	2003/4	380	3,720
	2004/5	540	7,310
Occupational therapist	2003/4	86,380	775,390
	2004/5	88,680	820,800
Physiotherapist	2003/4	26,200	171,510
	2004/5	10,030	81,050
Social worker	2003/4	42,680	251,540
	2004/5	58,450	365,900
All	**2003/4**	**599,060**	**4,547,020**
	2004/5	**662,720**	**4,846,520**

Source: Information Centre 2006b, 2006c

2004; and the evidence suggests that these have been effective in reducing admissions (Glover *et al* 2006).

Three years' worth of data is available from HES, recording outpatient activity in mental health. As Figure 58, p 157, shows, activity is increasing, although this may be due to better recording.

Changes in statistical collection mean that published data in community-based mental health service activity are readily available only for 2003/4 and 2004/5 (from the Mental Health Minimum Dataset). Table 42, p 157, shows the scale of activity in terms of patients seen and contacts made by different staff groups and services. With only two years' worth of data no sensible observations can be made about trends.

Primary care: general practice and prescribing

GENERAL PRACTICE

Data on attendances at GP surgeries is not routinely collated by the NHS at national level. However, the General Household Survey (GHS) provides information on the average number of GP attendances each year, from which it is possible to estimate the number of consultations. As Figure 59, below, shows, the consultation rate has remained relatively stable since the early 1990s, fluctuating between 200 and 250 million a year.

The 2002 review assumed that by 2022, under the solid progress scenario, people under 65 would have an average of one additional GP visit per year over and above current average visits for this age group and that GP consultations per head among those aged 75 and over would match current use for those aged 65–74 age group. In the fully engaged scenario it was assumed that these changes would occur earlier, by 2012.

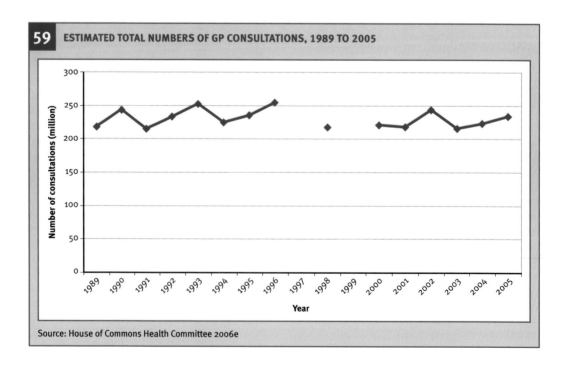

59 ESTIMATED TOTAL NUMBERS OF GP CONSULTATIONS, 1989 TO 2005

Source: House of Commons Health Committee 2006e

TABLE 43: AVERAGE NUMBER OF GP CONSULTATIONS PER PERSON PER YEAR BY AGE, 1985 TO 2005

Age groups	Unweighted	Weighted						
	1985	1998	2000	2001	2002	2003	2004	2005
0–4	7	6	5	6	5	5	5	5
5–15	3	3	2	3	2	2	2	2
16–44	4	4	4	4	4	4	4	4
45–64	4	5	5	5	5	5	5	5
65–74	5	6	6	5	7	6	6	6
75+	6	6	7	6	8	7	7	7
Average for all age groups	4	4	4	4	5	4	4	4

Source: Office for National Statistics 2006a

Since 1985 the average number of NHS GP consultations has risen from five to six for the 'young old' (65–74) and from six to seven for the 'old old' (75 and over). However, these rates have remained unchanged since 2003 (*see* Table 43, above).

These longer-term trends have taken two decades to emerge; and, given that the 2002 review predicated its projections on a more responsive health service, with greater personal engagement in health, it is difficult to predict future trends.

PRESCRIBING

A total of 752 million prescription items were dispensed in the community in England in the year to December 2006, representing a rise of almost 22 per cent on 2002 and a 4.4 per cent increase on the previous year (*see* Table 44, below). The cost to the NHS of dispensing prescriptions in 2006 was £8.2 billion.

TABLE 44: TRENDS IN NUMBERS OF PRESCRIPTION ITEMS ISSUED PER HEAD, 2000 TO 2006

Year	Prescription items (million)	Prescription items per head
2000	551.8	11.2
2001	587.0	11.9
2002	617.0	12.4
2003	649.7	13.0
2004	686.1	13.7
2005	720.3	14.3
2006	752.0	na
% change 2002–6	21.9%	na
% change 2005–6	4.4%	na

Source: Department of Health 2006d; Information Centre 2007d

TABLE 45: TOP TEN INCREASES IN VOLUMES OF PRESCRIPTION DRUGS DISPENSED, 2002 TO 2006

Prescription drugs	Change 2002–6		Change as a % of total net change
	Number (thousand)	Percentage	
Lipid-regulating drugs	24,493.8	139.1	18.3
Hypertension and heart failure	18,151.0	61.3	13.6
Antiplatelet drugs	11,177.7	51.7	8.4
Ulcer-healing drugs	8,957.9	43.5	6.7
Drugs used in diabetes	8,130.6	40.0	6.1
Nitrates, calcium channel blockers and other antianginal drugs	6,713.5	24.0	5.0
Thyroid and antithyroid drugs	5,672.2	47.7	4.2
Diuretics	5,396.8	16.8	4.0
Beta-adrenoceptor blocking drugs	4,938.8	22.0	3.7
Antidepressant drugs	4,708.6	17.9	3.5
All prescriptions			
Gross increase	144,067.0		
Gross decrease	10,538.9		
Net change: all prescriptions	133,528.1		100.0

Source: King's Fund analysis; Information Centre 2007d

A more detailed breakdown of the change in prescribing activity is presented in Table 45, above. Of the total net increase in prescription items of 133.5 million between 2002 and 2006, three-quarters is accounted for by just 10 drugs, with lipid-regulating drugs accounting for more than 18 per cent of the net change.

SUMMARY: MENTAL HEALTH AND PRIMARY CARE ACTIVITY

- Between 1998/9 and 2005/6, the number of consultant episodes and admissions where the primary diagnosis related to mental illness fell by 10 per cent and 17 per cent, respectively.
- GP attendances are not routinely recorded nationally. However, in Great Britain it is estimated that there were around 250 million NHS GP consultations in 2005, an increase of just over a third since the early 1980s.
- Prescriptions dispensed rose by more than a fifth (135 million items) between 2002 and 2006, and prescription items per head rose by 16 per cent.
- In the community in England, increases in just 10 drugs (six related to the cardiovascular system) accounted for three quarters of the net rise in prescription items between 2002 and 2006, with lipid-regulating drugs (including statins) accounting for the largest single share (18.3 per cent) of the total net rise in prescription items.
- Over this period, the number of statins dispensed rose by 138 per cent, compared with a rise of 22 per cent for all prescriptions. Lower-cost statins (particularly simvastatin) have seen the largest increases in volumes dispensed

TABLE 46: USE OF NHS DIRECT SERVICES, 1998/9 TO 2005/6

Year	Calls received (thousand)	Visits to NHS Direct website[1] (thousand)
1998/9	110	0
1999/2000	1,650	0
2000/1	3,420	1,500[2]
2001/2	5,213	2,028
2002/3	6,319	3,972
2003/4	6,405	6,542
2004/5	6,586	9,285
2005/6	6,810	13,537

Source: Department of Health 2006d
[1] NHS Direct Online was launched in December 1999.
[2] Figure for 2000/1 is an estimate.

Other services: NHS Direct, walk-in centres and ambulance services

NHS DIRECT

NHS Direct has handled more than 36 million calls since it was launched in March 1998, and currently receives around half a million calls a month. NHS Direct Online was launched in December 1999 and the website currently receives about 1.5 million visits a month (*see* Table 46, above).

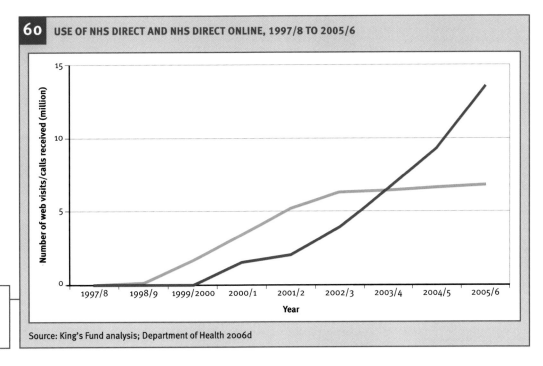

60 USE OF NHS DIRECT AND NHS DIRECT ONLINE, 1997/8 TO 2005/6

KEY
— Website visits
— Calls received

Source: King's Fund analysis; Department of Health 2006d

Between 2002/3 and 2005/6 the number of calls received by NHS Direct rose by only 8 per cent, while visits to the website rose by 241 per cent. Figure 60, p 161, illustrates the rapid increase in the use of NHS Direct Online and also reveals a plateau effect for calls to NHS Direct.

Since December 2004, NHS Direct has also been available through NHS Direct Interactive digital TV. Roll-out of the service onto other digital platforms (such as Freeview) during 2006 was expected to increase coverage to all digital households – around 85 per cent of the population.

The latest usage information, as of 16 February 2007, indicates that:
- NHS Direct Online has around 24 million visitors a year
- NHS Direct receives 7 million calls a year
- NHS Direct Interactive is available through digital TV to 16 million households (NHS Direct 2007).

WALK-IN CENTRES

Walk-in centres offer access to a range of NHS services, including advice, information and treatment, without need for an appointment. By May 2006, 75 centres had opened in England, and in 2005/6 more than 2.5 million visits were made – an average of just over 100 daily visits per centre (*see* Table 47, below).

One of the purposes of walk-in centres was to relieve pressure on and improve access to GPs (Department of Health 1999b). However, a recent study (Maheswaran *et al* 2007) found no evidence that these centres reduced waiting times for access to primary care. Although there had been a demonstrable increase in the number of practices achieving the target waiting time of less than 48 hours to see a GP, there was no evidence that walk-in centres had contributed to this improvement.

TABLE 47: VISITS TO WALK-IN CENTRES[1], 2000/1 TO 2005/6

Year	Number of sites open[2]	Total number of visits for the year[3]	Average daily number of visits for the average number of centres open
2000/1	39	574,000	57
2001/2	42	1,143,000	78
2002/3	42	1,372,000	90
2003/4	43	1,582,000	103[4]
2004/5	63	2,068,000	106[5]
2005/6	72	2,510,000	101[6]

Source: Department of Health 2006d
[1] Includes all visits, including non-accident and emergency attendances
[2] Total number open as at end of period
[3] Figures are collated from monthly returns and include some estimates for missing returns.
[4] Excludes NHS walk-in centres opened after December 2003
[5] Excludes NHS walk-in centres opened after December 2004
[6] Data source changed to QMAE.

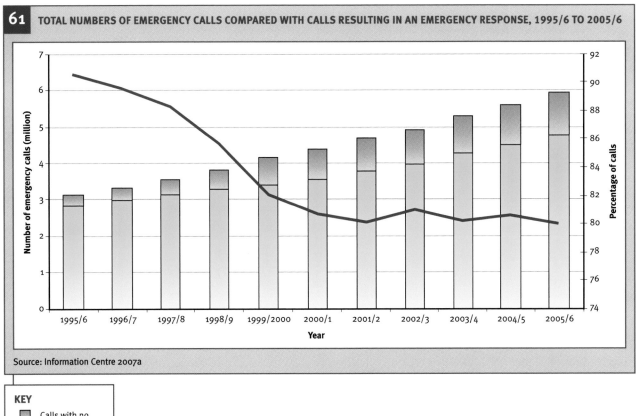

61 TOTAL NUMBERS OF EMERGENCY CALLS COMPARED WITH CALLS RESULTING IN AN EMERGENCY RESPONSE, 1995/6 TO 2005/6

Source: Information Centre 2007a

KEY

■ Calls with no response

□ Calls resulting in a response

— Percentage of calls resulting in a response

AMBULANCE SERVICES

The ambulance service cost nearly £1 billion in 2005/6. Calls to the service have nearly doubled since 1995/6 (*see* Figure 61, above), although calls resulting in a response (that is, an emergency ambulance arriving at the scene of an incident) have fallen from around 90 per cent to 80 per cent.

However, some three-quarters of ambulance journeys are planned rather than being in response to emergency calls. And since 2000/1, the total number of ambulance journeys made has been falling because of reductions in planned journeys (*see* Figure 62, overleaf).

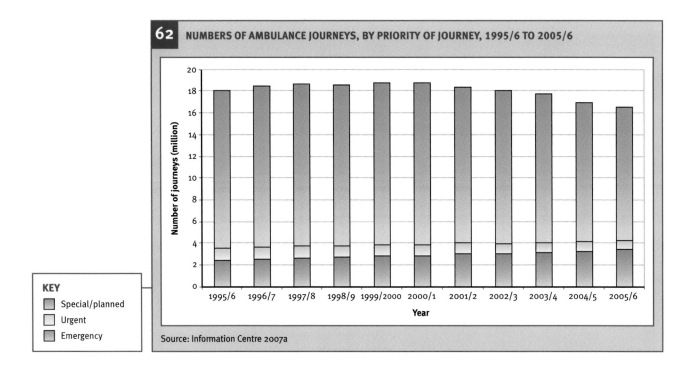

62 | NUMBERS OF AMBULANCE JOURNEYS, BY PRIORITY OF JOURNEY, 1995/6 TO 2005/6

KEY
- Special/planned
- Urgent
- Emergency

Source: Information Centre 2007a

SUMMARY: OTHER NHS SERVICES

- NHS Direct has handled more that 36 million calls since it was launched in 1998, and currently receives around 0.5 million calls a month. Calls now seem to have reached a plateau of just under 7 million a year.

- NHS Direct Online, launched in 1999, has seen a rapid increase in use and currently receives about 1.5 million visits per month.

- By May 2006 there were 75 walk-in centres in England. In 2005/6 more than 2.5 million visits were made to these centres, with an average of just over 100 visits per centre per day.

- The number of ambulance journeys in England fell from around 18 million to 16.5 million in the 10 years to 2005/6. However, the number of calls to the service nearly doubled – to almost 6 million – over this period, although the percentage of calls resulting in a response fell from around 90 to 80 per cent.

9 Outcomes and determinants of health

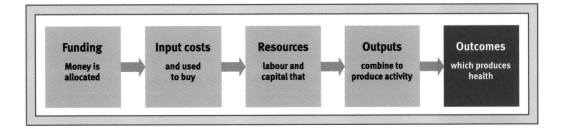

The ultimate objective of any health care system is to improve people's quality and length of life. But many factors unconnected with health services also have a considerable impact on health, and it is difficult to isolate the particular contribution of health care. In the absence of any routine data on changes in health status as a result of NHS interventions, we have to rely on less direct measures of population heath. As the 2001 interim Wanless report (Wanless 2001) noted, although health is influenced by many factors, including lifetime consumption of goods, services and education, as well as genetic history and lifestyle behaviour, the impact of health services may be less marginal than has been argued previously.

Two further measures are also relevant. First, health services not only act directly to restore current ill health but also intervene in less direct ways to influence known determinants of health – such as smoking, diet and other lifestyle behaviours. Second, while the process of care will contribute to the eventual (health) outcome, there are measures of process – reduced waiting, for example – which have an intrinsic value of their own.

Recent progress relating to key health determinants of health is analysed below; aspects of the care process, such as patient safety and experience, are then considered and finally population health outcome measures, such as life expectancy and cancer survival rates are discussed.

Health determinants: smoking, obesity, exercise and diet

Smoking, obesity and physical activity all have an impact on the overall level of population health in the United Kingdom. An underpinning assumption of the 2002 review was that public health and its impact on public engagement in health was crucial to determining which of the three scenario projections would ultimately be realised (Wanless 2002). The importance of public health in achieving the most optimistic 2002 review scenario was expanded on in the 2004 review; this concluded that the activity currently under way could put the nation on course for the solid progress scenario, as far as public health is concerned, but that a step change would be needed to move to the fully engaged path (Wanless 2004).

HEALTH PROMOTION EXPENDITURE

The 2002 review estimated that health promotion expenditure in England at the time – covering smoking, diet, blood pressure, exercise, obesity and alcohol, among other factors – was around £250 million. All three scenarios projected an increase in health promotion spend, with the fully engaged scenario seeing the largest and most rapid rise in expenditure, doubling to around £500 million by 2007/8 and enabling public health targets to be met and exceeded. Solid progress envisaged public health targets being met as expenditure rose in line with spending on GP and hospital care. The worst outcomes occurred in the slow progress scenario, where health promotion expenditure increased

TABLE 48: REAL COST OF DEPARTMENT OF HEALTH PUBLIC HEALTH CAMPAIGNS

Campaign	Real cost (£ million)[1]								
	1997/8	1998/9	1999/2000	2000/1	2001/2	2002/3	2003/4	2004/5	2005/6
Antibiotics	–	0.29	1.34	–	0.80	0.59	0.99	–	0.36
Campaign against living miserably (CALM)	0.55	0.13	0.55	0.68	0.39	0.58	0.42	0.42	0.30
Drugs[2]	–	–	–	–	–	–	1.70	2.48	3.02
Flu	0.26	0.31	0.09	4.56	1.49	2.40	1.89	2.13	2.15
Hepatitis C	–	–	–	–	–	–	0.15	0.66	1.19
Immunisation	–	–	–	–	1.72	2.36	3.53	2.93	1.25
Mental health (Mind Out)	–	–	–	–	1.00	1.01	1.57	–	–
Teenage pregnancy (Sexwise)	0.88	0.93	1.32	4.06	2.52	1.97	2.09	–	–
Sexual health	–	–	–	–	0.31	1.50	1.55	1.20	0.58
Smoking	–	–	16.59	14.49	12.68	11.56	22.73	25.05	28.30
TB awareness	–	–	–	–	0.31	0.09	0.01	0.19	–
Fruit/veg consumption ('5-a-day')	–	–	–	0.53	0.52	0.48	1.00	0.85	0.85
Total	1.69	1.66	19.87	24.32	21.74	22.54	37.63	35.90	38.00

Source: Adapted from *Hansard* 2007a
[1] 2002/3 prices
[2] Departmental contribution to the Frank substance misuse campaign has been jointly funded by the Department of Health, Home Office and Department for Education and Skills.

only in line with population growth and inflation. This scenario envisaged minimal public engagement and, at best, limited change in such public health outcomes as smoking, exercise and diet.

It is impossible to measure trends in public health or spending on health promotion in relation to the 2002 review's recommendations, since there are no official figures to analyse. However, some indication of spending can be gleaned from the Department of Health's National Programme Budget Project (NPBP) initiative. The NPBP includes a programme budget category called 'healthy individuals', which aims to capture expenditure on people who have no current health problems but are involved in programmes for preventing illness and promoting good health.

In 2005/6, gross cash expenditure on this programme in England was around £2.46 billion, up from £2.17 billion in 2004/5 (an increase of 13.4 per cent); this was, in turn, an increase of 7.4 per cent over spending of £2.02 billion in 2003/4 (Department of Health 2005c and 2006e) . These figures should be viewed with some caution, particularly when compared with the 2002 review's original estimate of current spending on health promotion at around £250 million. It is important to note that this programme's definition of health promotion spend is different from the one used by the 2002 review, and also that some health promotion expenditure is undertaken by other stakeholders, including the private sector. Furthermore, NPBP data will be subject to some uncertainty, particularly for its first year and for this particular programme.

A further source of information is expenditure on Department of Health public health campaigns. Table 48, opposite, shows that £38 million was spent on departmental public health campaigns in 2005/6, of which almost two thirds was related to smoking (Hansard 2007a). At 2002/3 prices, Department of Health expenditure on public health campaigns increased in real terms by £15.46 million between 2002/3 and 2005/6 – a real increase of

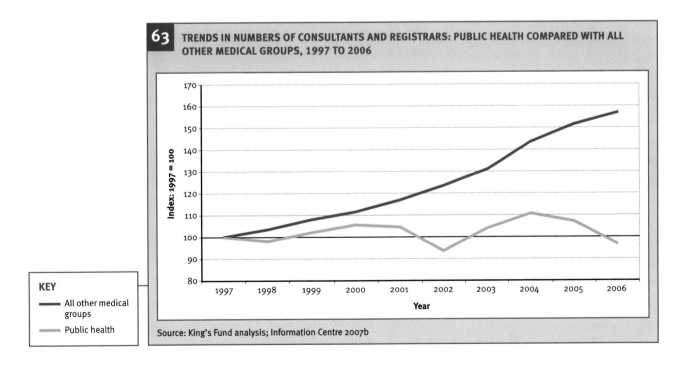

63 TRENDS IN NUMBERS OF CONSULTANTS AND REGISTRARS: PUBLIC HEALTH COMPARED WITH ALL OTHER MEDICAL GROUPS, 1997 TO 2006

KEY
—— All other medical groups
—— Public health

Source: King's Fund analysis; Information Centre 2007b

almost 70 per cent. Between 2004/5 and 2005/6, the real cash increase in expenditure was £2.1 million, representing a real increase of almost 6 per cent.

Another indication of the priority given to public health and health promotion comes from employment trends among NHS medical staff. Figure 63, p 167, shows that, while senior medical staff numbers have risen by nearly 60 per cent since 1997, numbers of public health consultants and registrars have, uniquely, declined overall.

The lack of robust data makes it very difficult to assess whether or not expenditure on health promotion has followed any of the original Wanless trajectories. NPBP data suggests a cash increase between 2003/4 and 2005/6 of around £440 million – up by more than a fifth in cash terms and around 16 per cent in real terms. However, over this period the real increase in departmental spend on public health campaigns was only 1 per cent. And, as the Chief Medical Officer's 2005 annual report noted, local public health budgets have been regularly 'raided' to find funding to reduce hospital deficits or to meet productivity targets. It is hard to disagree with Sir Liam Donaldson's assessment that public health spending is 'way off' the fully engaged and more in line with slow uptake (Donaldson 2006).

EVIDENCE ABOUT KEY DETERMINANTS OF HEALTH

The health of individuals and the population as a whole is influenced by a range of factors, some relating to direct intervention by health services and others to lifestyle choices. Individual health is also a consequence of genetic inheritance, income, housing, employment and education. Although all of these factors are important, this section considers four key determinants in detail: smoking, obesity, diet and physical activity.

Solid progress in the 2002 review envisaged that public engagement with health determinants would be achieved in line with government targets. The fully engaged scenario assumed that these targets would be attained more quickly than planned before being exceeded or maintained, while slow uptake assumed that health determinants would remain largely unchanged. The 2004 review outlined the framework and processes required to encourage public engagement with health. However, progress in implementing the recommended framework has been slow and, in some respects, non-existent.

SMOKING

The adverse health impacts of smoking are well known. As Figures 64 and 65, opposite, demonstrate, smoking could have been responsible for more than 1.4 million hospital admissions in England in 2004/5 (a rising trend since 1995/6), while deaths attributable to smoking accounted for around 18 per cent of all deaths in 2004.

By comparison with other European countries, the prevalence of smoking among men in the United Kingdom is relatively low (*see* Figure 66, p 170).

The proportion of UK women who smoke is relatively high (*see* Figure 67, p 170). However, while some European countries – such as France, Greece and Germany – saw increases in the prevalence of smoking between 1994–8 and 2002–5, the UK prevalence has fallen.

The 2002 review envisaged that reductions in the prevalence of smoking in the solid progress scenario would be in line with the government's public health targets. Under the

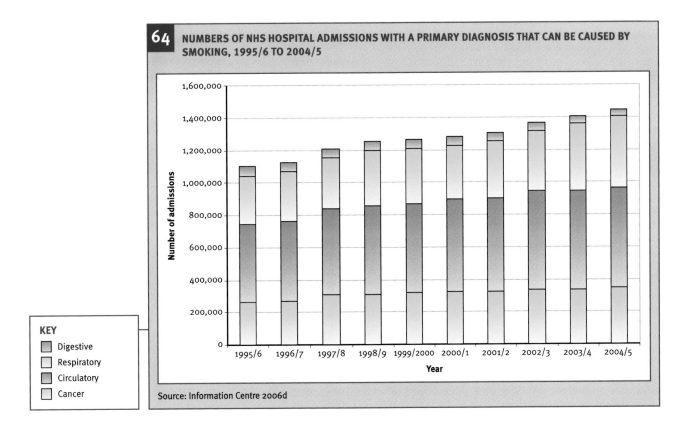

64 NUMBERS OF NHS HOSPITAL ADMISSIONS WITH A PRIMARY DIAGNOSIS THAT CAN BE CAUSED BY SMOKING, 1995/6 TO 2004/5

KEY
- Digestive
- Respiratory
- Circulatory
- Cancer

Source: Information Centre 2006d

fully engaged scenario, these targets would be realised more rapidly and then exceeded, while the slow progress scenario saw little change in the prevalence of smoking.

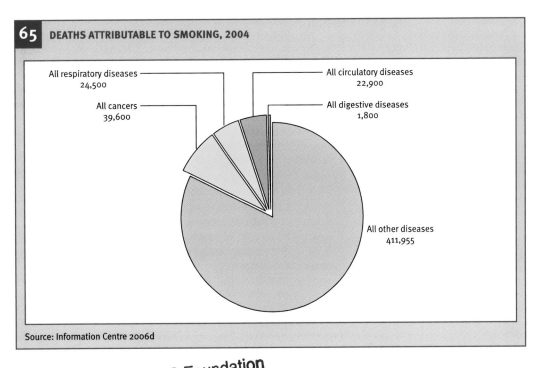

65 DEATHS ATTRIBUTABLE TO SMOKING, 2004

All respiratory diseases
24,500

All cancers
39,600

All circulatory diseases
22,900

All digestive diseases
1,800

All other diseases
411,955

Source: Information Centre 2006d

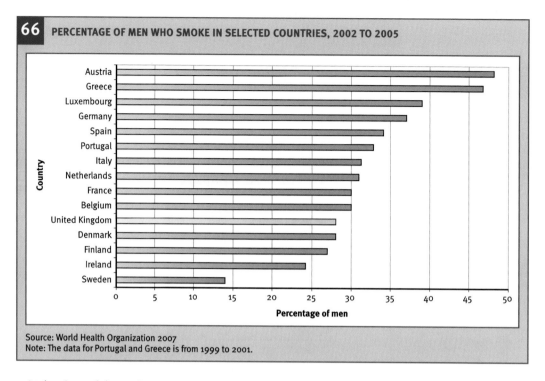

66 PERCENTAGE OF MEN WHO SMOKE IN SELECTED COUNTRIES, 2002 TO 2005

Source: World Health Organization 2007
Note: The data for Portugal and Greece is from 1999 to 2001.

At the time of the review, government strategy was formalised in the 1998 White Paper, *Smoking Kills: A White Paper on tobacco* (Department of Health 1998b), which specified three targets:

■ to reduce smoking among children, from 13 per cent to 11 per cent by 2005 and to 9 per cent or less by 2010

■ to reduce adult smoking in all social classes, with the overall rate falling from 28 per cent to 26 per cent by 2005 and to 24 per cent or less by 2010

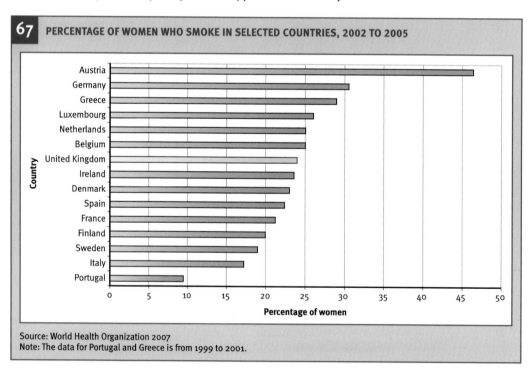

67 PERCENTAGE OF WOMEN WHO SMOKE IN SELECTED COUNTRIES, 2002 TO 2005

Source: World Health Organization 2007
Note: The data for Portugal and Greece is from 1999 to 2001.

■ to reduce the proportion of pregnant women smokers from 23 per cent to 18 per cent by 2005 and to 15 per cent by 2010.

In 2004 the Department of Health agreed a new Public Service Agreement (PSA) target with the Treasury to reduce adult smoking rates to 21 per cent or less by 2010, with a reduction to 26 per cent or less among routine and manual groups.

The last 30 years have witnessed a substantial decline in the proportion of adults in England who smoke cigarettes; however, much of this decline occurred before the mid-1990s. The 2005 General Household Survey (Office for National Statistics 2006a) reported that 24 per cent of adults in England were cigarette smokers in that year, 1 per cent less than in 2004. Smoking prevalence among adults in the routine and manual socio-economic groups was, at 31 per cent, the same as in 2002. The proportion of children aged 11–15 considered to be regular smokers was 9 per cent in 2005 – 1 per cent less than in 2002.

Early results from the 2005 Infant Feeding Survey (Bolling 2006) found that the proportion of women in England who smoked throughout pregnancy fell from 19 per cent in 2000 to 17 per cent in 2005, with the UK average falling from 20 per cent to 17 per cent over the same period. The relevant 2005 figures for other UK countries were 22 per cent in Wales, 20 per cent in Scotland and 18 per cent in Northern Ireland.

The impact of socio-economic grouping was significant: smoking prevalence among pregnant women in routine and manual groups was 29 per cent, compared with 24 per cent among those who had never worked, 12 per cent for those in 'intermediate occupations' and just 7 per cent for those in managerial and professional groups. There

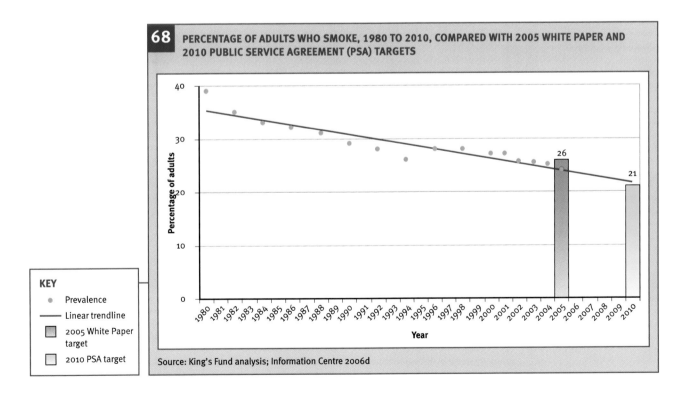

68 PERCENTAGE OF ADULTS WHO SMOKE, 1980 TO 2010, COMPARED WITH 2005 WHITE PAPER AND 2010 PUBLIC SERVICE AGREEMENT (PSA) TARGETS

KEY
- Prevalence
— Linear trendline
▪ 2005 White Paper target
▫ 2010 PSA target

Source: King's Fund analysis; Information Centre 2006d

TABLE 49: PROGRESS TOWARDS 1998 WHITE PAPER SMOKING REDUCTION TARGETS, BY GROUP, 2005

Group	Percentage of smokers			
	1998 baseline	2005 target	2010 target	2005 actual
Children	13	11	9	9
Adults	28	26	24	24
Pregnant women	23	18	15	17

Source: Bolling 2006; Goddard 2006; Information Centre 2006d

was also a clear correlation between smoking and age, with 45 per cent of mothers aged 20 or under smoking in pregnancy, compared with 9 per cent of those aged 35 and over.

In England, all of the original 1998 White Paper's intermediate 2005 public health targets for smoking have been met, and for children and adults the 2010 targets were met in 2005 (*see* Table 49, above).

More demanding targets were formalised as Public Service Agreements in 2004 and, although England seems on track to achieve the headline population targets (*see* Figure 68, p 171), large variations remain between socio-economic groups. Evidence of progress in reducing these inequalities is weak, at best. Between 2001 and 2005 there was an 11 per cent reduction in the prevalence of all adult smokers, compared with a 6 per cent reduction for routine and manual group adults (Goddard 2006). Although the evidence is not conclusive, these trends suggest that the PSA target to reduce the prevalence of

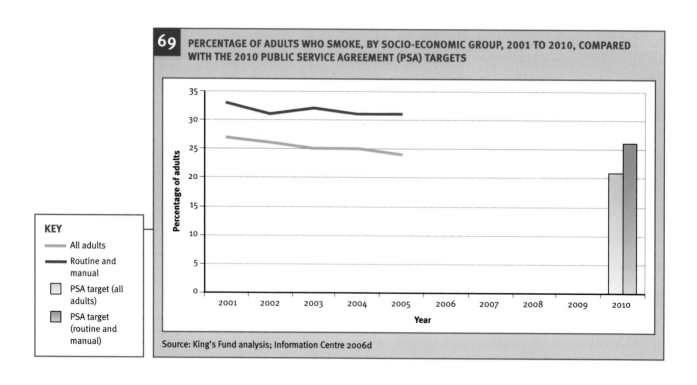

69 PERCENTAGE OF ADULTS WHO SMOKE, BY SOCIO-ECONOMIC GROUP, 2001 TO 2010, COMPARED WITH THE 2010 PUBLIC SERVICE AGREEMENT (PSA) TARGETS

KEY
All adults
Routine and manual
PSA target (all adults)
PSA target (routine and manual)

Source: King's Fund analysis; Information Centre 2006d

smoking in routine and manual groups to 26 per cent or less by 2010 may not be achieved (*see* Figure 69, opposite). In this case, the gap between this group and the rest of the population would probably increase.

Progress to date in realising national smoking targets in England places achievements firmly on a solid progress trajectory. However, the more aspirational targets set since the 2002 review, while less demanding than the fully engaged scenario are more demanding than solid progress.

OBESITY

Obesity is responsible for more than 9,000 premature deaths a year in England and is an important risk factor for a number of chronic diseases, including heart disease, stroke, some cancers and type 2 diabetes (Department of Health 2007h). The Health Committee estimated the economic cost of obesity at between £3.3 and £3.7 billion in 2002, with around 30 per cent of these costs falling directly on the NHS. Increasing levels of obesity will mean higher costs in future.

The National Audit Office has emphasised the health gains of reducing obesity: for example, one million fewer obese people in England could mean around 15,000 fewer

TABLE 50: PREVALENCE OF ADULT MALE OBESITY ACROSS THE EU-15 COUNTRIES (RANKED BY PERCENTAGE OF OBESE MALES)

Country	Year of data collection	Percentage overweight but not obese	Percentage obese	Combined overweight and obese (%)
Austria	2005/6	42.3	23.3	65.6
England	2004	43.9	22.7	66.6
Germany*	2002/3	52.9	22.5	75.4
Ireland	1997–9	46.3	20.1	66.4
Greece (ATTICA)	2001/2	53.0	20.0	73.0
Finland	1997	48.0	19.8	67.8
Luxembourg	na	45.6	15.3	60.9
Sweden (Göteborg)	2002	43.5	14.8	58.3
Portugal	2003/4	44.1	14.5	58.6
Belgium	1994–7	49.0	14.0	63.0
Spain	1990–2000	45.0	13.4	58.4
Denmark*	2001	40.1	11.8	51.9
France*	2006	35.6	11.8	47.4
Netherlands	1998–2002	43.5	10.4	53.9
Italy	2003	42.1	9.3	51.4

Source: International Association for the Study of Obesity 2007
Note: Age range and year of data in surveys may differ; data is not age standardised; and self-reported surveys (*see* below) may underestimate true prevalence.
* Figures are self-reported.

TABLE 51: PREVALENCE OF ADULT FEMALE OBESITY ACROSS THE EU-15 COUNTRIES (RANKED BY PERCENTAGE OF OBESE FEMALES)

Country	Year of data collection	Percentage overweight but not obese	Percentage obese	Combined overweight and obese (%)
England	2004	34.7	23.8	58.5
Germany*	2002/3	35.6	23.3	58.9
Austria	2005/6	32.4	20.8	53.2
Finland	1997	33.0	19.4	52.4
Ireland	1997–9	32.5	15.9	48.4
Spain	1990–2000	32.2	15.8	48.0
Greece (ATTICA)	2001/2	31.0	15.0	46.0
Portugal	2003/4	31.9	14.6	46.5
Luxembourg	na	30.7	13.9	44.6
Belgium	1994–7	28.0	13.0	41.0
France*	2006	23.3	13.0	36.3
Denmark*	2001	26.9	12.5	39.4
Sweden (Göteborg)	2002	26.6	11.0	37.6
Netherlands	1998–2002	28.5	10.1	38.6
Italy	2003	25.8	8.7	34.5

Source: International Association for the Study of Obesity 2007
Note: Age range and year of data in surveys may differ; data is not age standardised; and self-reported surveys (*see* below) may underestimate true prevalence.
* Figures are self-reported.

people with coronary heart disease, 34,000 fewer people developing type 2 diabetes and 99,000 fewer people with high blood pressure. For definitions of obesity, *see* box, below.

The 2002 review's solid progress scenario assumed that the rising prevalence of obesity would first slow and then go into reverse, so that by 2005 the Health of the Nation target for obesity (still the most recent target set, although by then wildly ambitious) would be

---

OBESITY DEFINED

Obesity is commonly defined by reference to the body mass index (BMI), which is calculated as weight in kilograms divided by height in metres squared. A BMI ‹18.5 is classified as underweight, 18.5-25 as healthy weight, 25-30 as overweight and ›30 as obese. A BMI of ›35 is classified as 'morbidly obese' and ›40 as extreme obesity. Children are defined as overweight and obese if their BMI falls above the 85th and 95th centile respectively of the reference curve for their age and gender.

It should be noted that, while BMI provides an indication of possible adverse health effects, the association is not perfect. Other weight/mass/body fat measures (such as amount and location of internal fat) can be better indicators but are less easily measurable for the whole population.

met, with just 6 per cent of men and 8 per cent of women classified as obese. As with smoking, the fully engaged scenario assumed that the Health of the Nation obesity target would be achieved more rapidly and then maintained, while the slow uptake scenario assumed no change in the prevalence of obesity.

International comparisons of the prevalence of overweight and obesity have recently been collated by the International Association for the Study of Obesity (IASO). Although the data is not directly comparable, Tables 50 and 51, p 173 and opposite, emphasise the problem facing England. Across the EU 15, England ranks second only to Austria in terms of adult male obesity and is top of the list for women.

The IASO has also collated international information on the proportions of overweight children. As with adults, England performs poorly, ranking fourth (behind Spain, Greece and Portugal) in terms of the percentage of boys classified as overweight and third (behind Spain and Portugal) for girls (*see* Table 52, below).

Since the 2002 review, the prevalence of obesity has continued to rise (*see* Figures 70 and 71, overleaf). Consequently, a PSA target for obesity was set for the first time in July 2004 with the aim of '...halting the year-on-year rise in obesity among children aged under 11 by 2010 in the context of a broader strategy to tackle obesity in the population as a whole' (HM Treasury 2004).

TABLE 52: PREVALENCE OF OVERWEIGHT CHILDREN ACROSS THE EU-15 COUNTRIES (RANKED BY PERCENTAGE OF OVERWEIGHT BOYS)

Country	Year of data collection	Age range (years)	Percentage overweight	
			Boys	Girls
Spain	2000/2	13–14	35.0	32.0
Greece	2003	13–17	29.6	16.1
Portugal	2002/3	7–9	29.5	34.3
England	2004	5–17	29.0	29.3
Belgium	1998–9	5–15	27.7	26.8
Italy	1993–2001	5–17	26.6	24.8
Austria	2003	8–12	22.5	16.7
France	2000	7–9	17.9	18.2
Sweden	2001	6–11	17.6	27.4
Finland*	1999	12, 14 and 16	17.2	10.1
Denmark	1996/7	5–16	14.1	15.3
Germany	1995	5–17	14.1	14.0
Netherlands	1997	5–17	8.8	11.8
Luxembourg	na	na	na	na
Ireland*	2001/2	10–16	13.7	13.7

Source: International Association for the Study of Obesity 2007
Note: Age range and year of data in surveys may differ; data is not age standardised; and self-reported surveys (*see* below) may underestimate true prevalence.
* Figures are self-reported.

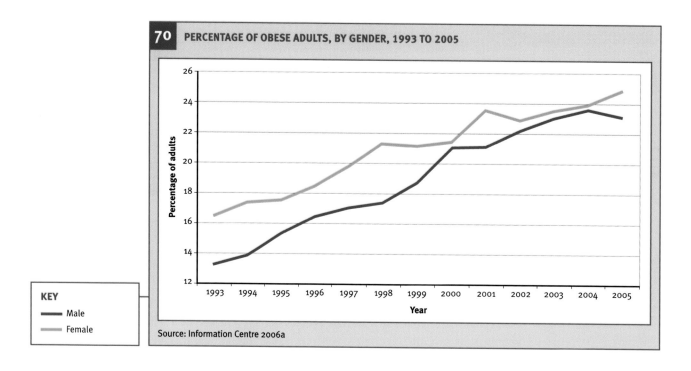

70 PERCENTAGE OF OBESE ADULTS, BY GENDER, 1993 TO 2005

KEY
Male
Female

Source: Information Centre 2006a

Data collected in the Health Survey for England (The Information Centre 2006a) shows the rise in the prevalence of obesity in England. Between 1995 and 2005 the proportion of adult males classified as obese rose by 51 per cent to stand at 23.1 per cent of the male adult population, while prevalence among women rose by 42 per cent to 24.8 per cent. Obesity prevalence in children (aged 2–15) has shown similar increases over this period, with the prevalence of obese boys rising by 65 per cent and obese girls by 51 per cent to stand at 18 and 18.1 per cent of their respective populations (Figure 71, opposite).

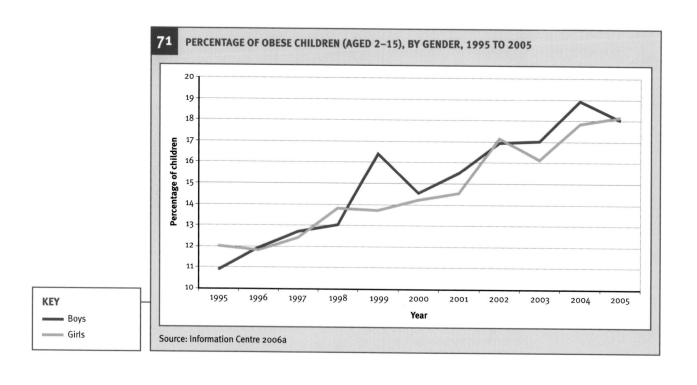

71 PERCENTAGE OF OBESE CHILDREN (AGED 2–15), BY GENDER, 1995 TO 2005

KEY
Boys
Girls

Source: Information Centre 2006a

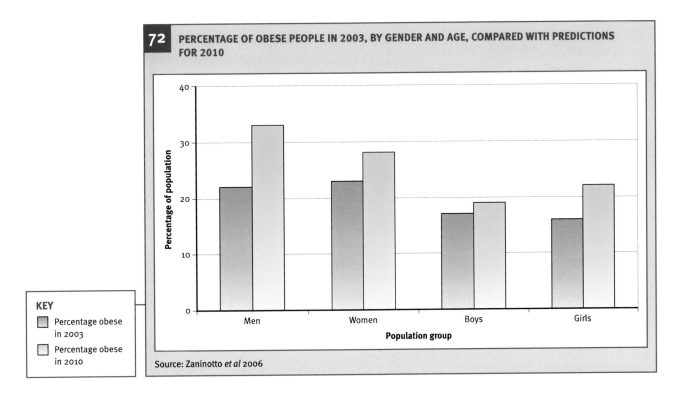

72 PERCENTAGE OF OBESE PEOPLE IN 2003, BY GENDER AND AGE, COMPARED WITH PREDICTIONS FOR 2010

KEY
- Percentage obese in 2003
- Percentage obese in 2010

Source: Zaninotto *et al* 2006

The 2006 National Centre for Social Research report *Forecasting Obesity to 2010* (Zaninotto *et al* 2006), prepared for the Department of Health, suggests a continuing rising trend in obesity to 2010 (*see* Figure 72, above). The report estimates that in 2010 around 6.7 million men (33 per cent) will be obese, increasing from around 4.3 million in 2003. The corresponding rise for women over the same period is estimated at 1.2 million, bringing the projected proportion of obese women in 2010 to 28 per cent. Obesity among children is also projected to rise, with the number of obese boys rising from around 750,000 in 2003 to nearly 800,000 in 2010 (equivalent to nearly a fifth of all boys aged 2–15). But the largest increases are expected among girls, with around a 6 per cent rise in obesity rates between 2003 and 2010, when some 910,000 girls (more than a fifth of those aged 2–15) are expected to be obese. The proportion of obese children aged 2–11 is also forecast to rise by 2010.

It should not come as a surprise to learn that the Health of the Nation targets for 2005 have not been met. The number of obese people in England looks set to rise up to 2010 (and possibly beyond). If this were to happen, it would seems unlikely that the 2004 PSA obesity target for children could be achieved by 2010. Even if this target *were* met and the upward trend in child obesity were to level off, the health benefits would not be realised until the middle of the century. This is a worse performance than slow uptake.

PHYSICAL ACTIVITY

Physical activity and diet are both areas where greater population engagement is required to halt the rising prevalence of obesity and combat other ill health effects of sedentary lifestyles. As with other determinants of health, the 2002 review defined a solid progress path as one where existing government targets and recommendations for physical activity were met. Again, the fully engaged path saw targets being achieved sooner, then exceeded, while slow uptake saw physical activity levels remaining largely unchanged.

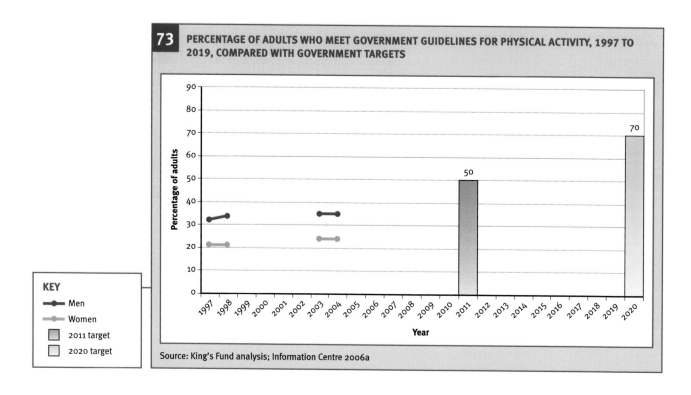

73 PERCENTAGE OF ADULTS WHO MEET GOVERNMENT GUIDELINES FOR PHYSICAL ACTIVITY, 1997 TO 2019, COMPARED WITH GOVERNMENT TARGETS

KEY
- Men
- Women
- 2011 target
- 2020 target

Source: King's Fund analysis; Information Centre 2006a

Since 1996, the government has recommended that adults should participate in at least 30 minutes of moderately intense activity on five days a week, and this recommendation was restated by the Chief Medical Officer in his 2004 report *At Least Five a Week* (Department of Health 2004b). The target in England is for 70 per cent of adults to have achieved physical activity levels in line with this recommendation by 2020, with an interim target of 50 per cent by 2011 (Department of Health Strategy Unit 2002).

Although physical activity levels remain low in England, Health Survey for England data shows that the proportion of adults meeting the physical activity guidelines has been rising. More than a third of men and a quarter of women met the current physical activity guidelines in 2004 – respective increases of just under a third and around a fifth since 1997 (*see* Figure 73, above). The government may achieve its interim target (which would represent solid progress at best) but this will require sustained effort up to and beyond 2011.

The *At Least Five a Week* report also restated the recommendation that all children and young people aged 5–18 should participate in at least one hour a day of moderate physical activity; however, the children's physical activity target in England relates to the proportion of school children spending at least two hours a week on high-quality sport. Targets have been formalised in a PSA – shared with the Departments for Education and Skills, and Culture, Media and Sport – to increase this proportion from 25 per cent in 2002 to 75 per cent in 2006, and 85 per cent in 2008.

Progress towards the children's physical activity targets has been significant. The School Sport Survey 2005/6 (TNS 2006) found that 80 per cent of pupils in partnership schools (accounting for 80 per cent of schools in England) participate in at least two hours of high-quality physical education and school sport in a typical week – a rise of 11 per cent on the previous year. This means that the 2006 school sport PSA target has actually been *exceeded* by 5 per cent. Since the survey was undertaken *all* schools in England have come within a school sports partnership (Department for Education and Skills 2006). Additionally, 70 per cent of boys and 61 per cent of girls aged 2–15 met the government's physical activity guideline in 2002.

DIET

As with physical activity, diet is seen as a factor in the challenge to reduce levels of obesity. The 2002 review's solid progress scenario assumed that diet would improve in line with government targets, changing most rapidly in the fully engaged scenario and very little under slow uptake (Wanless 2002).

The Department of Health's 2005 publication *Choosing a Better Diet: A food and health action plan* (Department of Health 2005a), provides the following six dietary objectives for England:

- increase average consumption of a variety of fruit and vegetables to at least five portions per day
- increase the average intake of dietary fibre to 18 g per day
- reduce average intake of salt to 6g per day by 2010
- reduce average intake of saturated fat to 11 per cent of food energy
- maintain the current trend for reducing average intake of total fat to 35 per cent of food energy
- reduce the average intake of added sugar to 11 per cent of food energy.

Crucially, five of these are recommendations rather than targets. Only salt intake is referred to as a target, with a defined time frame for delivery, in the Food Standards Agency's (FSA) strategic plan for 2005–2010. Furthermore, in March 2006 the FSA published voluntary salt reduction targets for food manufacturers and retailers to encourage a reduction in the amount of salt in processed foods. Although there are many dietary objectives, here the focus is on just two: salt intake and fruit and vegetable consumption.

Salt intake

Findings from the Expenditure and Food Surveys show that between 2001 and 2004 the average intake of sodium per person per day in England was 3.1g, excluding sodium from table salt. This equates to around 7.7g of salt, which is almost 2 per cent above recommended levels, even excluding the consumption of table salt.

More recent research, using urinary sodium tests, carried out in 2005/6 (National Centre for Social Research 2006) shows that salt consumption in Great Britain is falling, but remains 50 per cent higher than the recommended 6g per day. Average adult salt intake in Great Britain (and in England) was found to be 9g per day, compared with 9.5g in 2001. Men consumed an average 10.2g per day compared with 11g in 2001, while average intake among women fell from 8.1g to 7.6g per day over the same period.

Fruit and vegetables

The Health Survey for England indicates that mean consumption of fruit and vegetables per day in 2005 was 3.7 pieces for adults and 3.1 for children. The proportion of adults and children consuming five or more pieces of fruit or vegetables a day in 2005 was 28 per cent and 17 per cent respectively. These findings show an improvement in both mean daily

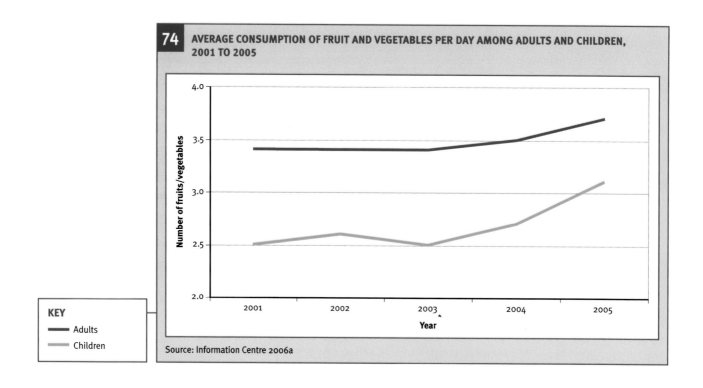

74 AVERAGE CONSUMPTION OF FRUIT AND VEGETABLES PER DAY AMONG ADULTS AND CHILDREN, 2001 TO 2005

KEY
— Adults
— Children

Source: Information Centre 2006a

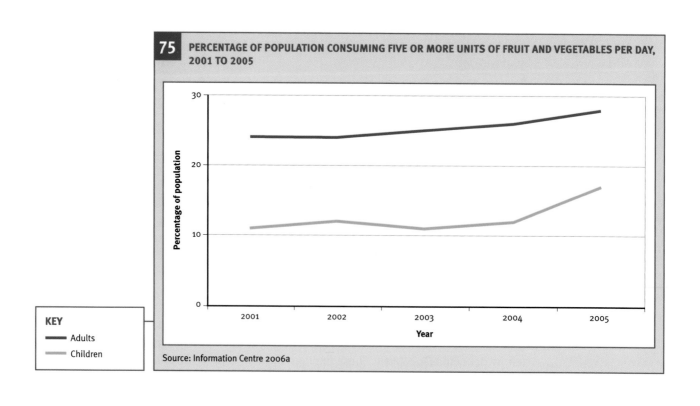

75 PERCENTAGE OF POPULATION CONSUMING FIVE OR MORE UNITS OF FRUIT AND VEGETABLES PER DAY, 2001 TO 2005

KEY
— Adults
— Children

Source: Information Centre 2006a

consumption and the proportion consuming five or more a day by comparison with 2001 (*see* Figures 74 and 75, opposite).

Thus, progress has been made since 2002 in reducing salt intake and increasing fruit and vegetable consumption – but it has been slow. Salt intake remains significantly higher than the target of 6g per day, while fruit and vegetable consumption remains well below the aspirational five-a-day target, especially for children. Although this is better than slow uptake, it seems likely to fall short of solid progress.

Given the lack of accurate information on public health expenditure since the 2002 review, it is impossible to assess whether the fully engaged aspirations for a doubling in public health spending by 2007/8 have been met. More fundamentally, it is also extremely difficult to determine the extent to which the observed changes in some of the key determinants of health are attributable to public health activities. Furthermore, optimistic targets, such as those relating to obesity, make it more difficult to assess engagement levels in accordance with the 2002 review scenarios. Nevertheless, the evidence to date suggests that the population is on a path that lies somewhere between slow uptake and solid progress and is therefore well short of full engagement.

SUMMARY: HEALTH DETERMINANTS

- The solid progress scenario in the 2002 review envisaged that public engagement with health determinants (including smoking, physical activity, diet and others) would be achieved in line with government targets. The fully engaged scenario assumed faster attainment of these targets, while slow uptake saw them largely unachieved.
- A lack of robust time series information on public health expenditure makes it difficult to assess whether expenditure on health promotion has followed any of the 2002 review trajectories. National Programme Budget Project data shows a cash increase between 2003/4 and 2005/6 of around £440 million for the 'healthy individuals' programme budget category – a rise of more than a fifth in cash terms and around 16 per cent in real terms.
- All the intermediate public health smoking targets set out in 1998 in *Smoking Kills: A White Paper on tobacco* have been met, and it is likely that the 2010 targets will also be achieved. More demanding PSA targets have now been set and, although England seems on track to achieve the overall target for smoking reduction, socio-economic variations in the prevalence of smoking seem set to remain and may even widen.
- The Health of the Nation obesity targets will not be met, and have since been surpassed with a loosely worded PSA target. The numbers of obese people in England are expected to rise between 2003 and 2010, so the PSA target to halt the year-on-year rise in obesity among children aged under 11 by 2010 is unlikely to be met.
- Physical activity targets for adults and children are likely to be achieved, although sustained effort will be required. However, progress has been slow in improving the population's diet, and the salt intake target of 6g per day by 2010 is unlikely to be attained.
- The evidence rules out a fully engaged scenario of public engagement in improving the determinants of health. Public engagement falls somewhere between solid progress and slow uptake.

Process outcomes: safety, choice, access and satisfaction

Health improvements are not the only beneficial outcomes of extra investment in health care. Other non-health outcomes, such as improved safety, shorter waiting times and greater choice, are also of value to patients.

Below four key process outcomes are reviewed:
- patient safety
- choice and privacy
- access and waiting times
- patient experience.

PATIENT SAFETY

Activities geared towards improving the safety of NHS patients are wide-ranging. The 2002 review saw the main driver for improvements in safety as increased time spent by NHS staff on clinical governance activities. The review assumed that by 2010/1, 10 per cent of staff time would be devoted to clinical governance, with the following benefits emerging relatively quickly:
- 15 per cent reduction in hospital-acquired infections (HAI) in acute care by 2012/3
- 10 per cent reduction in other adverse incidents in acute care by 2012/3
- 25 per cent reduction in the clinical negligence bill arising from incidents in obstetrics and gynaecology by 2005 (Wanless 2002).

In addition to the health benefits of better patient safety in the NHS, there are significant financial savings to be made, since the costs to the NHS of dealing with patient safety incidents is high. These include an estimated £2 billion a year for extra time spent in hospital, £1 billion for associated infections and more than £400 million for clinical negligence claims (Healthcare Commission 2006c).

Incidents involving patient safety

The National Patient Safety Agency (NPSA) is responsible for co-ordinating efforts to improve the safety of NHS patients in England and Wales. A central part of the NPSA's role is the national reporting and learning system (NRLS), which collates reports of incidents affecting patient safety.

TABLE 53: PERCENTAGE OF NHS STAFF WITNESSING POTENTIALLY HARMFUL ERRORS, NEAR MISSES OR INCIDENTS IN THE LAST MONTH, BY GROUPS AT RISK OF BEING HARMED, 2003 TO 2005

Groups at risk of being harmed	Percentage of NHS staff witnessing errors, near misses or incidents		
	2003	2004	2005
Patients	35	35	32
Staff	36	31	27
Either	47	44	40

Source: Healthcare Commission 2006b

The NPSA's Autumn 2006 *Quarterly National Reporting and Learning System data summary* reports that for the quarter up to the end of June 2006, NHS trusts reported 788,188 incidents to the NRLS in England and Wales. However, the total number of incidents would have been higher than this because many trusts have only recently started using the NRLS. The majority of incidents reported to the NRLS (68 per cent) involved no harm to patients and a further 25 per cent involved only minor or minimal harm. However, 5 per cent involved moderate (but no permanent) harm, 0.9 per cent involved severe permanent harm and 0.4 per cent involved the death of a patient.

The lack of historical data makes it difficult to assess how the number of incidents involving the safety of patients has changed in recent years. However, evidence from the Healthcare Commission's annual survey of NHS staff (Healthcare Commission 2006b) suggests that the situation has been improving (*see* Table 53, opposite).

Given the current limitations of the NRLS and the absence of a robust time series of data, it is difficult to assess progress towards the 2002 review's assumption of a 10 per cent reduction in non-HAI adverse incidents in acute care by 2012/3. Previous work (Department of Health 2000a) has suggested that in England alone there may be around 850,000 adverse events each year in the NHS; and a survey of all NHS trusts in England in 2004/5 by the National Audit Office estimated that there had been 1.3 million incidents

TABLE 54: CLAIMS RECEIVED AND DAMAGES PAID UNDER CLINICAL NEGLIGENCE SCHEME FOR TRUSTS (CNST) IN TOTAL AND IN OBSTETRICS, 1995/6 TO 2006/7

Incident year	Number of obstetrics claims received	Number of claims received	Damages paid on settled obstetrics claims	Damages paid on all settled claims	Percentage of damages paid on obstetrics claims of all damages paid
1995/6	943	6,056	109,992,847	231,701,442	47.5
1996/7	975	5,958	114,298,044	219,068,052	52.2
1997/8	956	6,099	87,834,687	198,269,595	44.3
1998/9	913	6,196	71,266,303	204,880,312	34.8
1999/2000	782	5,622	65,123,682	169,943,116	38.3
2000/1	753	5,515	27,306,108	131,087,657	20.8
2001/2	641	5,069	11,456,127	104,175,586	11.0
2002/3	664	5,220	8,929,192	53,794,385	16.6
2003/4	609	4,591	2,966,080	21,882,270	13.6
2004/5	412	3,046	1,283,844	8,982,119	14.3
2005/6	238	1,821	309,507	1,877,238	16.5
2006/7*	29	352	0	113,786	–
Total	**7,915**	**55,545**	**500,766,421**	**1,345,775,557**	**37.2**

Source: NHS Litigation Authority 2007
Notes: In each case, the incident date has been used rather than the date the claim was made as this reflects what was happening in trusts at the time. This means that the numbers per year could change as new claims continue to come in, particularly in the more recent years. The payment figures given are for the damages paid to the claimant; they do not include cost payments. Finally, the claims information relates to claims settled in a particular year, however, the money paid out is usually made over a longer period of time. The payments shown for a particular year therefore do not correspond with the incidents occurring in the same year. For example, the figure of £2,966,080 against 2003/4 is made up of whole or partial damages payments to a number of different claimants whose claims were settled in that year but which relate to incidents occurring up to eight years previously.
* as at 28 February 2007

involving patient safety, including an estimated 300,000 involving healthcare-associated infections. Information collected by the NRLS on the percentage of incidents occurring in acute/general hospitals and the percentage related to infection control suggests that in 2000 around 601,000 non-HAI adverse events occurred in acute care in England and around 719,000 in 2004/5. Based on these figures, it would take a significant drop to around 594,000 adverse incidence in acute care in 2012/3 to realise the 10 per cent reduction envisaged by the 2002 review.

The review also assumed a reduction in the clinical negligence bill by 2005, driven by a 25 per cent reduction in the number of negligent incidents in obstetrics and gynaecology. Table 54, p 183, shows how many claims have been made under the Clinical Negligence Scheme for Trusts (CNST) in each year since 1995, as well as the number of obstetrics claims and the totals paid out in compensation. However, the significant time lag between the occurrence of potentially negligent acts and final settlement of claims for compensation (which can be anything up to 21 years in the case of birth injury, or indefinitely if there is brain damage), makes it impossible to establish the outcomes of negligent incidents in obstetrics and gynaecology in 2005, the 2002 review target date for 25 per cent reduction.

Hospital cleanliness

The two main sources of information on hospital cleanliness are surveys of patients and data collected by the patient environment action teams (PEAT). The PEAT reviews have reported progressive improvements in cleanliness of hospitals in England over the past few years. However, the proportion of hospitals classified as 'poor' or 'unacceptable' more than doubled between 2004 and 2006 (*see* Table 55, below).

TABLE 55: NATIONAL RESULTS FOR QUALITY OF PATIENT ENVIRONMENT (CLEANLINESS) IN HOSPITALS, 2000 TO 2006

		Percentage of hospitals			
Old ratings system					
Year		**Green (good)**	**Yellow (acceptable)**	**Red (poor)**	
2000 (Autumn)		22.3	41.7	35.5	
2001 (Spring)		40.5	53.4	6.1	
2001 (Autumn)		43.7	56.3	0.0	
2002		60.0	40.0	0.0	
2003		78.7	21.3	0.0	
New ratings system					
Year	**Excellent**	**Good**	**Acceptable**	**Poor**	**Unacceptable**
2004	10.0	38.5	49.2	2.0	0.3
2005	10.3	44.8	40.1	4.6	0.2
2006	14.2	49.8	31.1	4.8	0.2

Source: National Patient Safety Agency 2007; Department of Health 2007c; NHS Estates 2007

TABLE 56: NUMBER OF HOSPITALS IN THE FOUR CLEANLINESS BANDS BY TYPE OF HOSPITAL, 2005

Cleanliness band	Type of hospital			
	NHS acute	Independent acute	NHS mental health and community	Independent mental health
Band 1: 91–100% High standards of cleanliness across the board; only a few instances where cleanliness is below standard	11	7	11	4
Band 2: 71–90% Isolated failures in cleanliness rather than a systemic problem; clear room for improvement	22	4	11	6
Band 3: 51–70% More likelihood of a systemic problem in managing cleaning services, lack of cleanliness is widespread and standards are unsatisfactory	4	0	5	7
Band 4: ≤50% Serious, widespread problems in relation to cleanliness; improvements need to be made immediately	0	0	6	0

Source: Healthcare Commission 2005a

In December 2005 the Healthcare Commission published *A Snapshot of Hospital Cleanliness in England: Findings from the Healthcare Commission's rapid inspection programme* (Healthcare Commission 2005a). The report showed cleanliness scores – the maximum being 100 per cent – grouped into four bands, with the best-performing hospitals in band 1 and the worst in band 4 (*See* Table 56, above).

Owing to the structure and the small size of the sample, it is not appropriate to extrapolate the findings across the NHS as a whole. However, the snapshot does reveal some interesting conclusions.

■ Roughly one-third of hospitals in both the NHS and independent sectors demonstrated high standards of cleanliness.
■ A higher proportion failed to perform as well as they could and were placed in band 2.
■ There was evidence of poor standards of cleanliness in a significant proportion of hospitals, suggesting systemic problems.
■ Standards were markedly poorer in mental health hospitals than acute hospitals.

The Healthcare Commission's third national survey of NHS staff (Healthcare Commission 2006b) included questions about hygiene and infection control. Three-fifths of staff (61 per cent) said that hot water, soap and paper towels, or alcohol rubs were always available when staff needed them and 28 per cent said they were available most of the time (*see* Table 57, overleaf). Fewer staff knew whether or not the same materials were available for patients and visitors. Staff were also asked whether or not they believed their trusts did

TABLE 57: RESPONSES OF NHS STAFF TO SURVEY QUESTION REGARDING THE AVAILABILITY OF CLEANING MATERIALS TO DIFFERENT GROUPS

Group	Are hot water, soap and paper towels, or alcohol rubs, available when they are needed?				
	Always (%)	Most of the time (%)	Sometimes (%)	Never (%)	Don't know (%)
Staff	61	28	6	0	5
Patients/users of service	52	25	6	1	16
Visitors to the trust	50	25	7	1	17

Source: Healthcare Commission 2006b

enough to promote hand washing. Although more than half the respondents (57 per cent) believed their trusts did enough to promote the importance of hand washing to staff, only 43 per cent believed that the same applied to patients, service users and visitors.

Health care-associated infections

The operating framework for 2007/8 allows primary care trusts to set local targets for reducing HAIs in their contracts with providers. These targets apply both to methicillin-resistant *Staphylococcus aureus* (MRSA) infection rates (which have fallen from a peak in 2003/4 but are still only slightly lower than in 2001, when surveillance became mandatory), and to *Clostridium difficile* rates (which increased by a quarter between 2004 and 2006). There are currently no national targets for *C difficile*, although the government has set a PSA target for hospital providers to reduce MRSA rates by 50 per cent by 2008, compared with the baseline rates of 2003/4. However, the latest progress report by the Health Protection Agency (2006) reports little movement towards the target.

According to the Health Protection Agency, 7,087 MRSA bacteraemia episodes were reported in England during 2005/6, a reduction of 8 per cent from the 2003/4 high. However, the Health Protection Agency (2006) warned that '...it would be premature to state that this indicates the beginning of a downturn in trend'. Nevertheless, while the overall figures show modest progress, some trusts, such as acute teaching hospitals, have made significant improvements. London still has the highest numbers of MRSA cases, but has still seen sizeable reductions. Trusts within the Yorkshire and the Humber region are also showing marked reductions. The latest commentary from the Health Protection Agency (April 2007) referred to 1,542 reports of MRSA bacteraemia between October and December 2006, representing a 7 per cent decrease on the previous quarter, when 1,652 reports were received (Health Protection Agency 2007).

The Health Protection Agency (HPA) commented:

> *...a significant proportion of the bacteraemia were likely to be present on admission. We cannot yet say whether these MRSA infections reflect acquisition previously in the same hospital, another hospital or nursing home, or community acquisition unrelated to health care. The suspicion in this country is that most of these cases are associated with healthcare activities and do not indicate true community acquisition. However, this requires further investigation.*
> (HPA 2006)

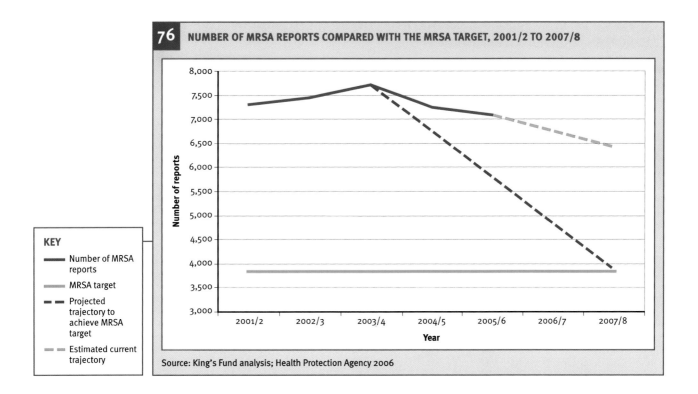

76 NUMBER OF MRSA REPORTS COMPARED WITH THE MRSA TARGET, 2001/2 TO 2007/8

KEY
— Number of MRSA reports
— MRSA target
▬ ▬ Projected trajectory to achieve MRSA target
▬ ▬ Estimated current trajectory

Source: King's Fund analysis; Health Protection Agency 2006

In 2004, the government set a target for hospital providers to reduce MRSA rates by 50 per cent by 2008, compared with the baseline rates of 2003/4 (*see* Figure 75). However, a leaked government memo, circulated to ministers in October 2006, suggested that the NHS was not on track to meet the MRSA target:

> *Although the numbers are coming down, we are not on course to hit that target and there is some doubt about whether it is in fact achievable ... The opinion of DH infection experts is that we will succeed in reducing MRSA bloodstream infections by a third, rather than a half – and even if we had a longer period of time, it may not be possible to get down to a half.*

The memo also warned that another bug, *Clostridium difficile*, was now '...endemic throughout the health service, with virtually all trusts reporting cases' and that 2004 saw twice as many deaths from this infection as from MRSA. Mandatory surveillance of *C difficile*-associated disease (CDAD) in people aged 65 years and over has been included in the health care-associated infection surveillance system for acute trusts in England since January 2004. In 2006, 55,681 cases of CDAD were reported through mandatory surveillance, compared with 44,314 cases in 2004, representing a rise of just over a quarter (Health Protection Agency 2007).

The European Antimicrobial Resistance Surveillance System (EARSS) is an international network of national surveillance systems that collects antimicrobial susceptibility data for public health action. These data reinforce the United Kingdom's poor performance in dealing with MRSA. Table 58, overleaf, shows the proportion of methicillin-resistant infections among all *Staphylococcus aureus* bloodstream infections for various European countries, highlighting the high rates of MRSA occurring in the United Kingdom. Within the last seven years no fewer than 12 European countries have reported a significant increase

TABLE 58: RATES OF MRSA* AMONG STAPHYLOCOCCUS AUREUS BLOODSTREAM INFECTIONS FOR VARIOUS EUROPEAN COUNTRIES, 1999 TO 2005

Country	Percentage of MRSA						
	1999	2000	2001	2002	2003	2004	2005
France	na	na	33	33	29	29	27
Germany	8	12	16	18	18	20	21
Netherlands	‹1	‹1	‹1	‹1	1	1	‹1
Sweden	‹1	‹1	‹1	‹1	‹1	‹1	1
United Kingdom	33	39	44	44	43	44	44

Source: EARSS 2007
* methicillin-resistant Staphylococcus aureus bacteraemia

in the proportion of MRSA. However, two European countries (Slovenia and France) have successfully reduced the proportion of MRSA among *Staphylococcus aureus* bloodstream infections over the past five or six years.

The 2002 review assumed there would be a 15 per cent reduction in HAIs in acute care by 2012/3. Although the government's more ambitious targets seem unlikely to be met, based on current progress, the review's target seems achievable (Wanless 2002).

CHOICE AND PRIVACY

Enhanced patient choice is a key element of the government's health system reforms. Since January 2006, all patients referred by their GP for a specialist consultation at a hospital outpatient department should have been offered a choice of at least four hospitals, including NHS and private; and from 2008 the government intends that all patients needing elective care will be offered the choice of any accredited hospital, public or private, anywhere in England.

To assess the implementation of choice at primary care trust (PCT) level, the Department of Health (2007u) has commissioned a series of national patient choice surveys. Four such surveys have so far been undertaken, the first relating to referrals made in May/June 2006 and the most recent for referrals made in November and early December 2006. The fourth survey showed an increase in the proportion of patients who recalled being offered a choice of hospital for their first outpatient appointment (41 per cent, compared with 30 per cent in the first); and 35 per cent of patients were aware before they visited their GP that they had a choice of hospitals for their first appointment, compared with 29 per cent in the first survey. In the last survey, 78 per cent of patients who were offered choice were satisfied with the process, with only five per cent dissatisfied – similar proportions to those in the first survey. Figure 77, opposite, shows changes in the proportion of patients in England offered choice between September and November 2006.

Research by the Picker Institute (Coulter 2005) found that in 2005 36 per cent of respondents to the primary care survey had been referred to a specialist; of these:
■ 26 per cent were given a choice of hospital

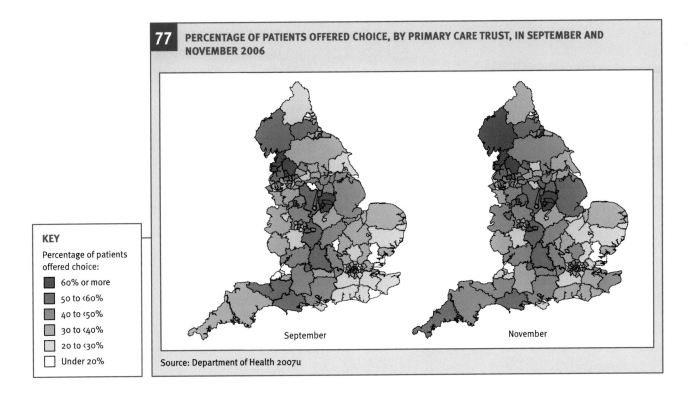

77 PERCENTAGE OF PATIENTS OFFERED CHOICE, BY PRIMARY CARE TRUST, IN SEPTEMBER AND NOVEMBER 2006

KEY

Percentage of patients offered choice:

- 60% or more
- 50 to <60%
- 40 to <50%
- 30 to <40%
- 20 to <30%
- Under 20%

September

November

Source: Department of Health 2007u

- 17 per cent would have liked a choice but said they were not offered one (compared with 16 per cent in 2004)
- 57 per cent were not given a choice but did not mind (compared with 58 per cent in 2004).

The research also found a slight reduction in numbers of patients having to stay in mixed wards, but with a substantial minority still complaining about lack of privacy. There is some evidence of improved privacy in accident and emergency (A&E) departments: the proportion of patients saying they had sufficient privacy for treatment discussions rose from 70 per cent in 2002 to 72 per cent in 2004, and for examinations from 78 per cent to 80 per cent. However, in 2004 as in 2002, 31 per cent of inpatients complained of insufficient privacy for treatment discussions and 13 per cent said there was not enough privacy for physical examinations. Cancer patients appear more satisfied in these respects, with 85 per cent in 2004 saying they had sufficient privacy for treatment discussions and 97 per cent saying the same for physical examinations – improvements of 4 per cent and 5 per cent respectively since 2000.

ACCESS AND WAITING TIMES

Improving access to health care by reducing waiting lists and times has been a concern of governments for many decades and has arguably become the dominant policy issue over the past 10 years. The benefits to patients of reduced waiting times manifest themselves not only in improved health outcomes, but also in improvements in the patient experience.

Following the achievement of the Labour Party's 1997 election manifesto promise to reduce numbers waiting for hospital treatment after an initial appointment with a consultant by 100,000, subsequent efforts have been directed at reducing waiting times.

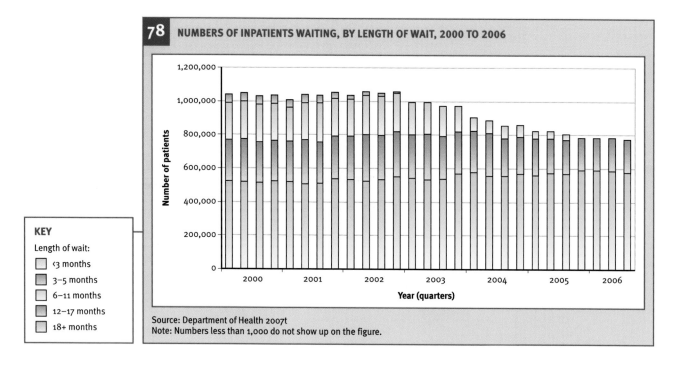

78 NUMBERS OF INPATIENTS WAITING, BY LENGTH OF WAIT, 2000 TO 2006

KEY

Length of wait:

- ☐ <3 months
- ☐ 3–5 months
- ☐ 6–11 months
- ☐ 12–17 months
- ☐ 18+ months

Source: Department of Health 2007t
Note: Numbers less than 1,000 do not show up on the figure.

The NHS Plan, for example, promised that by the end of 2005 no one would wait more than six months on an inpatient list or 13 weeks on an outpatient list. It also promised that no one would wait more than 48 hours for an appointment with a GP or more than four hours before being treated, admitted or discharged in a hospital A&E department. Other maximum waiting time targets – such as for patients with suspected cancer – have been set since the Plan was published.

The 2002 review echoed these goals but suggested that even shorter waiting times would be desirable over the coming decades. The review outlined a series of waiting time reductions up to 2022/3, by which time maximum inpatient and outpatient waits would be no longer than two weeks.

Trends in inpatient and outpatient waiting times since have shown considerable improvement, as shown by Figures 78, above, and 79, opposite. By April 2007, 40 per cent of outpatients were waiting less than four weeks from GP referral to their first appointment, with a further 30 per cent waiting up to eight weeks. Picker Institute patients surveys (Coulter 2005) also show improvements in access to health services. In 2004, 83 per cent of outpatients had their first appointment within three months of referral, compared with 75 per cent in 2003.

A further key target concerned waits in A&E departments; Figure 80, opposite, shows how, across all trusts, the proportion of patients seen within four hours has risen from around three quarters of patients in 2002 to nearly 98 per cent in 2006.

The outstanding waiting times target is the maximum 18-week wait from GP referral to a bed in hospital, if needed. Historic data on this particular wait is not available as it is only in the last year that an important part of patients' waiting experience – the wait for diagnostic tests – has begun to be recorded.

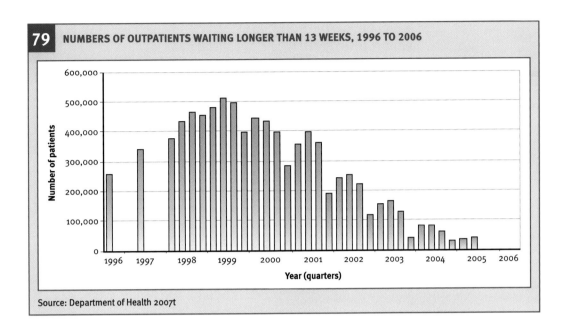

79 **NUMBERS OF OUTPATIENTS WAITING LONGER THAN 13 WEEKS, 1996 TO 2006**

Source: Department of Health 2007t

Figures 81 and 82, overleaf, show that at the end of 2006 numbers waiting for various tests stood at around 800,000 (virtually unchanged since January 2006), with very little change over the year in the distribution of waiting times for those still waiting.

The latest departmental milestone is for 85 per cent of trusts to have achieved the 18-week target by March 2008 and the remainder by December 2008.

Except where speed of treatment is imperative (such as for suspected cancer and heart disease, where particularly short waiting time targets have been set) the impact of reduced waiting times on aggregate patient health may be less substantial than had been

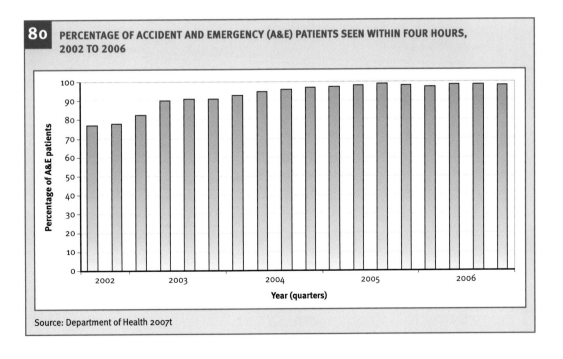

80 **PERCENTAGE OF ACCIDENT AND EMERGENCY (A&E) PATIENTS SEEN WITHIN FOUR HOURS, 2002 TO 2006**

Source: Department of Health 2007t

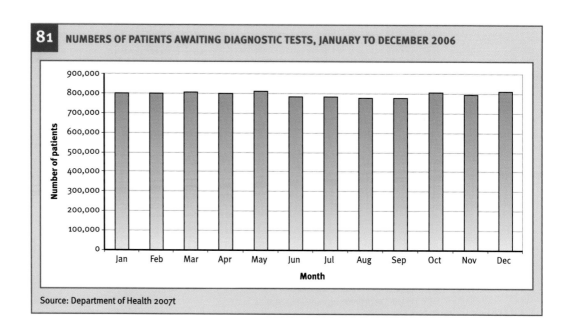

81 NUMBERS OF PATIENTS AWAITING DIAGNOSTIC TESTS, JANUARY TO DECEMBER 2006

Source: Department of Health 2007t

assumed. This is partly because the government's maximum waiting time targets affect relatively few patients because most are treated within target times and partly because the effects of waiting are less damaging than might be supposed; for waiting lists do not

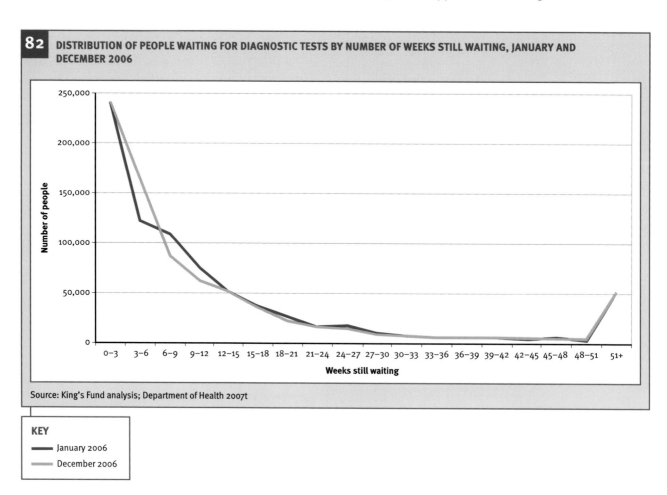

82 DISTRIBUTION OF PEOPLE WAITING FOR DIAGNOSTIC TESTS BY NUMBER OF WEEKS STILL WAITING, JANUARY AND DECEMBER 2006

Source: King's Fund analysis; Department of Health 2007t

KEY
— January 2006
— December 2006

operate on a simple first-come-first-served basis and patients can and do move up the queue if, for example, their symptoms deteriorate. While there is relatively little research in this area, various studies have found little or no relationship between length of wait and health-related quality of life (for example, Hirvonen *et al* 2006; Derrett *et al* 1999), although some suggest that shorter waits lead to larger health-related quality of life gains (for example Mahon *et al* 2002). However, there is an undoubted value to patients in improving the process of care even if, for many, it has a minimal impact on their eventual health status.

Finally, it is surprising, given that waiting times are such a major strand of government health policy, that there is no readily available data on the costs and benefits of meeting successive waiting time targets since 2000.

PATIENT EXPERIENCE OF CARE

By May 2007, around 1.4 million patients had participated in the national patient survey programme. Analysis of the surveys – which probe patient experience rather than satisfaction – indicates that most patients are very appreciative of their care, particularly in areas of the NHS that have been subject to co-ordinated action (Coulter 2005; The Picker Institute Europe 2005; Healthcare Commission 2005b and 2007b). There are, however, some areas of concern, including a lack of patient involvement with their own care, lack of privacy during treatment and a decline in the perceived cleanliness of hospitals.

In 2005 and 2006, 77 per cent of inpatients rated their care as excellent or very good, compared with 74 per cent in 2002. Additionally, 78 per cent of outpatients and 70 per cent of people attending A&E departments rated their care as excellent or very good in 2004, the former statistic unchanged and the latter up by 4 per cent on 2003.

Patients have also reported improved access to health care. In 2003, 75 per cent of outpatients had their first appointment within three months of referral, compared with 83 per cent in 2004. In 2000, 70 per cent of cancer patients saw a specialist within one month of referral; four years later, this proportion had increased to 80 per cent. Finally, in 2002 67 per cent of patients admitted to hospital as emergencies were allocated a bed within four hours of arrival; by 2005 this had improved to 75 per cent (although it fell to 72 per cent in 2006).

In 1998, 87 per cent of GPs' patients said they had sufficient time with their doctors; however, in 2004 only 74 per cent of primary care patients said they had enough time with the doctor or nurse. Furthermore, between 2003 and 2005 the proportion of patients reporting that they were seen by their GP without an appointment halved (to 7 per cent).

However, this downward trend has not been demonstrated across all NHS services. In 2004, 75 per cent of outpatients and 66 per cent of A&E patients said they had sufficient time with the doctor or nurse. By comparison with the previous year, this represented no change for outpatients but an improvement of 4 per cent for those attending A&E.

Although most patients report that staff treat them with respect and dignity most of the time, many have expressed concern that they are less involved than they would like to be in decisions about their care and treatment. In 2004, this concern was expressed by:
- 47 per cent of inpatients
- 30 per cent of outpatients

- 36 per cent of A&E patients
- 32 per cent of primary care patients
- 39 per cent of patients with coronary heart disease
- 59 per cent of patients with mental health problems.

SUMMARY: PROCESS OUTCOMES

- Despite a lack of detailed historical data to assess levels of patient safety, the Healthcare Commission's annual survey of NHS staff suggests that the NHS, as a whole, has been improving. In 2005, 32 per cent of staff had seen at least one error, near miss or incident that could have hurt patients, down from 35 per cent in 2003.

- The European Antimicrobial Resistance Surveillance System (EARSS) annual report (2005) indicates that the United Kingdom has one of the highest rates of MRSA infection in Europe.

- A PSA target commits hospital providers to reducing MRSA rates by 50 per cent by 2008; but the latest progress report by the Health Protection Agency (2006) notes little movement towards this target.

- The 2002 review assumed there would be a 15 per cent reduction in hospital-acquired infections (HAI) in acute care by 2012/3 (Wanless 2002). Although the more ambitious PSA target for reducing MRSA is unlikely to be met, current progress suggests the review target may be achieved. This does not take account of other HAIs, such as *C difficile*, which may pose a larger threat to patient safety in future.

- Patient choice is a key element of the government's health system reforms. Since January 2006, all patients referred to a hospital outpatient department should have been offered a choice of at least four hospitals. The national patient choice surveys reveal that 35 per cent of patients recalled being offered choice in July 2006, compared with 30 per cent in May/June of that year.

- Improving access to health care by reducing waiting lists and times has been a concern of governments for many decades, and none more so than the current Labour administration. The 2002 review endorsed the waiting time reduction targets of the NHS Plan and went further by assuming that the maximum inpatient and outpatient wait in 2022/3 would be no more than two weeks (Wanless 2002).

- Trends in inpatient and outpatient waiting times since the review have shown considerable improvement. Although reductions in numbers of patients waiting long periods has improved patients' experience of care, it is unlikely to have had any substantial impact on health outcomes (except where speed of treatment is important, such as with suspected cancer and coronary heart disease, which are subject to very short wait targets). No data is readily available to quantify the costs and benefits of what has been a major strand of government health policy since 2000.

- Patient surveys also show evidence of recent improvements in access to health services. In 2004, 83 per cent of outpatients had their first appointment within three months of referral, compared with 75 per cent in 2004.

- Through its involvement with the national patient survey programme in England, the Picker Institute has concluded that the patient experience and the quality of NHS care has been improving over time, particularly in areas of the NHS that have been subject to co-ordinated action. There are, however, considerable variations in the quality of care in different sectors and institutions across England.

Additionally, in 2004, 12 per cent of outpatients and 16 per cent of A&E patients reported receiving conflicting information from staff, a proportion unchanged since previous surveys. However, complaints about conflicting information were highest among inpatients, at 31 per cent, and this rose to 35 per cent in 2006.

The proportion of patients reporting that their care environment met their expectations has declined slightly since 2002. In that year, 56 per cent of inpatients thought their ward was very clean; but this proportion fell to 54 per cent in 2004 and to 53 per cent in 2006. Furthermore, in 2006 only 47 per cent of inpatients reported that toilets and bathrooms were very clean, compared with 48 per cent in 2004 and 51 per cent in 2002. In primary care, 72 per cent of patients reported that their local surgery or health centre was very clean in 2005, 2 per cent down on 2003.

The 2002 review made a general assumption that patient expectations of the health service would continue to rise and, specifically, that age discrimination in the service would be reduced. Although, there is very little robust assessment of progress in these areas, there is some evidence that support these assumptions.

For example, the Healthcare Commission's (2006a) progress report on the National Service Framework for Older People concluded that explicit age discrimination had declined in the health service, citing improvements in access to cardiac procedures and hip and knee replacements. However, it found that explicit age discrimination remained a feature of mental health services and that there was still evidence of ageism across the health service.

Rising patient expectations are very difficult to assess accurately; however, if patient involvement is used as a proxy, it does seem that expectations are rising. The Picker Institute's assessment of its research between 1998 and 2005 indicates that 'Patients want more information, more involvement in decisions that affect them, and more support for self-care' (The Picker Institute Europe 2005). Furthermore, work commissioned by the Department of Health found that '... people's expectations about what kind of services they want, and how they want to use them, are changing. People increasingly expect to be given more of a say about the health and social care services they use' (Opinion Leader Research 2006).

Health outcomes: life expectancy, mortality and cancer survival

As previous chapters have shown, the NHS collects large amounts of data about its activity and outputs but none about the change in the health status of the patients it treats. Routine information on population health is available, however, and that is the focus of this section. The problem is that changes in, say, mortality rates cannot necessarily be attributed to interventions by the NHS because a wide variety of factors contribute to mortality, often over many decades. There are numerous measures of the health of the population, but this section focuses on five: self-reported health status, life expectancy at birth, infant mortality, premature mortality and cancer survival rates. The most up-to-date figures have been used wherever possible, but some of these are up to two years old.

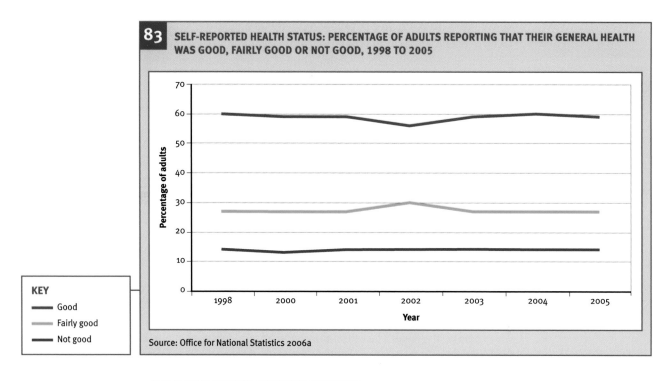

83 SELF-REPORTED HEALTH STATUS: PERCENTAGE OF ADULTS REPORTING THAT THEIR GENERAL HEALTH WAS GOOD, FAIRLY GOOD OR NOT GOOD, 1998 TO 2005

KEY
— Good
— Fairly good
— Not good

Source: Office for National Statistics 2006a

SELF-REPORTED HEALTH STATUS

In the 2005 General Household Survey (ONS 2006a) 59 per cent of the adult population of Great Britain reported their health status as good, 27 per cent as fairly good and 14 per as not good. These proportions have remained largely unchanged since 1998 (*see* Figure 83, above).

In the same survey, 33 per cent of the population of Great Britain reported that they had a longstanding illness, which was 'limiting' for 19 per cent. These proportions have also seen little change from 1998 (*see* Figure 84, below).

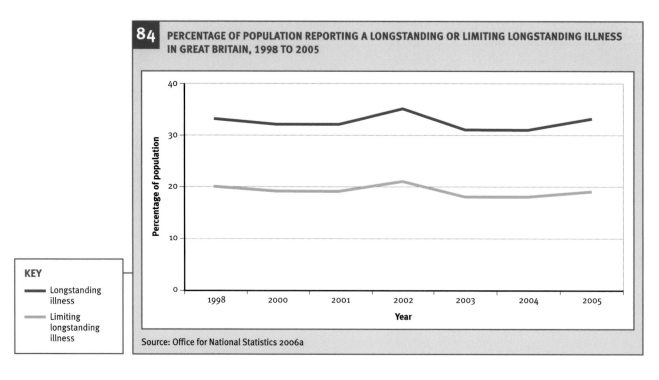

84 PERCENTAGE OF POPULATION REPORTING A LONGSTANDING OR LIMITING LONGSTANDING ILLNESS IN GREAT BRITAIN, 1998 TO 2005

KEY
— Longstanding illness
— Limiting longstanding illness

Source: Office for National Statistics 2006a

LIFE EXPECTANCY AT BIRTH

Life expectancy at birth is a very broad measure of population health, with many contributory factors. There have been large increases in life expectancy across most countries in the world over the past 40 years, with a strong convergence towards the average. The latest year for which all comparable data is available is 2003. In the United Kingdom, female life expectancy rose from 79.7 years in 1998 to 80.7 years in 2003 – an increase of 1.3 per cent. For males, life expectancy rose from 74.8 to 76.2 years over the same period – an increase of 1.9 per cent. The United Kingdom's performance over this period exceeded that of the population-weighted EU 15 average, which rose by 1 per cent for females and 1.7 per cent for males.

Despite this progress, as Table 59, below, shows, male life expectancy at birth in the United Kingdom is low in relation to comparator countries, including Australia, Canada, France, Germany, Netherlands, New Zealand and Sweden. Female life expectancy in the United Kingdom is lower than the EU 15 average and is the lowest of the seven comparable countries (*see* Table 60, overleaf).

Between 1998 and 2003, of the seven comparator countries, Australia saw the highest percentage increases in life expectancy for both genders (1.6 per cent for females and 2.5 per cent for males), with the Netherlands showing the smallest increases for both genders (0.4 per cent for females and 1.3 per cent for males).

The 2002 review projected that life expectancy at birth in the United Kingdom would continue to increase under all three scenarios, with slow uptake demonstrating the smallest rise by 2022 (*see* Table 61, overleaf). Because of evidence that past projections had tended to underestimate future numbers of elderly people, the Government Actuary's Department (GAD) principal life expectancy assumptions were used in the slow uptake scenario rather than the solid progress scenario. Solid progress used GAD's 'high' life expectancy assumptions, while fully engaged used the even higher assumptions prepared

TABLE 59: TRENDS IN MALE LIFE EXPECTANCY AT BIRTH IN SELECTED COUNTRIES, 1998 TO 2003

Country	Life expectancy (years)						% change 1998–2003
	1998	1999	2000	2001	2002	2003	
Australia	75.9	76.2	76.6	77.0	77.4	77.8	2.5
Canada	76.0	76.2	76.7	77.0	77.2	77.4	1.8
France	74.8	75.0	75.3	75.5	75.8	75.9	1.5
Germany	74.5	74.7	75.0	75.5	75.4	75.7	1.6
Netherlands	75.2	75.3	75.5	75.8	76.0	76.2	1.3
New Zealand	75.2	76.0	76.3	76.3	76.3	77.0	2.4
Sweden	76.9	77.1	77.4	77.6	77.7	77.9	1.3
United Kingdom	74.8	75.0	75.4	75.7	75.9	76.2	1.9
EU 15	74.9	75.1	75.5	75.8	75.9	76.2	1.7

Source: Organisation for Economic Co-operation and Development 2007

TABLE 60: TRENDS IN FEMALE LIFE EXPECTANCY AT BIRTH IN SELECTED COUNTRIES, 1998 TO 2003

Country	Life expectancy (years)						% change 1998–2003
	1998	1999	2000	2001	2002	2003	
Australia	81.5	81.8	82.0	82.4	82.6	82.8	1.6
Canada	81.5	81.7	81.9	82.1	82.1	82.4	1.1
France	82.4	82.5	82.7	82.9	83.0	82.9	0.6
Germany	80.6	80.7	81.0	81.3	81.2	81.4	1.0
Netherlands	80.6	80.5	80.5	80.7	80.7	80.9	0.4
New Zealand	80.4	80.9	81.1	81.1	81.1	81.3	1.1
Sweden	81.9	81.9	82.0	82.1	82.1	82.5	0.7
United Kingdom	79.7	79.8	80.2	80.4	80.5	80.7	1.3
EU 15	81.1	81.2	81.5	81.7	81.8	81.9	1.0

Source: Organisation for Economic Co-operation and Development 2007

by Eurostat (Wanless 2002). GAD projections (as of December 2006) for life expectancy at birth in the year 2022 have moved close to the three life expectancy trajectories used in the 2002 review (*see* Figures 85 and 86, opposite).

INFANT MORTALITY

The United Kingdom has a high infant mortality rate by comparison with the EU 15 average and comparator countries (*see* Table 62, p 200). The infant mortality rate in 2003 was 5.3 deaths per 1,000 live births, 7 per cent lower than in 1998. However, this compared with a 16 per cent reduction for the EU 15 as a whole, with Greece and Portugal showing large reductions of 40 and 32 per cent, respectively. More recent data for the United Kingdom shows that since 2003 infant mortality rates have gone down slightly – to 5.0 per thousand in 2006.

TABLE 61: UK LIFE EXPECTANCY PROJECTIONS IN 2022

Projection	Life expectancy at birth in 2022 (years)	
	Men	Women
2002 Wanless: solid progress	80.0	83.8
2002 Wanless: slow uptake	78.7	83.0
2002 Wanless: fully engaged	81.6	85.5
Latest GAD principal projection	80.3	84.0
Latest GAD low life expectancy variant	79.1	83.3
Latest GAD high life expectancy variant	81.5	84.8

Source: Government Actuary's Department 2006
Notes: The life expectancy data used to produce GAD projections are based on historic mortality rates and projected mortality rates from the 2004-based national population projections.

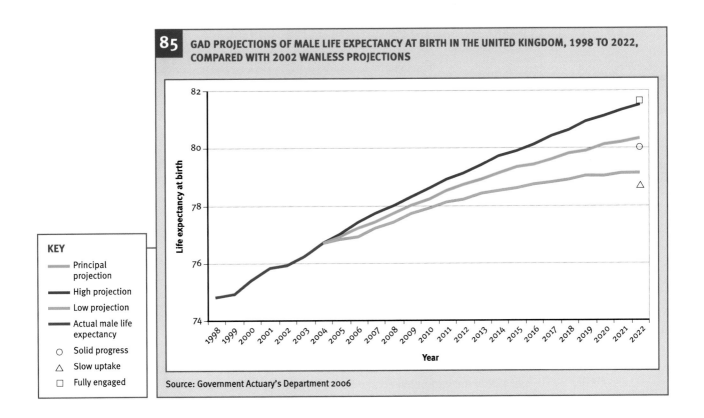

85 GAD PROJECTIONS OF MALE LIFE EXPECTANCY AT BIRTH IN THE UNITED KINGDOM, 1998 TO 2022, COMPARED WITH 2002 WANLESS PROJECTIONS

KEY
— Principal projection
— High projection
— Low projection
— Actual male life expectancy
○ Solid progress
△ Slow uptake
□ Fully engaged

Source: Government Actuary's Department 2006

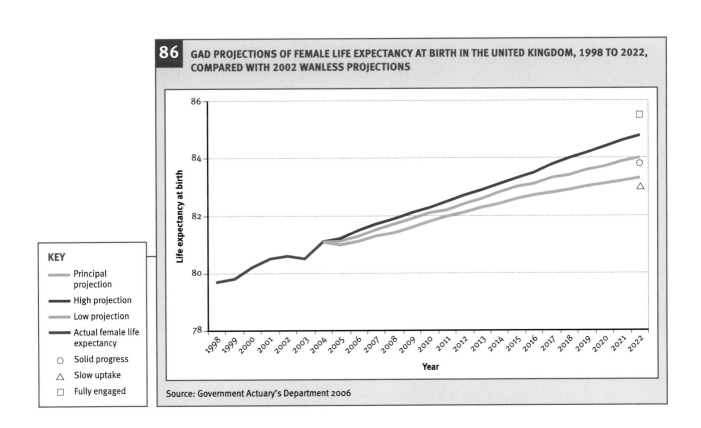

86 GAD PROJECTIONS OF FEMALE LIFE EXPECTANCY AT BIRTH IN THE UNITED KINGDOM, 1998 TO 2022, COMPARED WITH 2002 WANLESS PROJECTIONS

KEY
— Principal projection
— High projection
— Low projection
— Actual female life expectancy
○ Solid progress
△ Slow uptake
□ Fully engaged

Source: Government Actuary's Department 2006

TABLE 62: TRENDS IN INFANT MORTALITY AT BIRTH IN SELECTED COUNTRIES, 1998 TO 2003

Country	Infant mortality (deaths per 1,000 live births)						% change 1998–2003
	1998	1999	2000	2001	2002	2003	
Australia	5.0	5.7	5.2	5.3	5.0	4.8	-4.0
Canada	5.3	5.3	5.3	5.2	5.4	5.3	0.0
France	4.6	4.3	4.4	4.5	4.1	4.0	-13.0
Germany	4.7	4.5	4.4	4.3	4.2	4.2	-10.6
Netherlands	5.2	5.2	5.1	5.4	5.0	4.8	-7.7
Sweden	3.6	3.4	3.4	3.7	3.3	3.1	-13.9
United Kingdom	5.7	5.8	5.6	5.5	5.2	5.3	-7.0
EU 15	5.1	4.8	4.7	4.6	4.4	4.3	-16.2

Source: Organisation for Economic Co-operation and Development 2007

PREMATURE MORTALITY

Potential years of life lost (PYLL) is a measure of premature mortality, calculated by measuring the gap between age at death and a specified age limit – often 70 years. Mortality is considered premature when it could have been prevented if:

■ appropriate medical knowledge had been applied

■ known public health principles had been in force *or*

■ risky behaviour had been less prevalent.

The United Kingdom does not compare well with comparator countries in terms of potential years of life lost per 100,000 of the population. For males in 2002, the PYLL (excluding self-harm) ranked better than the EU-15 average; but between 1998 and 2002 the PYLL for UK males fell by only 5 per cent, a rate of decline that was lower than for all comparable countries and the EU 15 (*see* Table 63, opposite). In 2002 the PYLL for UK females was higher than for all comparator countries (where data was available) and also higher than the EU-15 average (*see* Table 64, opposite).

It is also possible to look at PYLL in relation to specific diseases and causes of illness. PYLL data for 2002 indicates that the United Kingdom continues to compare poorly with comparator countries for ischaemic heart, cerebrovascular and respiratory diseases. However, the United Kingdom performs relatively better for malignant neoplasms (cancer), ranking higher than France and the Netherlands (*see* Table 65, p 202).

CANCER SURVIVAL RATES

Post-diagnosis survival rates refer to the length of time people survive after a disease has been diagnosed. Survival rates for cancer, which accounts for around a quarter of all deaths in the United Kingdom, have been improving, although they still lag behind those of comparator European countries. The EUROCARE-3 study (Berrino *et al* 1999), based on people diagnosed with cancer between 1990 and 1994, showed that the age-standardised relative five-year survival rate for all cancers in England was notably lower than for France, Germany, the Netherlands and Sweden. The five-year survival rate for all cancers in England was 35.9 per cent for males and 46.8 per cent for females (*see* Figure 87, p 203);

TABLE 63: POTENTIAL LIFE YEARS LOST (PYLL) FOR ALL CAUSES EXCEPT SELF-HARM, FOR MALES AGED 0–69, IN SELECTED COUNTRIES, 1998 TO 2002

Country	PYLL per 100,000 population					% change 1998–2002
	1998	1999	2000	2001	2002	
Australia	4,284	4,267	4,065	3,811	3,677	-14
Canada	4,172	4,067	3,969	3,943	3,838	-8
France	5,254	5,211	5,079	5,079	4,861	-7
Germany	4,806	4,733	4,611	4,408	4,292	-11
Netherlands	4,102	4,026	3,977	3,918	3,766	-8
Sweden	3,452	3,345	3,297	3,293	3,093	-10
United Kingdom	4,573	4,508	na	4,385	4,334	-5
EU 15	4,859	4,781	4,664	4,543	4,410	-9

Source: Organisation for Economic Co-operation and Development 2007
Note: In the light of incomplete data, to derive a population weighted EU average we have used imputed data by assuming that data at time t is the same as that in time t-1. Imputed data has been used for Belgium (1998–2002), Denmark (2002) and the United Kingdom (2000).

this compares with male survival rates above 40 per cent and female survival rates above 50 per cent in the other comparator European countries (Coleman *et al* 2003; Sant *et al* 2003).

Despite its lower five-year survival rate, England seems to be catching up with comparator European countries. Between the EUROCARE-2 study (Berrino *et al* 1999), based on people diagnosed with cancer between 1985 and 1989, and the EUROCARE-3 study, the five-year survival rate in England for all cancers rose by 15.4 per cent for males and 9.6 per cent for females. By comparison with the comparator countries, this improvement was more

TABLE 64: POTENTIAL LIFE YEARS LOST (PYLL) FOR ALL CAUSES EXCEPT SELF-HARM, FOR FEMALES AGED 0–69, IN SELECTED COUNTRIES, 1998 TO 2002

Country	PYLL per 100,000 population					% change 1998–2002
	1998	1999	2000	2001	2002	
Australia	2,513	2,513	2,458	2,243	2,310	-8
Canada	2,631	2,602	2,535	2,502	2,532	-4
France	2,547	2,506	2,445	2,464	2,379	-7
Germany	2,599	2,564	2,503	2,422	2,409	-7
Netherlands	2,600	2,750	2,728	2,651	2,656	2
Sweden	2,128	2,028	2,041	2,057	1,999	-6
United Kingdom	2,901	2,871	No data	2,780	2,687	-7
EU 15	2,612	2,566	2,515	2,450	2,397	-8

Source: Organisation for Economic Co-operation and Development 2007
Note: In the light of incomplete data, to derive a population weighted EU average we have used imputed data by assuming that data at time t is the same as that in time t-1. Imputed data has been used for Belgium (1998–2002), Denmark (2002) and the United Kingdom (2000).

TABLE 65: POTENTIAL LIFE YEARS LOST (PYLL) FOR SELECTED DISEASES AND CAUSES OF ILLNESS, FOR PEOPLE AGED 0–69, IN SELECTED COUNTRIES, 2002

Country	PYLL per 100,000 population			
	Malignant neoplasms	Ischaemic heart diseases	Cerebrovascular diseases	Respiratory diseases
Australia	800	228	72	105
Canada	847	244	69	89
France	1,059	132	86	80
Germany	907	257	97	102
Netherlands	961	207	109	95
Sweden	724	224	83	83
United Kingdom	912	345	121	172

Source: Organisation for Economic Co-operation and Development 2007

pronounced for females than males, with improvements in female survival rates bettered only by Germany and significantly better than Sweden, France and the Netherlands, while improvements in male survival rates outperformed Sweden and Germany (*see* Figure 88, p 204).

A similar picture of lower cancer survival rates in England emerges when specific cancers are considered. Five-year survival rates in England for stomach, lung, breast (females only), prostate and kidney cancers are lower than in France, Germany, the Netherlands and Sweden. However, relative to comparator European countries England has shown the largest improvement in five-year survival for stomach cancer and breast cancer (females only), and has matched France and the Netherlands, with an increase in five-year survival for prostate cancer of more than 20 per cent between 1985–89 and 1990–94 (*see* Tables 66–70, pp 204–5, and Figures 89 and 90, p 206). However, since England started from a lower base than other countries, a larger proportionate improvement might have been expected.

The Office for National Statistics (2007a) has prepared more recent survival rates for England in relation to eight cancers, including breast, lung, prostate and stomach cancers. The latest data reports on one- and five-year cancer survival rates for adult patients in England who were diagnosed during 1997–99 and followed up to the end of 2004 (*see* Tables 71 and 72, p 207 and Figure 91, p 207). The evidence is that five-year survival rates for lung, prostate, stomach and breast cancer continue to improve. Between 2001 and 2004 five-year survival for lung cancer increased by 13.5 per cent for males and 26.3 per cent for females. Over this period, the five-year stomach cancer survival rate for both males and females also experienced double-digit growth.

A recent study published by the University of York (Martin *et al* 2007) used the Department of Health's National Programme Budget data to examine the link between expenditure and outcomes in two of the programme budget categories, one of them being cancer. The preliminary results show a strong positive link between expenditure and better health

COMPARATIVE INDEX OF FIVE-YEAR RELATIVE SURVIVAL RATES* FOR ALL CANCERS COMBINED, AMONG ADULTS (AGED 15–99) DIAGNOSED IN THE PERIOD 1990 TO 1994 AND FOLLOWED UP TO 1999, BY SEX, IN SELECTED EUROPEAN COUNTRIES

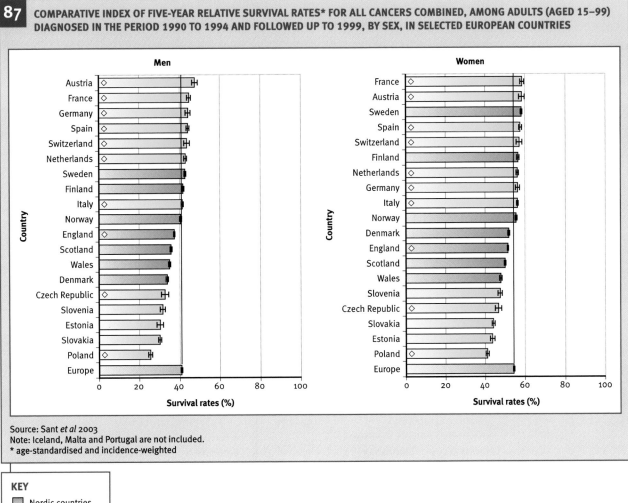

Source: Sant *et al* 2003
Note: Iceland, Malta and Portugal are not included.
* age-standardised and incidence-weighted

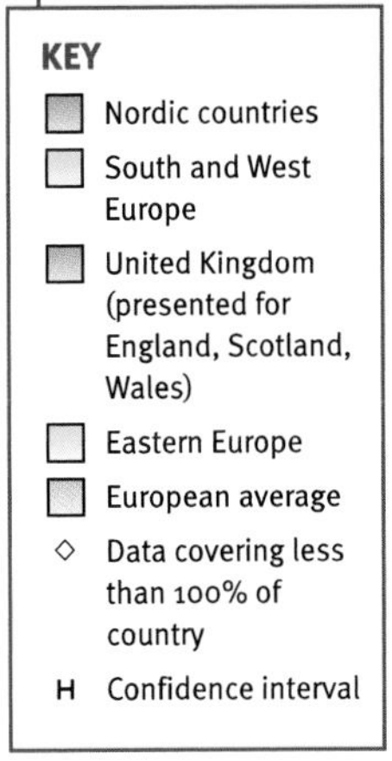

KEY

- ▣ Nordic countries
- ☐ South and West Europe
- ▨ United Kingdom (presented for England, Scotland, Wales)
- ☐ Eastern Europe
- ☐ European average
- ◇ Data covering less than 100% of country
- �muH Confidence interval

outcomes, as measured by standardised mortality rates, for cancer. Using a measure of 'years of life lost' as the health outcome, the researchers estimated the cost of a life year saved in cancer at about £13,100, although this has not been adjusted for quality. These findings are useful in challenging the widely held view that health care has relatively little impact on health. However, they need to be viewed with caution given the delayed impact of current health care activities on levels of cancer-related ill health.

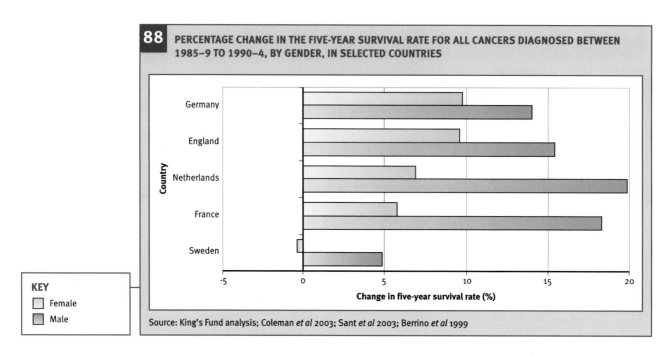

88 PERCENTAGE CHANGE IN THE FIVE-YEAR SURVIVAL RATE FOR ALL CANCERS DIAGNOSED BETWEEN 1985–9 TO 1990–4, BY GENDER, IN SELECTED COUNTRIES

KEY
☐ Female
☐ Male

Source: King's Fund analysis; Coleman *et al* 2003; Sant *et al* 2003; Berrino *et al* 1999

TABLE 66: FIVE-YEAR AGE-STANDARDISED RELATIVE SURVIVAL RATES FOR STOMACH CANCER IN SELECTED COUNTRIES

Country	Men			Women		
	Survival rates (%)		% change	Survival rates (%)		% change
	Eurocare-2	Eurocare-3		Eurocare-2	Eurocare-3	
England	11.2	12.8	14.3	12.7	15.2	19.7
France	23.8	21.4	-10.1	26.3	28.0	6.5
Germany	24.5	24.8	1.2	26.6	30.2	13.5
Netherlands	18.0	17.5	-2.8	21.6	24.6	13.9
Sweden	17.9	18.1	1.1	16.6	19.3	16.3

Source: Coleman *et al* 2003; Sant *et al* 2003; Berrino *et al* 1999

TABLE 67: FIVE-YEAR AGE-STANDARDISED RELATIVE SURVIVAL RATES FOR LUNG CANCER IN SELECTED COUNTRIES

Country	Men			Women		
	Survival rates (%)		% change	Survival rates (%)		% change
	Eurocare-2	Eurocare-3		Eurocare-2	Eurocare-3	
England	7.0	7.4	5.7	7.1	7.7	8.5
France	11.5	13.1	13.9	15.9	15.9	0.0
Germany	8.7	10.8	24.1	13.8	10.5	-23.9
Netherlands	11.7	11.7	0.0	10.8	12.4	14.8
Sweden	8.8	8.5	-3.4	9.6	11.5	19.8

Source: Coleman *et al* 2003; Sant *et al* 2003; Berrino *et al* 1999

TABLE 68: FIVE-YEAR AGE-STANDARDISED RELATIVE SURVIVAL RATES FOR BREAST CANCER AMONG WOMEN IN SELECTED COUNTRIES

Country	Survival rates (%)		% change
	Eurocare-2	Eurocare-3	
England	66.7	73.6	10.3
France	80.3	81.3	1.2
Germany	71.7	75.4	5.2
Netherlands	74.4	78.2	5.1
Sweden	80.6	82.6	2.5

Source: Coleman *et al* 2003; Sant *et al* 2003; Berrino *et al* 1999

TABLE 69: FIVE-YEAR AGE-STANDARDISED RELATIVE SURVIVAL RATES FOR PROSTATE CANCER AMONG MEN IN SELECTED COUNTRIES

Country	Survival rates (%)		% change
	Eurocare-2	Eurocare-3	
England	44.3	53.8	21.4
France	61.7	75.2	21.9
Germany	67.6	75.9	12.3
Netherlands	55.3	68.4	23.7
Sweden	64.7	67.4	4.2

Source: Coleman *et al* 2003; Sant *et al* 2003; Berrino *et al* 1999

TABLE 70: FIVE-YEAR AGE-STANDARDISED RELATIVE SURVIVAL RATES FOR KIDNEY CANCER IN SELECTED COUNTRIES

Country	Men			Women		
	Survival rates (%)		% change	Survival rates (%)		% change
	Eurocare-2	Eurocare-3		Eurocare-2	Eurocare-3	
England	39.4	42.3	7.4	36.9	41.4	12.2
France	57.4	62.9	9.6	56.3	65.0	15.5
Germany	47.3	61.0	29.0	54.6	65.5	20.0
Netherlands	53.4	53.1	-0.6	44.5	53.3	19.8
Sweden	48.7	51.1	4.9	48.0	53.8	12.1

Source: Coleman *et al* 2003; Sant *et al* 2003; Berrino *et al* 1999

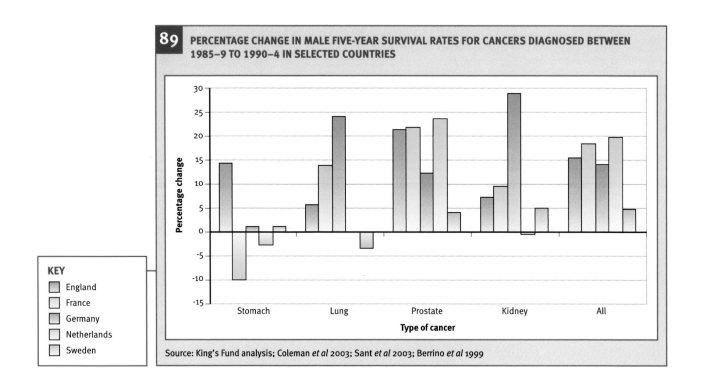

89 PERCENTAGE CHANGE IN MALE FIVE-YEAR SURVIVAL RATES FOR CANCERS DIAGNOSED BETWEEN 1985–9 TO 1990–4 IN SELECTED COUNTRIES

KEY
England
France
Germany
Netherlands
Sweden

Source: King's Fund analysis; Coleman *et al* 2003; Sant *et al* 2003; Berrino *et al* 1999

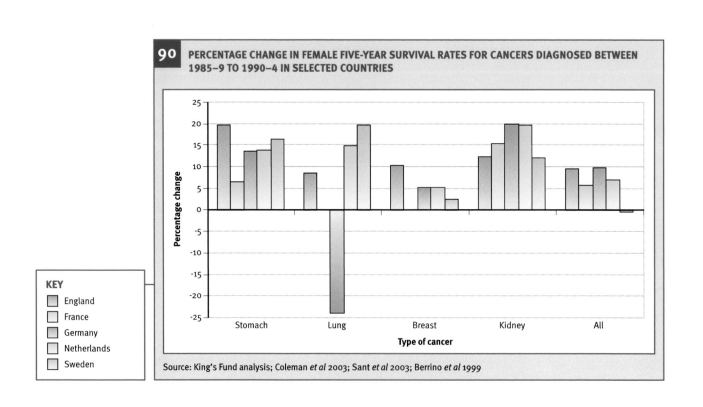

90 PERCENTAGE CHANGE IN FEMALE FIVE-YEAR SURVIVAL RATES FOR CANCERS DIAGNOSED BETWEEN 1985–9 TO 1990–4 IN SELECTED COUNTRIES

KEY
England
France
Germany
Netherlands
Sweden

Source: King's Fund analysis; Coleman *et al* 2003; Sant *et al* 2003; Berrino *et al* 1999

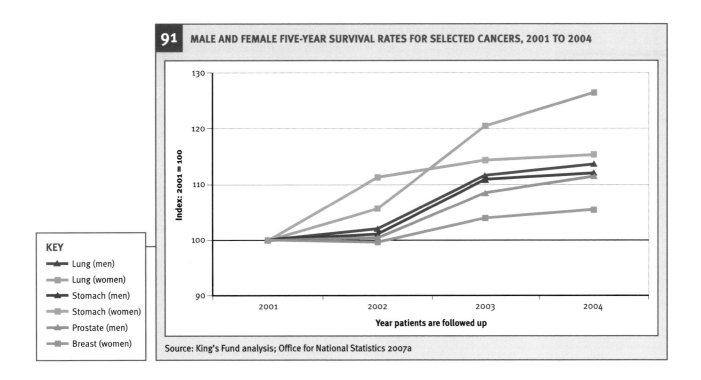

91 MALE AND FEMALE FIVE-YEAR SURVIVAL RATES FOR SELECTED CANCERS, 2001 TO 2004

KEY
- Lung (men)
- Lung (women)
- Stomach (men)
- Stomach (women)
- Prostate (men)
- Breast (women)

Source: King's Fund analysis; Office for National Statistics 2007a

TABLE 71: FIVE-YEAR AGE-STANDARDISED RELATIVE SURVIVAL RATES FOR CANCER AMONG MEN IN ENGLAND

Cancer	Survival rates (%)				% change: patients diagnosed 1994–6 to 1997–9
	Diagnosed 1994–6 and followed up until 2001	Diagnosed 1995–7 and followed up until 2002	Diagnosed 1996–8 and followed up until 2003	Diagnosed 1997–9 and followed up until 2004	
Lung	5.2	5.3	5.8	5.9	13.5
Prostate	60.2	60.4	65.3	67.1	11.5
Stomach	11.1	11.2	12.3	12.4	12.0

Source: Office for National Statistics 2007a

TABLE 72: FIVE-YEAR AGE-STANDARDISED RELATIVE SURVIVAL RATES FOR CANCER AMONG WOMEN IN ENGLAND

Cancer	Survival rates (%)				% change: patients diagnosed 1994–6 to 1997–9
	Diagnosed 1994–6 and followed up until 2001	Diagnosed 1995–7 and followed up until 2002	Diagnosed 1996–8 and followed up until 2003	Diagnosed 1997–9 and followed up until 2004	
Breast	74.9	74.6	77.8	78.9	5.4
Lung	5.4	5.7	6.5	6.8	26.3
Stomach	12.6	14.0	14.4	14.5	15.1

Source: Office for National Statistics 2007a

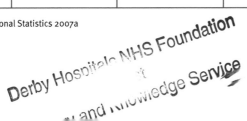

The Calman-Hine Report (1995) began the current process of transforming the organisation and delivery of cancer services in England. The NHS Plan (Department of Health 2000c) saw cancer services as high priority for the NHS, and the NHS Cancer Plan (Department of Health 2000d) was published later that year. Given the long time it takes for cancer to develop, it is difficult to make a direct causal connection between the activities of the NHS over the past 10 years (and particularly since 2002) and current improvements in many cancer survival rates. This will doubtless be an area for future research.

HEALTH INEQUALITIES

The 2002 review assumed that over time there would be differences in socio-economic inequalities in health across the three scenarios. The slow uptake scenario projected an unchanged picture of inequalities in health between groups of people, while the solid progress and fully engaged scenarios projected reductions in health inequalities. For example, in solid progress the gap in life expectancy between those in the poorest areas and the average was predicted to fall by 10 per cent, in line with government objectives, and more steeply in the fully engaged scenario (Wanless 2002).

The government's health inequalities PSA target is to reduce inequalities in health outcomes (as measured by infant mortality and life expectancy at birth) by 10 per cent by 2010. This target is underpinned by two more specific objectives to be achieved by 2010:

■ starting with children under 1 year, to reduce by at least 10 per cent the gap in mortality between routine and manual groups and the population as a whole

■ starting with local authorities, to reduce by at least 10 per cent the gap between the areas with the worst health and deprivation indicators and the population as a whole.

Both *Tackling Health Inequalities: 2003–05 data update for the national 2010 PSA target* (Department of Health 2006l) and the *Review of the Health Inequalities Infant Mortality PSA Target* (Department of Health 2007v) show that health inequalities, as measured by infant mortality and life expectancy, have not narrowed but have rather grown wider. Given past trends, this is not unexpected. Without successful interventions to reduce inequalities, it is likely that key health determinants, such as lifestyle and educational status, would continue to drive health outcomes further apart.

Although overall infant mortality rates have been declining, the *Review of the Health Inequalities Infant Mortality PSA Target* found higher-than-average infant mortality rates in 66 per cent of Spearhead (that is, high-deprivation, high-need areas) local authorities compared with only 27 per cent in non-Spearhead areas. It also found that for 2002–04 the overall infant mortality rate in England and Wales was 4.9 deaths per 1,000 live births, compared with 5.9 per thousand for those in the routine and manual groups. Furthermore, although infant mortality rates in the routine and manual group are continuing to decline, the gap between this group and the population as a whole has widened to 19 per cent from the target baseline in 1997–99 of 13 per cent. In the light of this, the 2010 target looks challenging.

Nationally, life expectancy has been increasing for both men and women, including those in the Spearhead areas, but it is increasing more slowly in the latter so the gap continues to widen, particularly for females. For males the relative gap is has grown from 2.57 per cent to 2.61 per cent and for females, from 1.77 per cent to 1.91 per cent (*see* Tables 73, above, and 74, below).

TABLE 73: MALE LIFE EXPECTANCY AT BIRTH, 1995–7 TO 2003–5

	1995–7	1996–8	1997–9	1998–2000	1999–2001	2000–2	2001–3	2002–4	2003–5
England average (years)	74.6	74.8	75.1	75.4	75.7	76.0	76.2	76.6	76.9
Average for Spearhead group (years)	72.7	72.9	73.1	73.4	73.7	74.1	74.3	74.6	74.9
Relative gap (%)	2.57	2.59	2.66	2.63	2.62	2.57	2.61	2.60	2.61

Source: Department of Health 2006l

For life expectancy, the 2003–05 data indicates that 11.4 per cent of Spearhead areas are on track to narrow the gap with England by 10 per cent by 2010 for both males and females; 24.3 per cent are on track to achieve the target for males only and 24.4 per cent are on track for females only, but 40 per cent of Spearhead areas are on track to achieve the PSA target for neither males nor females.

Although it can be argued that the targeted 10 per cent reduction in specific health inequalities is not ambitious, the latest evidence suggests that progress towards the targets, in terms of health outcomes, has not yet been realised. Much more will need to be achieved over the next five years for the government to fulfil its PSA promises on health inequalities.

While inequalities persist in terms of life expectancy and infant mortality, inequalities in morbidity also persist (*see* Figures 91 and 92), and, in the case of limiting longstanding illness, have grown wider in recent years (ONS 2006a).

Economic inequalities

The solid progress and fully engaged scenarios are, in part, underpinned by reductions in socio-economic inequality, with slow uptake seeing no change in inequality. The 2002 review briefly touched on the 'strong correlation between health inequality and socio-economic inequality', noting that '... changes in socio-economic inequalities could have an impact on health-related behaviours and ultimately demand for care'. However, it was the 2004 review that placed significant emphasis on this relationship.

TABLE 74: FEMALE LIFE EXPECTANCY AT BIRTH, 1995–7 TO 2003–5

	1995–7	1996–8	1997–9	1998–2000	1999–2001	2000–2	2001–3	2002–4	2003–5
England average (years)	79.7	79.8	80.0	80.2	80.4	80.7	80.7	80.9	81.1
Average for Spearhead group (years)	78.3	78.4	78.5	78.7	78.9	79.2	79.2	79.4	79.6
Relative gap (%)	1.77	1.83	1.85	1.87	1.85	1.86	1.87	1.90	1.91

Source: Department of Health 2006l

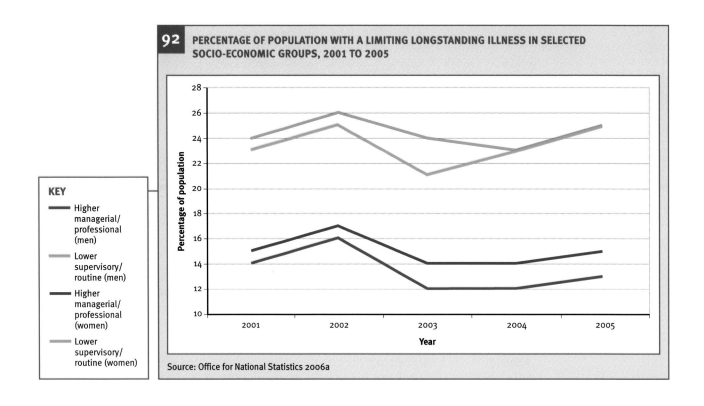

92 PERCENTAGE OF POPULATION WITH A LIMITING LONGSTANDING ILLNESS IN SELECTED SOCIO-ECONOMIC GROUPS, 2001 TO 2005

KEY
— Higher managerial/ professional (men)
— Lower supervisory/ routine (men)
— Higher managerial/ professional (women)
— Lower supervisory/ routine (women)

Source: Office for National Statistics 2006a

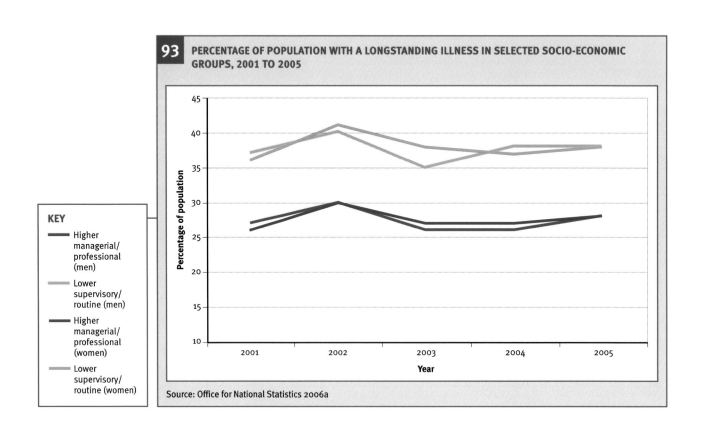

93 PERCENTAGE OF POPULATION WITH A LONGSTANDING ILLNESS IN SELECTED SOCIO-ECONOMIC GROUPS, 2001 TO 2005

KEY
— Higher managerial/ professional (men)
— Lower supervisory/ routine (men)
— Higher managerial/ professional (women)
— Lower supervisory/ routine (women)

Source: Office for National Statistics 2006a

Persistent socio-economic inequalities in the UK, combined with a greater severity of market failures affecting lower socio-economic groups, seem to have contributed to significant inequalities in health outcomes which, unless tackled, will present a significant barrier to many in society becoming fully engaged.
(Wanless 2004)

Two measures of socio-economic inequality are examined below to see how the position has changed since 2002.

The Gini coefficient

The Gini coefficient is one measure of income inequality. It is a value between zero and one, and the higher the number, the greater the degree of income inequality within a society. A value of zero means there is no income inequality within that society/community – in other words that everyone has the same income. By contrast, a value of one indicates a situation of extreme inequality whereby one person has all the income within that society/community.

Since 2002/3 there has been a reduction in the inequality of disposable income in the United Kingdom (ONS 2007b), with the Gini coefficient falling from 0.335 to 0.323 by 2004/5 (*see* Figure 94, below). Interestingly, in 2001/2 the United Kingdom's Gini coefficient stood at 0.360, the highest level since 1990, when it was 0.365. Overall, income inequality remains high by historical standards and the large increase that occurred in the second half of the 1980s has not been reversed.

Poverty

The most widely used measure of relative poverty is the number of people living in households with income below 60 per cent of the median. Data from the Institute for Fiscal Studies (Brewer *et al* 2007) shows that relative poverty has improved since 2002/3.

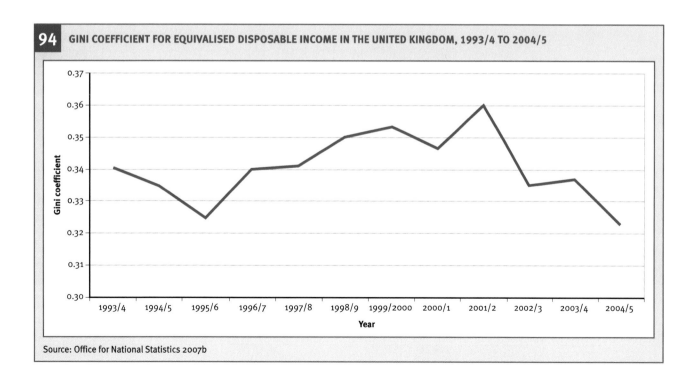

94 GINI COEFFICIENT FOR EQUIVALISED DISPOSABLE INCOME IN THE UNITED KINGDOM, 1993/4 TO 2004/5

Source: Office for National Statistics 2007b

TABLE 75: RELATIVE POVERTY: PERCENTAGE AND NUMBER OF INDIVIDUALS IN HOUSEHOLDS WITH INCOMES BELOW 60 PER CENT OF MEDIAN 'AFTER HOUSING COSTS' INCOME, 1996/7 TO 2005/6

Year	Children (%)	Children (millions)	Pensioners (%)	Pensioners (millions)	All (%)	All (millions)
1996/7[1]	34.1	4.3	29.1	26.6	25.3	14.0
1997/8[1]	33.2	4.2	29.1	25.9	24.4	13.6
1998/9[1]	33.9	4.3	28.6	26.3	24.4	13.6
1999/2000[1]	32.7	4.2	27.6	25.5	24.0	13.4
2000/1[1]	31.7	3.9	25.9	24.7	23.1	13.0
2001/2[1]	30.8	3.9	25.6	24.5	22.7	12.8
2002/3[2]	29.8	3.9	24.2	24.1	22.4	13.1
2003/4[2]	28.7	3.7	20.6	23.5	21.5	12.6
2004/5[2]	28.4	3.6	17.6	23.0	20.5	12.1
2005/6[2]	29.8	3.8	17.0	24.8	21.6	12.7
% change 2002/3 to 2005/6	*0.0%*	*-2.6%*	*-29.8%*	*2.9%*	*-3.6%*	*-3.1%*
% change 2004/5 to 2005/6	*4.9%*	*5.6%*	*-3.4%*	*7.8%*	*5.4%*	*5.0%*

Source: Institute for Fiscal Studies 2007
[1] GB figures
[2] UK figures

TABLE 76: RELATIVE POVERTY: PERCENTAGE AND NUMBER OF INDIVIDUALS IN HOUSEHOLDS WITH INCOMES BELOW 60 PER CENT OF MEDIAN 'BEFORE HOUSING COSTS' INCOME, 1996/7 TO 2005/6

Year	Children (%)	Children (millions)	Pensioners (%)	Pensioners (millions)	All (%)	All (millions)
1996/7[1]	26.7	3.4	24.6	2.4	19.4	10.8
1997/8[1]	26.9	3.4	25.3	2.5	19.6	10.9
1998/9[1]	26.0	3.3	26.8	2.7	19.3	10.8
1999/2000[1]	25.6	3.3	25.1	2.5	19.2	10.7
2000/1[1]	23.3	3.0	24.8	2.5	18.4	10.4
2001/2[1]	23.1	2.9	25.1	2.5	18.4	10.4
2002/3[2]	22.6	2.9	24.4	2.5	18.1	10.6
2003/4[2]	22.1	2.9	22.9	2.4	17.8	10.4
2004/5[2]	21.3	2.7	21.3	2.3	17.0	10.0
2005/6[2]	22.1	2.8	20.8	2.2	17.6	10.4
% change 2002/3 to 2005/6	*-2.2%*	*-3.4%*	*-14.8%*	*-12.0%*	*-2.8%*	*-1.9%*
% change 2004/5 to 2005/6	*3.8%*	*3.7%*	*-2.3%*	*-4.3%*	*3.5%*	*4.0%*

Source: Institute for Fiscal Studies 2007
[1] GB figures
[2] UK figures

However, 2005/6 saw the first rise since 1997–9 in the number and proportion of people living in relative poverty.

The number of people in poverty *after* housing costs fell by 3.1 per cent between 2002/3 and 2005/6, from 13.1 million to 12.7 million. Over this period the number of people in poverty *before* housing costs fell by 1.9 per cent (*see* Tables 75 and 76, opposite).

Socio-economic inequalities consist of complex interrelationships, and the measures examined here cannot tell the full story. However, these two measures imply that both income inequality and relative poverty have improved in the United Kingdom since publication of the 2002 review. Perhaps the Joseph Rowntree Foundation (Palmer *et al* 2006) summarised the situation correctly when it concluded that '... the overall picture is not so much a mixture of success and failure as one of success and neglect. Where Government has acted, change has happened. Where it has not, previous trends have continued'.

SUMMARY: HEALTH OUTCOMES

- The 2002 review saw health outcomes as the most important output of the National Health Service and, at the same time, the most difficult to measure.

- In the General Household Survey 2005, 59 per cent of the adult population of Great Britain reported their health status as good, 27 per cent as fairly good and 14 per cent as not good. These percentages have remained largely unchanged since 1998.

- Male life expectancy at birth in the United Kingdom rose by 1.9 per cent and female life expectancy by 1.3 per cent between 1998 and 2003. Over this period the EU 15 (population-weighted) average life expectancy for males rose by 1.7 per cent and for females by 1 per cent. Latest Government Actuary's Department projections for life expectancy at birth in 2022 have moved into line with the 2002 review's projections. GAD's most recent principal life expectancy projection is now close to that of the solid progress scenario.

- The UK's infant mortality rate in 2003 was 5.3 deaths per 1,000 live births, a reduction of 7 per cent since 1998. Over the same period, the EU 15 (population-weighted) average infant mortality rate fell by 16 per cent.

- The 2002 data on potential life years lost (PYLL) indicated continued under-performance by the United Kingdom by comparison with comparator countries for ischaemic heart, cerebrovascular and respiratory diseases; however, the United Kingdom ranks higher than France and the Netherlands for PYLL relating to cancer.

- The EUROCARE-3 study showed the age-standardised relative five-year survival rate for all cancers in England as notably lower than for France, Germany, the Netherlands and Sweden, although there are some signs of catch-up. Compared with its European comparator countries, between 1985–89 and 1990–94 England demonstrated the largest improvement in five-year survival for stomach cancer and breast cancer (females only) and has matched France and the Netherlands with an increase in five-year survival for prostate cancer of more than 20 per cent. More recent ONS data shows that survival rates for lung, prostate, stomach and breast cancer continued to improve in England between 2001 and 2004, but international comparisons are not yet available

- The 2002 review assumed varying movements in health inequalities between the three scenarios, with only solid progress and fully engaged seeing reductions in inequalities. The government PSA target is to reduce inequalities in health outcomes, as measured by infant mortality and life expectancy at birth, by 2010. However, recent departmental publications indicate that health inequalities, as measured by these two indicators, have actually widened. Given long-running trends, this might have been expected.

10 Productivity: efficiency and quality

A key assumption of the 2002 review was that productivity would improve over time – in other words that there would be more or better outputs/outcomes per unit of input.

This chapter tracks recent changes in NHS productivity in the light of the 2002 review's assumptions, taking account of quality outcomes as well as unit costs.

Although the 2002 review attempted to build up estimates of potential productivity improvement from individual productivity drivers (including greater and more innovative use of ICT, better use of the workforce and redirection of existing NHS resources to more cost-effective interventions), such an approach proved impractical. The eventual productivity assumptions were based partly on what the NHS might reasonably be expected to achieve. For example, it was assumed that the NHS should be able to at least match the productivity performance in the rest of the service sector of the economy, where quality-adjusted productivity had improved by an average of around 1.5 per cent a year over the previous two decades (Wanless 2002).

The 2002 review made an important distinction between two aspects of productivity improvement:
- those related to inputs – that is, reductions in unit costs
- those associated with outputs/outcomes – that is, improved quality.

The first of these is a reasonably straightforward measure of the ratio of the volume of an output to the costs of its production. This ratio may change as a result of changes in costs, volume or a combination of the two. However, 'quality' is more elusive, both conceptually and empirically. Although the quality of health care has health outcome as its primary measure, it also encompasses a range of other factors, including access/reduction in waiting times, patient safety and other process measures, such as professional–patient communication.

Although the concept of productivity is familiar, it is not easy to measure, or to understand the difference between productivity and efficiency (*see* box, below).

Before examining how these aspects of NHS productivity have changed since 2002, this section first sets out the implications of the 2002 review's productivity assumptions in more detail and reports on official measures of productivity.

INTERPRETING CHANGES IN PRODUCTIVITY AND EFFICIENCY

Productivity measures are simply a description of performance – in particular, the ratio of outputs to inputs. Definitions vary: inputs could be measured in terms of the total costs, or factors, or elements of factors (such as labour), that combine to produce an output; while outputs can be measured in terms of the final product – such as a car – or elements of that product – such as an engine.

This simple definition of productivity can be extended to embrace outcomes – the value consumers derive from consumption of a product. It is in these terms that the quality of the output is defined. Productivity improvements may thus be a result not just of increased outputs relative to inputs, but of increased *quality* of outputs. The NHS may treat fewer patients each year, but improvements in survival rates (a possible measure of quality) could imply an increase in productivity. Further adjustments to allow for improved quality of *inputs* can also change the final productivity measure.

Although the terms productivity and efficiency are often used interchangeably, they are based on different (but related) concepts. While productivity is a ratio of (quality-adjusted) outputs to (quality-adjusted) inputs, efficiency is measured as the ratio of outputs to given inputs *relative to a maximum feasible output (given the inputs)*. The NHS could improve its productivity from one year to the next; but at the same time it could become less efficient if there were an increase in what it was feasible to produce with given inputs because, for example, of technological or organisational changes (*see* Figure 95 below).

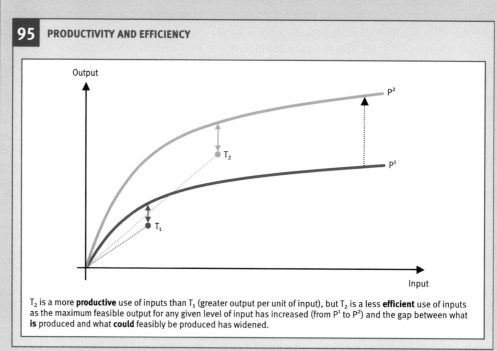

95 PRODUCTIVITY AND EFFICIENCY

T_2 is a more **productive** use of inputs than T_1 (greater output per unit of input), but T_2 is a less **efficient** use of inputs as the maximum feasible output for any given level of input has increased (from P^1 to P^2) and the gap between what **is** produced and what **could** feasibly be produced has widened.

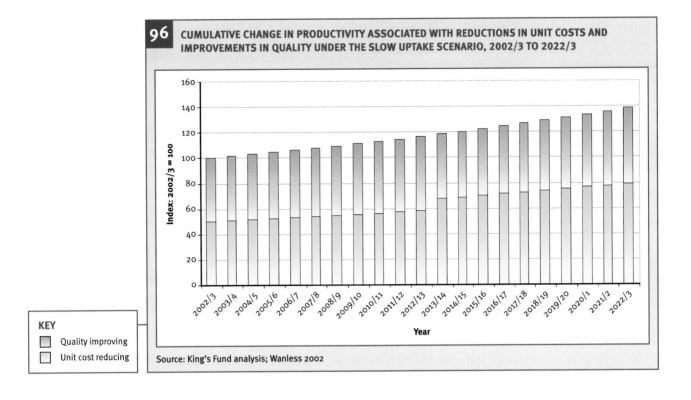

96 CUMULATIVE CHANGE IN PRODUCTIVITY ASSOCIATED WITH REDUCTIONS IN UNIT COSTS AND IMPROVEMENTS IN QUALITY UNDER THE SLOW UPTAKE SCENARIO, 2002/3 TO 2022/3

KEY
Quality improving
Unit cost reducing

Source: King's Fund analysis; Wanless 2002

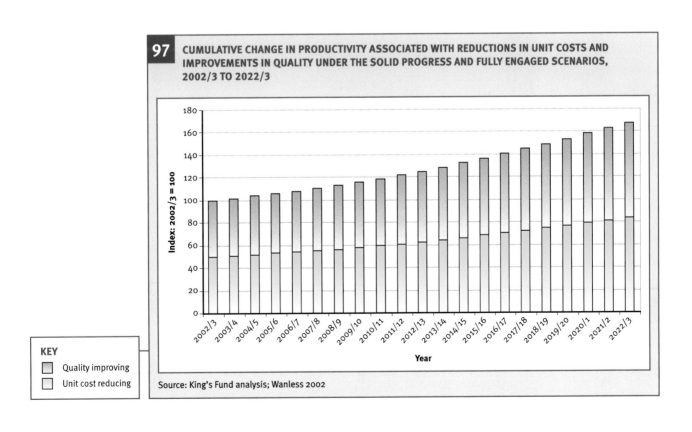

97 CUMULATIVE CHANGE IN PRODUCTIVITY ASSOCIATED WITH REDUCTIONS IN UNIT COSTS AND IMPROVEMENTS IN QUALITY UNDER THE SOLID PROGRESS AND FULLY ENGAGED SCENARIOS, 2002/3 TO 2022/3

KEY
Quality improving
Unit cost reducing

Source: King's Fund analysis; Wanless 2002

The 2002 review's productivity assumptions

The 2002 review took a macro or aggregate view of productivity improvement, expecting, in particular, that the NHS would increase its productivity year on year, at rates which varied between the three scenarios, as follows:

- solid progress: 2 to 2.5 per cent a year in the first decade, 3 per cent in the second
- slow uptake: 1.5 per cent a year in the first decade, 1.75 per cent in the second
- fully engaged: 2 to 2.5 per cent a year in the first decade, 3 per cent in the second.

Figures 96 and 97, p 217, show the cumulative impact of these assumptions over 20 years.

By 2022, in the solid progress and fully engaged scenarios, every unit of input is assumed to produce nearly 70 per cent more output than in 2002, with improvements split equally between enhanced quality and reductions in unit costs. The slow uptake scenario takes a more pessimistic view, with improvements in unit cost reduction averaging just under 1 per cent a year and quality improvements averaging 0.75 per cent, giving a total change in quality and unit cost-adjusted productivity of just over 40 per cent by 2022/3. The importance of these productivity assumptions becomes even more evident when they are converted into monetary terms and set against the 2002 review's final recommendations for health care spending up to 2022/3. Figures 98, 99 and 100 (below and opposite) show how much more expenditure the 2002 review would have had to recommend in order to achieve the same standards of service and other health care goals *if no productivity gains were made*. For the fully engaged (Figure 100) and solid progress scenarios (Figure 99) for example, the value of productivity gains by 2022/3 (at 2002/3 prices) amounts to £46.5 billion. *For both scenarios, this represents around half of the additional forecast growth in spending over and above the 2002/3 level of £68 billion.*

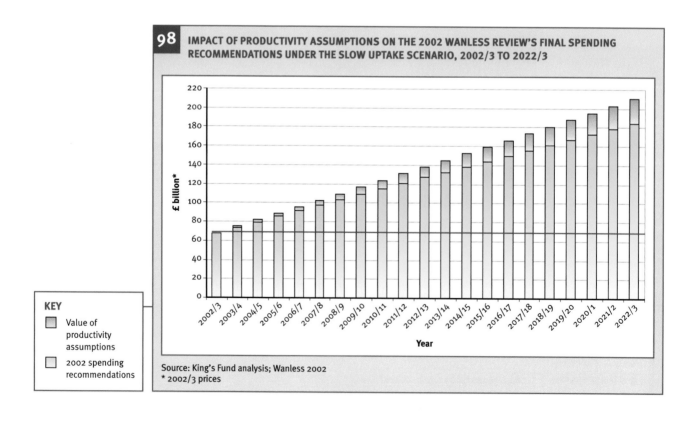

98 IMPACT OF PRODUCTIVITY ASSUMPTIONS ON THE 2002 WANLESS REVIEW'S FINAL SPENDING RECOMMENDATIONS UNDER THE SLOW UPTAKE SCENARIO, 2002/3 TO 2022/3

KEY
- Value of productivity assumptions
- 2002 spending recommendations

Source: King's Fund analysis; Wanless 2002
* 2002/3 prices

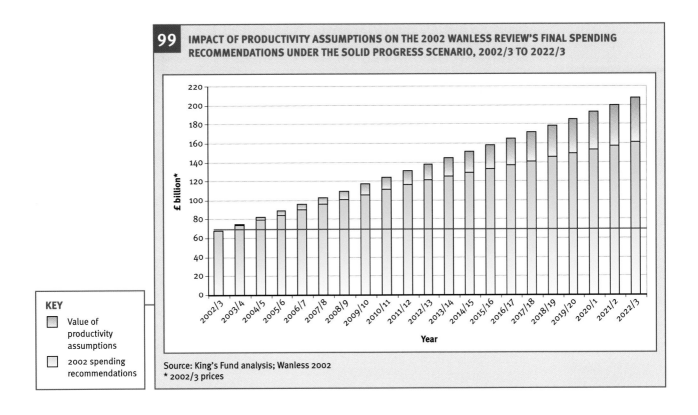

99 IMPACT OF PRODUCTIVITY ASSUMPTIONS ON THE 2002 WANLESS REVIEW'S FINAL SPENDING RECOMMENDATIONS UNDER THE SOLID PROGRESS SCENARIO, 2002/3 TO 2022/3

KEY

Value of productivity assumptions

2002 spending recommendations

Source: King's Fund analysis; Wanless 2002
* 2002/3 prices

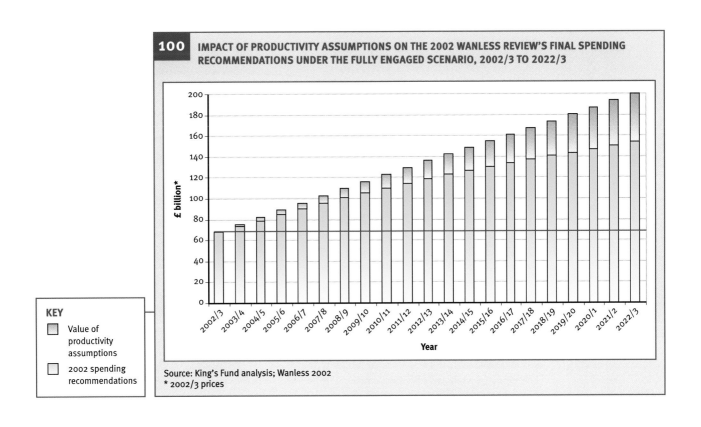

100 IMPACT OF PRODUCTIVITY ASSUMPTIONS ON THE 2002 WANLESS REVIEW'S FINAL SPENDING RECOMMENDATIONS UNDER THE FULLY ENGAGED SCENARIO, 2002/3 TO 2022/3

KEY

Value of productivity assumptions

2002 spending recommendations

Source: King's Fund analysis; Wanless 2002
* 2002/3 prices

How has NHS productivity changed since 2002?

AGGREGATE ONS/DH PRODUCTIVITY MEASURES

The 2002 review drew attention to the need for work on the measurement of productivity and for action to achieve success in accelerating productivity gains. Better measurement was considered crucial to the ability to forecast future spending, and improved productivity was considered crucial to the long-term sustainability of the health service. For many industries, not just health care, the measurement of output and the calculation and interpretation of productivity measures is problematic. Over the past few years the Department of Health and the Office for National Statistics have been working on developing more sophisticated ways of measuring the output of the NHS (Atkinson 2005; Office for National Statistics 2006b; Department of Health 2004f and 2005f) . There has been some progress in, for example, incorporating a wider range of NHS activity into the aggregate measure of NHS output, and adjusting output for changes in quality; but both parties acknowledge that further refinements are needed.

The latest measures of NHS productivity (Office for National Statistics 2006b) produce a wide range of estimates, depending on methods used to measure and value NHS inputs and outputs. Figure 101, opposite, shows that since 1999, depending on the assumptions made, changes in NHS productivity may be considered to have ranged from minus 7.5 per cent to plus 8.5 per cent.

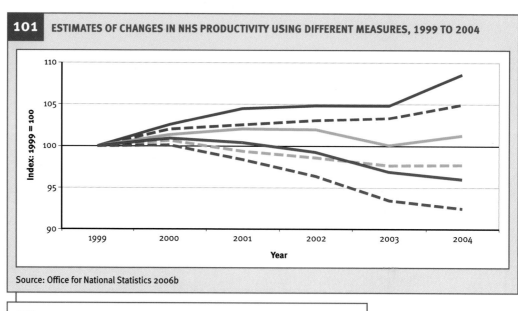

101 ESTIMATES OF CHANGES IN NHS PRODUCTIVITY USING DIFFERENT MEASURES, 1999 TO 2004

Source: Office for National Statistics 2006b

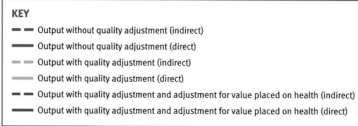

KEY

▬ ▬ Output without quality adjustment (indirect)
▬▬ Output without quality adjustment (direct)
▬ ▬ Output with quality adjustment (indirect)
▬▬ Output with quality adjustment (direct)
▬ ▬ Output with quality adjustment and adjustment for value placed on health (indirect)
▬▬ Output with quality adjustment and adjustment for value placed on health (direct)

While it is clearly desirable to adjust inputs for changes in the quality of labour and mix of labour inputs, and also adjust outputs for quality changes, the problem is how to make these adjustments. Furthermore, it is clear from figure 101, opposite, that adjusting NHS outputs to reflect increases in the value the public places on them is key to increasing the estimate of NHS productivity. This implies, counter-intuitively, that even if NHS output growth merely matched the growth in inputs, the annually increasing *value* placed on that output would produce an increase in productivity. Adjusting the value of NHS outputs in this way is contentious and, except in very specific cases, has been rejected by a panel of experts convened by a new ONS directorate, the UK Centre for Measurement of Government Activity (UKCeMGA), which has been taking forward the implementation of output and quality measurement principles noted by Atkinson (Simpkins 2007).

Given the current state of development of official NHS productivity measures, it is hard to draw definitive conclusions about changes in productivity. At best, and allowing for a degree of uncertainty, it could be concluded that productivity *possibly* improved between 1999 and 2004, largely owing to improvements in the quality of outputs.

TRIANGULATING INDICATORS OF PRODUCTIVITY

As ONS noted (Office for National Statistics 2006b), in the absence of an agreed robust productivity measure, cross-checking the range of results shown in Figure 101, opposite, by triangulation with other performance indicators can supplement our understanding of current productivity estimates. ONS examined four such indicators:

- average length of stay in hospital
- elective day case rates
- emergency readmissions
- public attitudes to health care.

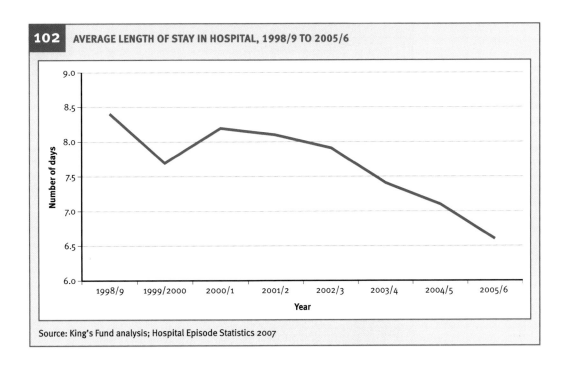

102 AVERAGE LENGTH OF STAY IN HOSPITAL, 1998/9 TO 2005/6

Source: King's Fund analysis; Hospital Episode Statistics 2007

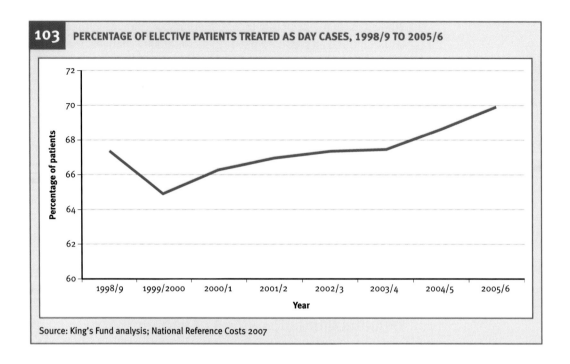

103 PERCENTAGE OF ELECTIVE PATIENTS TREATED AS DAY CASES, 1998/9 TO 2005/6

Source: King's Fund analysis; National Reference Costs 2007

Recent trends in these triangulation indicators are shown in figures 102–5, pp 221–3, which present a mixed picture of changes in productivity.

Historically, reducing length of stay in hospital has been a key driver of improved NHS productivity via a combination of increases in patient throughput/activity and reductions in beds. Recent patterns are a continuation of historic trends; since 1998/9, average

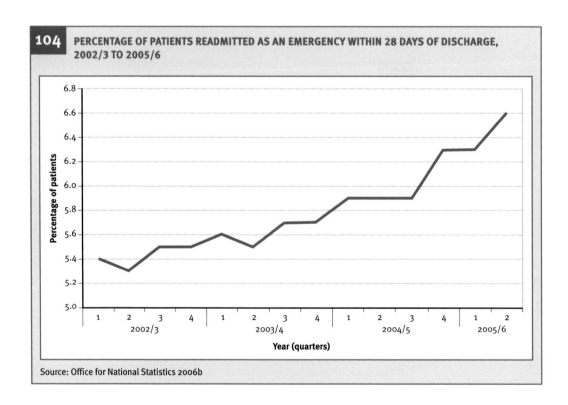

104 PERCENTAGE OF PATIENTS READMITTED AS AN EMERGENCY WITHIN 28 DAYS OF DISCHARGE, 2002/3 TO 2005/6

Source: Office for National Statistics 2006b

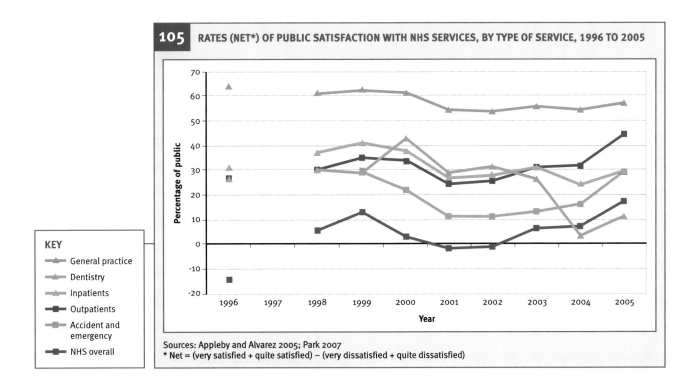

105 RATES (NET*) OF PUBLIC SATISFACTION WITH NHS SERVICES, BY TYPE OF SERVICE, 1996 TO 2005

KEY
- General practice
- Dentistry
- Inpatients
- Outpatients
- Accident and emergency
- NHS overall

Sources: Appleby and Alvarez 2005; Park 2007
* Net = (very satisfied + quite satisfied) – (very dissatisfied + quite dissatisfied)

length of stay has fallen by more than 20 per cent, suggesting an increase in productivity.

Treating patients on a day basis rather than as inpatients is another source of improved productivity; treatment tends to be less expensive and throughput increased. Recent trends indicate that in 2005/6 nearly 70 per cent of elective patients were treated as day cases, continuing an upward trend and, again, suggesting improved productivity.

Emergency readmission within 28 days of discharge after surgery is an indicative clinical quality measure. A trend for increased readmissions since 2002 suggests a deterioration in clinical quality, possibly due, in part, to early discharges linked to reduced lengths of stay in hospital.

Public attitudes to health care services provide a consumers' perspective on the NHS. Figure 105, above, suggests that net satisfaction with the NHS overall has improved since 2001 – particularly between 2004 and 2005 – and is now higher than at any time since 1996. Net satisfaction with outpatient and accident and emergency (A&E) services show significant improvement between 2001 and 2005, but trends remain relatively static for inpatient services. For some services, particularly general practice, satisfaction has traditionally been very high. However, as the ONS has noted (Office for National Statistics 2006b), surveys of satisfaction can be difficult to interpret, since drivers of satisfaction other than perceptions of the quality of NHS services can influence the results.

GERSHON EFFICIENCY GAINS

The 2004 Gershon Report (Gershon 2004) committed the Department of Health to achieving efficiency gains – half of them cash-releasing – to the value of £6.5 billion by March 2008. Five efficiency gain 'workstreams' were identified by Gershon.

- **Productive time** Modernising the provision of front-line services to make them more efficient; also improving the quality of patient care by exploiting the combined opportunities provided by new technology, process redesign and a more flexible, committed and skilled workforce.

- **Procurement** Making better use of NHS buying power at national level to obtain better value for money in the procurement of health care services, facilities management, capital projects, medical supplies and other consumables and pharmaceuticals.

- **Corporate services** Ensuring NHS organisations can share and rationalise back- office services, such as finance, ICT and human resources.

- **Social care** Improving commissioning of social care, and other cash-releasing and non-cash-releasing gains arising from the design of social care processes by local authorities.

- **Public funding and regulation** Reducing operating costs of the Department of Health, arm's length bodies, strategic health authorities and primary care trusts by reducing processes and functions, and restructuring, merging or abolishing existing organisations.

GERSHON QUALITY ASSURANCE MEASURES

Productive time
- meeting Public Service Agreement (PSA) targets on waiting times, health outcomes and patient satisfaction
- reduction in patient readmissions

Procurement
- no specific measures identified; reliance on quality standards in contracts being met

Social care
- local authorities' Annual Efficiency Statements must include one 'cross-check' quality assurance measure for each reported efficiency gain

Public funding and regulation (and central budgets)
- 'Quality of DH to be assured through existing measures of performance relating to Ministerial and Parliamentary support and customer queries' (DH ETN Dec 2005)
- arms-length bodies to be assured by meeting business plan targets etc as set out in their Annual Accountability Agreements
- no specific assurance measures for central budgets: 'DH and OGC will be working jointly to ensure that there are no resulting adverse impacts on front line quality' (DH ETN December 2005)

Corporate services
- no specific measures of assurance on Microsoft contract – reliance on contractual guarantees of improved functionality
- no assurance measures in place yet on Electronic Staff record
- No specific assurance measure for shared services contract (for outsourced finance admin etc); reliance on penalties in contract to assure quality.

TABLE 77: GERSHON EFFICIENCY GAINS (2008/9 PRICES)[1], 2004/5 TO 2006/7

Workstream		Efficiency gains (£ million)		
		2004/5	2005/6	2006/7 (Q2)
Productive time	Cumulative	508	963	1,292
	Annual	508	455	329
Procurement	Cumulative	333	1,319	1,893
	Annual	333	986	574
Corporate services	Cumulative	14	38	42
	Annual	14	24	4
Social care	Cumulative	0	179	306
	Annual	0	179	127
Public funding and regulation	Cumulative	13	77	167
	Annual	13	64	90
Total	Cumulative	868	2,576	3,700[2]
	Annual	868	1,708	1,124
Total (excluding social care)	Cumulative	868	2,397	3,394
	Annual	868	1,529	997
Savings as % total NHS spend				
at 2008/9 prices		1.25%	1.96%	1.18%
at current prices		1.13%	1.81%	0.92%

Source: Adapted from Department of Health 2005d
[1] Savings are recurrent gains against 2004 baseline
[2] £1,241 million of the £3,700 million gains are 'interim' – that is, yet to be validated.

For each of these workstreams a number of specific service/performance improvements were identified as sources of potential cash- or non-cash releasing efficiency gains. For all workstream efficiency gain measures, Gershon insisted that there should be no loss of 'quality' (and, where possible, improvements). Current assurance measures are shown in the box, opposite.

The 2006 Departmental Autumn Performance report (Department of Health 2006a) indicates that recurrent savings by mid-2006/7 total £3.7 billion (see Table 77, above).

Unfortunately, no data is provided by this report on any of the quality assurance measures mentioned in the box, opposite.

An investigation by the National Audit Office (2007a) of the reliability of reported efficiency gains across the whole Gershon programme indicated that nearly half of the gains reported by the Department of Health may be unreliable, for various reasons. The NAO used a traffic

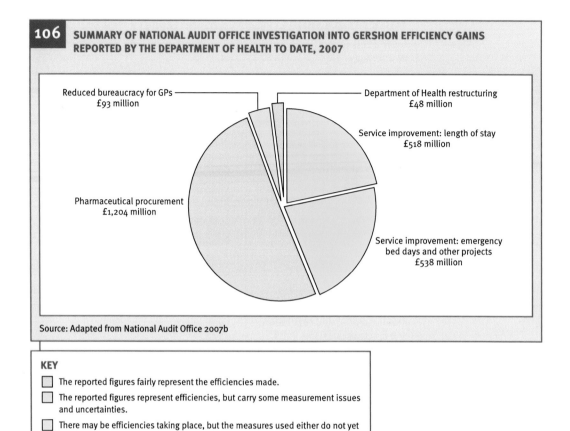

106 SUMMARY OF NATIONAL AUDIT OFFICE INVESTIGATION INTO GERSHON EFFICIENCY GAINS REPORTED BY THE DEPARTMENT OF HEALTH TO DATE, 2007

Reduced bureaucracy for GPs
£93 million

Department of Health restructuring
£48 million

Service improvement: length of stay
£518 million

Pharmaceutical procurement
£1,204 million

Service improvement: emergency bed days and other projects
£538 million

Source: Adapted from National Audit Office 2007b

KEY

☐ The reported figures fairly represent the efficiencies made.

☐ The reported figures represent efficiencies, but carry some measurement issues and uncertainties.

☐ There may be efficiencies taking place, but the measures used either do not yet demonstrate efficiencies, or the reported gains may be substantially incorrect.

light system to assess a total of £2.4 billion's worth of reported efficiency gains by the Department, and its findings are summarised in Figure 106, above.

While these official measures, productivity indicators and, in the case of Gershon, cost savings, provide one view of NHS productivity, the 2002 review emphasised the cost-reducing and quality-improving aspects of productivity. In this section and the next, the productivity experience of the NHS since 2002 is examined in some detail from the perspectives of cost and quality.

SUMMARY: 2002 REVIEW PRODUCTIVITY ASSUMPTIONS AND OFFICIAL PRODUCTIVITY MEASURES

- The 2002 review assumed that the NHS would increase its productivity year on year. The solid progress and fully engaged scenarios assumed productivity improvements of 2–2.5 per cent a year in the first decade and 3 per cent in the second. The slow uptake scenario projected lower productivity improvements of 1.5 per cent a year in the first decade and 1.75 per cent in the second.
- In monetary terms, the value of these productivity gains by 2022/3 (at 2002/3 prices) amounts to £46 billion in the solid progress and fully engaged scenarios. This represents around half of the additional forecast growth in spending over the 2002/3 level of £68 billion.
- The 2002 review made an important distinction between two aspects of productivity improvement: those related to inputs – that is, reductions in unit costs – and those associated with outputs/outcomes – that is, improved quality.
- There has been some progress in improving official measures of NHS productivity, although both the ONS and the Department of Health acknowledge that further refinements are needed. Depending on the methodology used, between 1999 and 2004 NHS productivity changed by anything from -4 per cent to +8.5 per cent.
- The National Audit Office investigation of progress on the 2004 Gershon efficiency savings programme, which committed the Department of Health to achieving £6.5 billion of cash-releasing savings/efficiency gains by March 2008, has concluded that nearly half of the reported gains are uncertain.
- A mixed picture of NHS productivity emerges when triangulation indicators, such as average length of stay in hospital, elective day case rates, emergency readmissions and public attitudes to health care, are examined.
- Official productivity measures make it hard to draw definitive conclusions about changes in productivity. At best, and allowing for a degree of uncertainty, it could be concluded that between 1999 and 2004 productivity has probably improved, largely because of improvements in the quality of outputs.

Unit costs of NHS services

The main data source for unit costs are the National Reference Costs data collection, which began in 1998. The accuracy and coverage of the reference costs has improved since then, extending to more areas of hospital and primary care trust (PCT) provider activity and covering around £36 billion of activity by 2005/6. Below unit costs in five NHS service areas are examined, which between them account for the majority of NHS spending:

- elective and emergency services
- outpatient services
- mental health services
- primary care and community services
- prescribing.

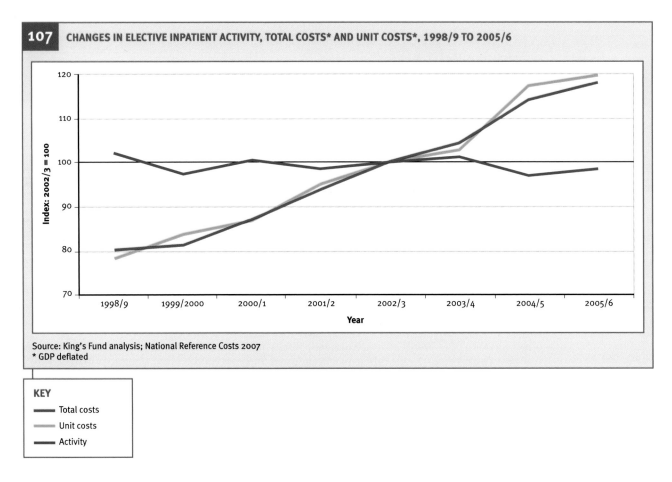

107 CHANGES IN ELECTIVE INPATIENT ACTIVITY, TOTAL COSTS* AND UNIT COSTS*, 1998/9 TO 2005/6

Source: King's Fund analysis; National Reference Costs 2007
* GDP deflated

KEY
— Total costs
— Unit costs
— Activity

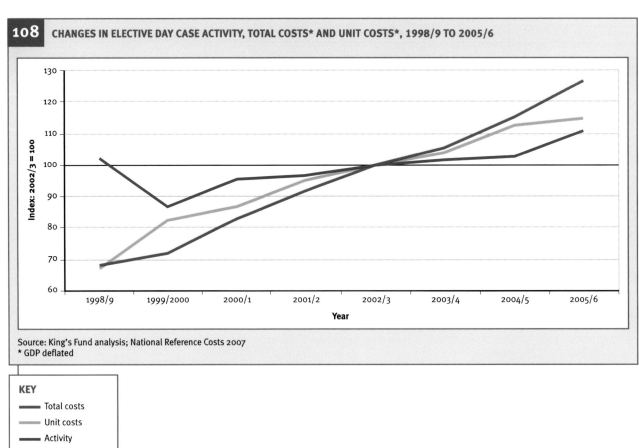

108 CHANGES IN ELECTIVE DAY CASE ACTIVITY, TOTAL COSTS* AND UNIT COSTS*, 1998/9 TO 2005/6

Source: King's Fund analysis; National Reference Costs 2007
* GDP deflated

KEY
— Total costs
— Unit costs
— Activity

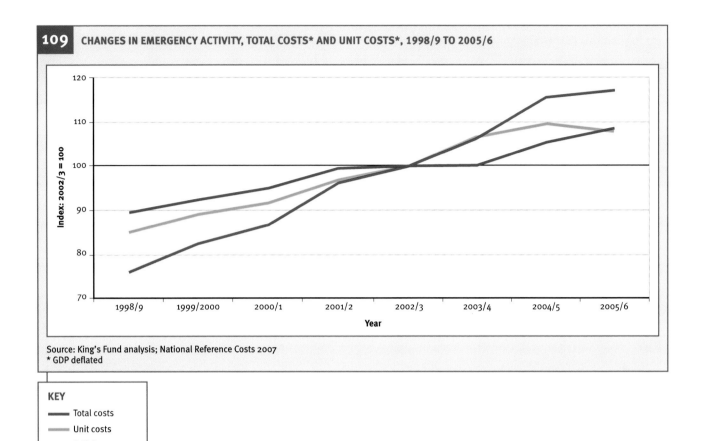

109 CHANGES IN EMERGENCY ACTIVITY, TOTAL COSTS* AND UNIT COSTS*, 1998/9 TO 2005/6

Source: King's Fund analysis; National Reference Costs 2007
* GDP deflated

KEY
Total costs
Unit costs
Activity

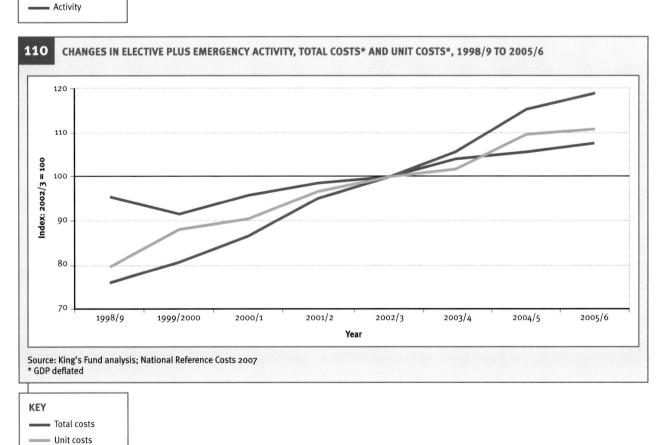

110 CHANGES IN ELECTIVE PLUS EMERGENCY ACTIVITY, TOTAL COSTS* AND UNIT COSTS*, 1998/9 TO 2005/6

Source: King's Fund analysis; National Reference Costs 2007
* GDP deflated

KEY
Total costs
Unit costs
Activity

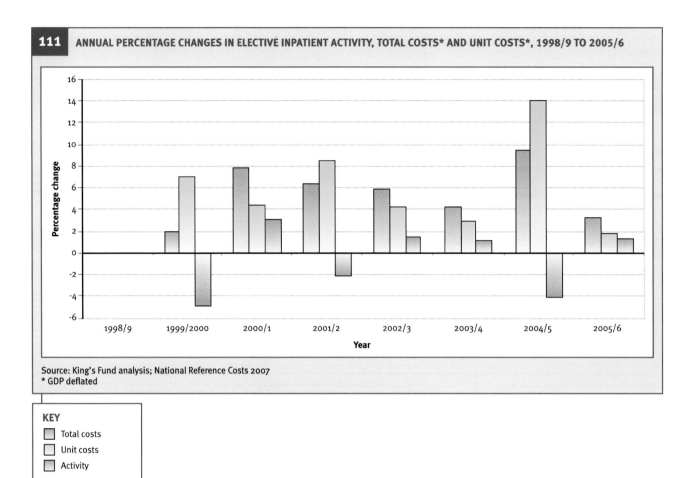

111 ANNUAL PERCENTAGE CHANGES IN ELECTIVE INPATIENT ACTIVITY, TOTAL COSTS* AND UNIT COSTS*, 1998/9 TO 2005/6

Source: King's Fund analysis; National Reference Costs 2007
* GDP deflated

KEY
- Total costs
- Unit costs
- Activity

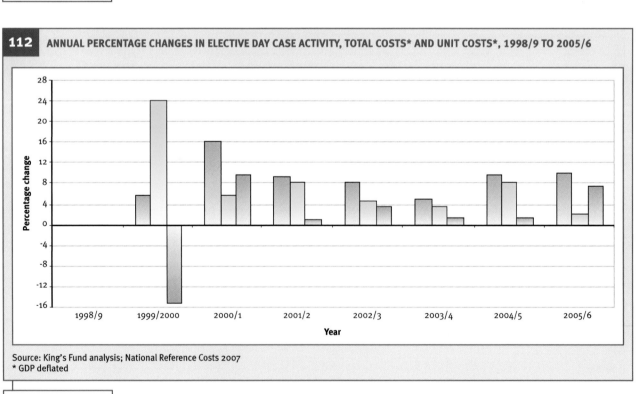

112 ANNUAL PERCENTAGE CHANGES IN ELECTIVE DAY CASE ACTIVITY, TOTAL COSTS* AND UNIT COSTS*, 1998/9 TO 2005/6

Source: King's Fund analysis; National Reference Costs 2007
* GDP deflated

KEY
- Total costs
- Unit costs
- Activity

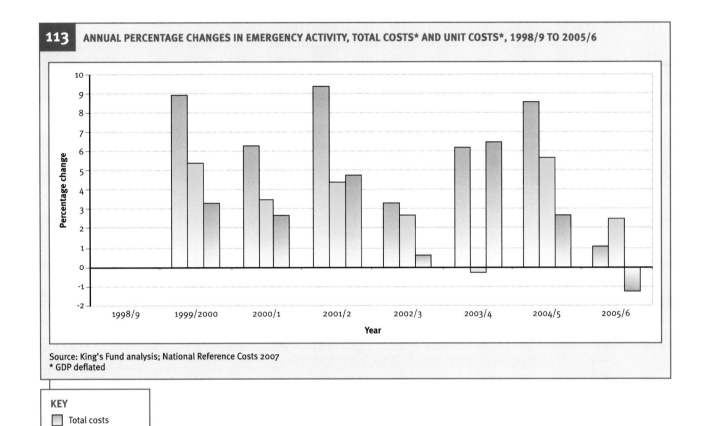

113 ANNUAL PERCENTAGE CHANGES IN EMERGENCY ACTIVITY, TOTAL COSTS* AND UNIT COSTS*, 1998/9 TO 2005/6

Source: King's Fund analysis; National Reference Costs 2007
* GDP deflated

KEY
☐ Total costs
☐ Unit costs
☐ Activity

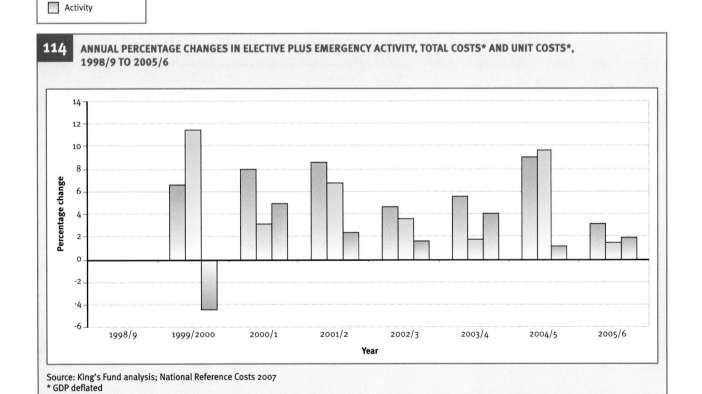

114 ANNUAL PERCENTAGE CHANGES IN ELECTIVE PLUS EMERGENCY ACTIVITY, TOTAL COSTS* AND UNIT COSTS*, 1998/9 TO 2005/6

Source: King's Fund analysis; National Reference Costs 2007
* GDP deflated

KEY
☐ Total costs
☐ Unit costs
☐ Activity

TABLE 78: ELECTIVE AND EMERGENCY ACTIVITY AND COSTS[1] COMBINED, 1998/9 TO 2005/6

	1998/9	1999/2000	2000/1	2001/2	2002/3	2003/4	2004/5	2005/6
Total cost (£)	8,904,452,554	9,442,120,449	10,138,137,011	11,114,043,803	11,720,182,438	12,376,643,401	13,490,788,559	13,909,775,154
% change		6.04	7.37	9.63	5.45	5.60	9.00	3.11
Index	76	81	87	95	100	106	115	119
Unit cost (£)	849	942	963	1,030	1,068	1,084	1,167	1,179
% change		10.90	2.25	6.98	3.68	1.51	7.63	1.08
Index	80	88	90	96	100	102	109	110
Activity (FCE[2])	10,485,816	10,026,369	10,528,884	10,789,038	10,973,379	11,416,002	11,561,689	11,793,703
% change		-4.38	5.01	2.47	1.71	4.03	1.28	2.01
Index	96	91	96	98	100	104	105	107

Source: King's Fund analysis; National Reference Costs 2007
[1] Costs deflated using GDP deflator
[2] FCE = Finished consultant episode

ELECTIVE AND EMERGENCY SERVICES

In 2005/6 elective (inpatient and day case) and non-elective (emergency) activity accounted for around £15 billion of NHS spending. Trends since 1999 for inpatients, day cases and emergencies in total spending, activity and unit costs are detailed in Figures 107–110, pp 228–9 (index trends) and 111–114, pp 230–1 (percentage annual changes); all costs have been adjusted using the GDP deflator.

Overall, as Table 78, above, shows for elective and emergency activity combined, the trend that emerges is of rising total spending – increasing by 56 per cent, from £8.9 billion to £13.9 billion (at 2002/3 prices) between 1998/9 and 2005/6. In part this was due to a 12 per cent increase in activity (10.5 million finished consultant episodes, rising to 11.8 million). But the bulk of the increase was due to increases in input costs. Average unit costs rose by 39 per cent between 1998/9 and 2005/6 – from £849 to £1,179 per case (at 2002/3 GDP-deflated prices).

These aggregate average unit costs can change not only because of actual changes in unit costs (that is, increases in input prices) and/or the total volume of outputs, but also

TABLE 79: PERCENTAGE REDUCTIONS IN UNIT COSTS EXPECTED UNDER DIFFERENT SCENARIOS, 2002/3 TO 2022/3

Scenario	% reduction in unit costs pa 2002/3–2012/13	% reduction in unit costs pa 2013/14–2022/3
Slow uptake	0.75	1.0
Solid progress	1.0	1.5
Fully engaged		

Source: Wanless 2002

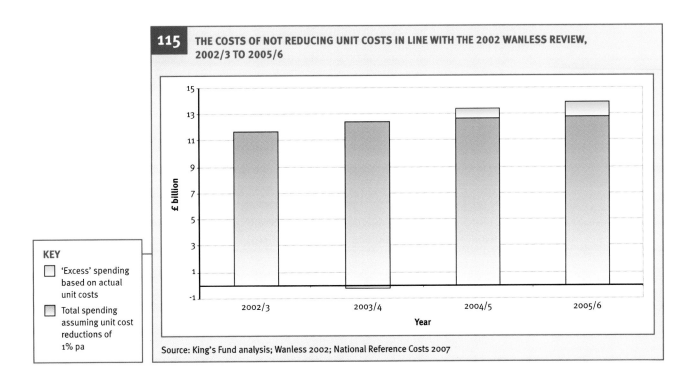

115 THE COSTS OF NOT REDUCING UNIT COSTS IN LINE WITH THE 2002 WANLESS REVIEW, 2002/3 TO 2005/6

KEY

☐ 'Excess' spending based on actual unit costs

▨ Total spending assuming unit cost reductions of 1% pa

Source: King's Fund analysis; Wanless 2002; National Reference Costs 2007

because of changes in the output mix; for example, increases in the proportion of relatively more costly activity, such as inpatient activity, can increase overall unit costs even if unit costs for individual activities remain unchanged. Between 1998/9 and 2005/6 the share of inpatient activity fell by 2.3 per cent, and by 1.6 per cent for day cases. However, emergency activity has increased its share by nearly 4 per cent. Separating out these effects (by keeping the mix of activity constant) shows, however, that of the 38 per

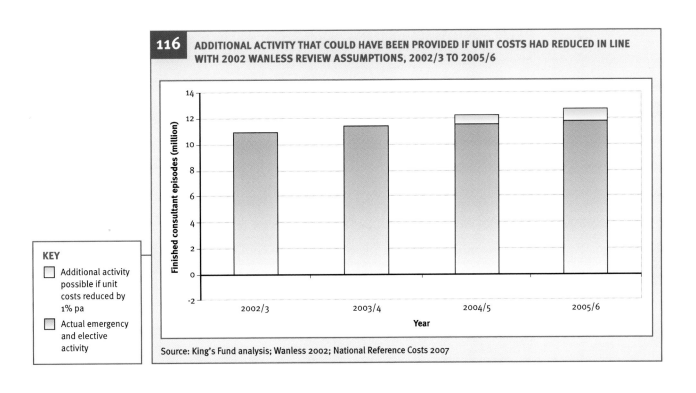

116 ADDITIONAL ACTIVITY THAT COULD HAVE BEEN PROVIDED IF UNIT COSTS HAD REDUCED IN LINE WITH 2002 WANLESS REVIEW ASSUMPTIONS, 2002/3 TO 2005/6

KEY

☐ Additional activity possible if unit costs reduced by 1% pa

▨ Actual emergency and elective activity

Source: King's Fund analysis; Wanless 2002; National Reference Costs 2007

cent rise in unit costs between 1998/9 and 2005/6, only 0.3 per cent was estimated to be due to changes in case-mix.

The effect of these unit cost increases in relation to the 2002 review's assumptions (see Table 75) of reductions in unit costs are illustrated in Figures 115 and 116, p 233.

Figure 115 shows the level of spend that would have been incurred to achieve the same actual level of activity each year if the unit cost reductions assumed by the 2002 review had occurred each year (from 2003/4). The 'excess' spending is the difference between this figure and actual spend, and suggests, for example, that in 2005/6, the same level of activity (of around 11.8 million finished consultant episodes) could have been produced for around 8 per cent less expenditure – equivalent to a saving of more than £1 billion on a total actual spend of £13.9 billion (at 2002/3 prices).

Another way of looking at this is in terms of the extra activity that could have been provided if the actual total spend remained the same and unit cost reductions had been spent entirely on increasing the number of patients treated. On this basis, in 2005/6 the NHS could have increased activity levels by nearly 9 per cent – treating an additional 1 million emergency and elective patients (see Figure 116, p 233).

The impacts on total costs and activity of failing to achieve unit cost reductions are illustrative only, but they emphasise the importance of productivity improvements and the real impact such improvements (or the lack of them) can have on patient care.

OUTPATIENT SERVICES

In 2005/6, total expenditure on outpatient services amounted to around £5.8 billion. Trends since 1999 for an aggregate of first, subsequent and 'undefined' outpatient activity

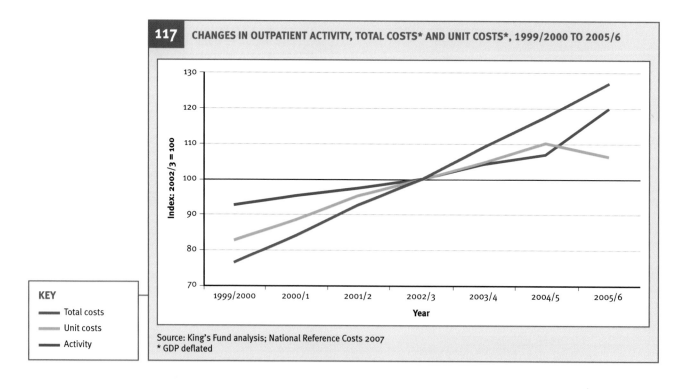

117 CHANGES IN OUTPATIENT ACTIVITY, TOTAL COSTS* AND UNIT COSTS*, 1999/2000 TO 2005/6

KEY
— Total costs
— Unit costs
— Activity

Source: King's Fund analysis; National Reference Costs 2007
* GDP deflated

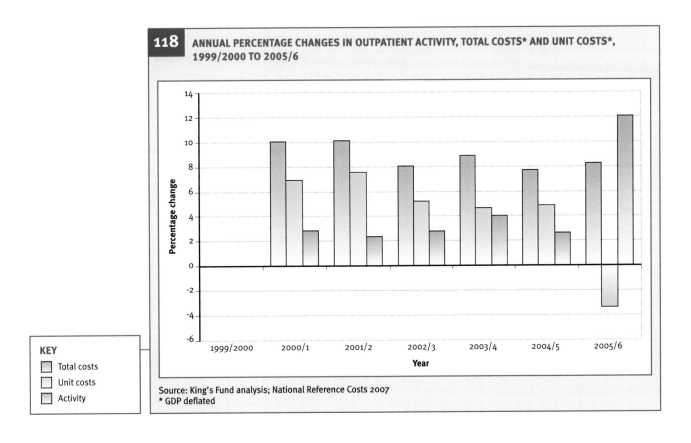

118 ANNUAL PERCENTAGE CHANGES IN OUTPATIENT ACTIVITY, TOTAL COSTS* AND UNIT COSTS*, 1999/2000 TO 2005/6

KEY
- Total costs
- Unit costs
- Activity

Source: King's Fund analysis; National Reference Costs 2007
* GDP deflated

in total spending, activity and unit costs are detailed in Figures 117, opposite (index trends) and 118, above (percentage annual changes) and in detail in Table 80, opposite: all cost figures have been adjusted using the GDP deflator.

TABLE 80: OUTPATIENT ACTIVITY AND COSTS¹ 1999/2000 TO 2005/6

	1999/2000	2000/1	2001/2	2002/3	2003/4	2004/5	2005/6
Total cost (£)	3,227,618,701	3,551,239,158	3,911,583,283	4,227,538,007	4,602,562,270	4,955,826,425	5,366,501,276
% change		10.03	10.15	8.08	8.87	7.68	8.29
Index	76.3	84.0	92.5	100.0	108.9	117.2	126.9
Unit cost (£)	77.25	82.63	88.89	93.49	97.86	102.64	99.18
% change		6.95	7.58	5.18	4.68	4.88	-3.37
Index	82.6	88.4	95.1	100.0	104.7	109.8	106.1
Activity (FCE²)	41,779,508	42,980,114	44,006,575	45,220,247	47,031,029	48,283,435	54,107,395
% change		2.87	2.39	2.76	4.00	2.66	12.06
Index	92.4	95.0	97.3	100.0	104.0	106.8	119.7

Source: King's Fund analysis; National Reference Costs 2007
¹ Costs deflated using GDP deflator
² FCE = Finished consultant episode

TABLE 81: UNIT COSTS AND CHANGE IN UNIT COSTS FOR MENTAL HEALTH SERVICES, 2004/5 TO 2005/6

Services	Unit cost 2005/6 (£)	% change in real unit cost 2004/5–2005/6
Inpatient	248	6.8
Specialist services: inpatient	401	-2.4
Outpatient first attendance	259	-0.4
Community-based first attendance	248	8.7
Specialist services: outpatient first attendance	246	-22.3
Specialist services: community-based first attendance	260	-28.4
Outpatient follow-up attendance	144	5.7
Community-based follow-up attendance	122	8.0
Specialist services: outpatient follow-up attendance	149	0.4
Specialist services: community-based follow-up attendance	135	-3.5
Domiciliary visit	211	9.2
Secure unit	474	7.7
Specialist teams	149	-12.4
Day care facilities	108	0.7

Source: National Reference Costs 2007
Note: Unit costs are based on various activity units depending on the service area.

MENTAL HEALTH SERVICES

The multi-activity nature of mental health services, coupled with significant changes in NHS services and in data collection, means that this sector of the NHS does not easily lend itself to the sort of analysis carried out above for hospital services. The following, inevitably partial, analysis of unit costs is based on National Reference Cost data.

These data suggest that around £4.5 billion was spent on mental health services across England in 2005/6. This is somewhat less than the total reported by the National Programme Budget data set, which includes such additional expenditure as prescribing related to mental health. Table 81, above, shows the real change in unit cost for various mental health services between 2004/5 and 2005/6 (the only period for which data are fully comparable). Of the 14 different categories of mental health services, six saw a reduction in unit costs between 2004/5 and 2005/6. However, the eight that saw an *increase* in unit costs accounted for 80 per cent of the total cost of mental health services in England in 2005/6.

Figures 119–122, pp 237–8, provide a historical analysis of selected mental health services, which, in 2005/6 accounted for 77 per cent of total mental health spend. They show that for 77 per cent of mental health spending in England, real unit costs rose by between 19 and 33 per cent between 2002/3 and 2005/6. These figures do not include specialist services for inpatients, outpatients and specialist team services, many of which showed a fall in unit costs in the single year to 2005/6 (*see* Table 81, above).

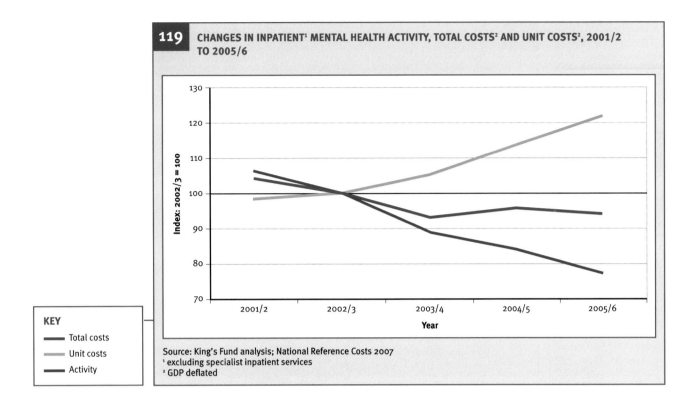

119 CHANGES IN INPATIENT[1] MENTAL HEALTH ACTIVITY, TOTAL COSTS[2] AND UNIT COSTS[2], 2001/2 TO 2005/6

KEY
— Total costs
— Unit costs
— Activity

Source: King's Fund analysis; National Reference Costs 2007
[1] excluding specialist inpatient services
[2] GDP deflated

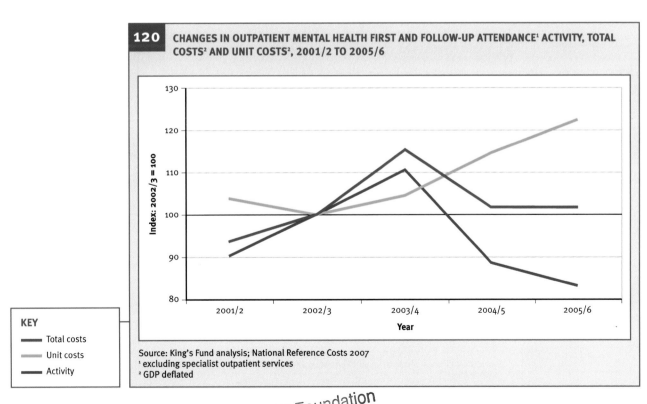

120 CHANGES IN OUTPATIENT MENTAL HEALTH FIRST AND FOLLOW-UP ATTENDANCE[1] ACTIVITY, TOTAL COSTS[2] AND UNIT COSTS[2], 2001/2 TO 2005/6

KEY
— Total costs
— Unit costs
— Activity

Source: King's Fund analysis; National Reference Costs 2007
[1] excluding specialist outpatient services
[2] GDP deflated

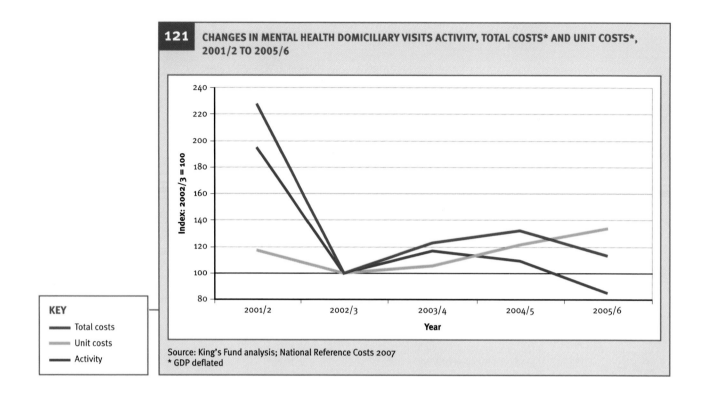

121 CHANGES IN MENTAL HEALTH DOMICILIARY VISITS ACTIVITY, TOTAL COSTS* AND UNIT COSTS*, 2001/2 TO 2005/6

KEY
— Total costs
— Unit costs
— Activity

Source: King's Fund analysis; National Reference Costs 2007
* GDP deflated

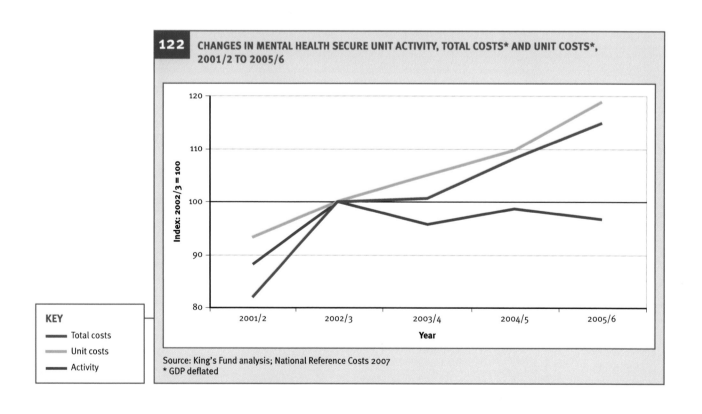

122 CHANGES IN MENTAL HEALTH SECURE UNIT ACTIVITY, TOTAL COSTS* AND UNIT COSTS*, 2001/2 TO 2005/6

KEY
— Total costs
— Unit costs
— Activity

Source: King's Fund analysis; National Reference Costs 2007
* GDP deflated

Overall, unit costs for mental health services in England have been on an upward trend since 2002/3. However, changes in unit costs should be interpreted with caution since the service has undergone significant transformation over the period examined, and many specialist mental health services have shown a recent improvement in unit cost performance, albeit based on one year's data.

PRIMARY CARE SERVICES

It is even more difficult to construct any meaningful cost measure for general medical services than it is for mental health services. But, given the increased costs associated with the new GP contract, there is clearly a need to quantify value for money, and not just in unit cost terms.

PRESCRIBING

The cost to the NHS of dispensing prescriptions in 2006 was £8.2 billion – a rise of 3.3 per cent on 2005. However, since 2002 total spending has increased by 22 per cent, while the cost per prescription has fallen by around 1.8 per cent (*see* Table 82, below). In real terms, the cost per prescription has fallen by the much greater margin of 12 per cent (*see* Figure 123, overleaf), mostly because of reduced costs (largely for statins) between 2004 and 2006.

Ranking drugs dispensed in 2006 by the value of the change in their costs (that is, the change in unit cost between 2002 and 2006 multiplied by the change in the volume of prescriptions), as in Table 83, overleaf, shows that the unit cost reduction of lipid-regulating drugs contributed around 55 per cent of the total net reduction in prescribing costs over this period (*see* below for details).

TABLE 82: PRESCRIPTION COSTS, 2000 TO 2006

Year to December	Prescription items (million)	Total cost (£ million)	Real cost at 2002 prices (£ million)	Cost per prescription (£)	Real cost per prescription at 2002 prices (£)	Prescription items per head
2000	551.8	5,584.6	5,894.0	10.12	10.68	11.2
2001	587.0	6,116.6	6,305.8	10.42	10.74	11.9
2002	617.0	6,846.7	6,846.7	11.10	11.10	12.4
2003	649.7	7,510.1	7,293.2	11.56	11.23	13.0
2004	686.1	8,079.6	7,636.1	11.78	11.13	13.7
2005	720.3	7,936.6	7,363.6	11.02	10.22	14.3
2006	752.0	8,196.8	7,401.1	10.90	9.77	na
% change 2002–6	21.9%	19.7%	8.1%	-1.8%	-12.0%	na
% change 2005–6	4.4%	3.2%	0.5%	-1.1%	-4.4%	na

Source: Department of Health 2006d; Information Centre 2007d

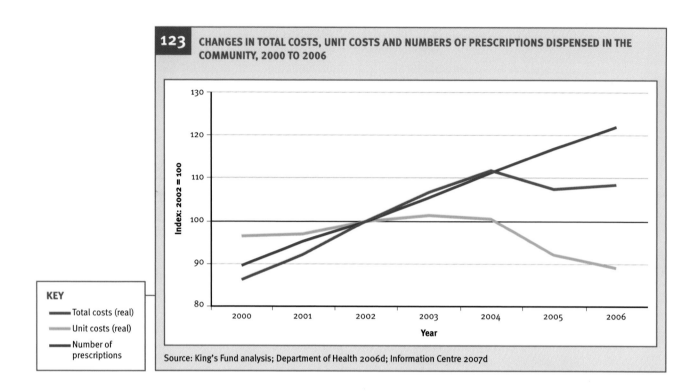

123 CHANGES IN TOTAL COSTS, UNIT COSTS AND NUMBERS OF PRESCRIPTIONS DISPENSED IN THE COMMUNITY, 2000 TO 2006

KEY
— Total costs (real)
— Unit costs (real)
— Number of prescriptions

Source: King's Fund analysis; Department of Health 2006d; Information Centre 2007d

TABLE 83: TOP TEN PRESCRIPTION DRUGS DISPENSED IN 2006, RANKED BY VALUE OF THE CHANGE IN UNIT COSTS, 2002 TO 2006

British National Formulary section name	Change in unit cost (£)	Change in volume (thousands)	Value of change in unit cost × volume (£)
Lipid-regulating drugs	-17.65	24,494	-432,382
Mucolytics	-410.37	334	-136,938
Hypertension and heart failure	-6.61	18,151	-120,028
Ulcer-healing drugs	-10.16	8,958	-90,987
Drugs affecting bone metabolism	-10.90	3,447	-37,579
Nitrates, calcium channel blockers and other antianginal drugs	-4.65	6,714	-31,234
Cytotoxic drugs	40.79	-671	-27,350
Antidepressant drugs	-5.07	4,709	-23,891
Other health supplements	-11.36	719	-8,170
Drugs for dementia	-11.34	529	-5,994
Net change: all prescriptions	**-0.190**	**133,528**	**-779,548**

Source: King's Fund analysis; Information Centre 2007d

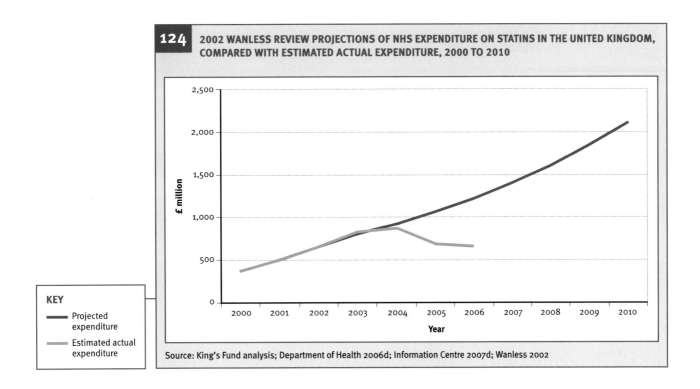

124 2002 WANLESS REVIEW PROJECTIONS OF NHS EXPENDITURE ON STATINS IN THE UNITED KINGDOM, COMPARED WITH ESTIMATED ACTUAL EXPENDITURE, 2000 TO 2010

KEY
━━━ Projected expenditure
━━━ Estimated actual expenditure

Source: King's Fund analysis; Department of Health 2006d; Information Centre 2007d; Wanless 2002

Lipid-regulating drugs: statins

The 2002 review noted that a significant aspect of the cost of improving quality in the treatment and prevention of coronary heart disease was new and more effective drug treatments, including statins. The 2002 review projected an increase in NHS expenditure on statins in the UK from around £700 million in 2002/3 to £2.1 billion by 2010,

TABLE 84: COST, REAL COST AND NUMBER OF STATINS DISPENSED IN THE COMMUNITY, 2000 TO 2006

Year to December	Number of statins dispensed (million)	Cost of statins (£ million)	Real cost of statins at 2002 prices (£)	Real cost per statin dispensed (£)
2000	9.4	308.4	325.5	34.6
2001	12.6	420.6	433.6	34.4
2002	16.7	552.2	552.2	33.1
2003	21.6	694.1	674.1	31.2
2004	28.1	738.2	697.6	24.8
2005	33.8	578.3	535.9	15.9
2006	39.7	554.1	501.0	12.6
% change 2002–6	*137.7%*	*0.3%*	*-9.3%*	*-61.8%*
% change 2005–6	*17.5%*	*-4.2%*	*-6.5%*	*-20.4%*

Source: Department of Health 2006d; Information Centre 2007d
Note: The GDP deflator has been used to create the real cost figures. However, as the deflator is only available for fiscal years and not calendar years we have applied the 2002/3 deflator for the calendar year 2000, for example. Overall statin data includes Atorvastatin, Fluvastatin Sodium, Pravastatin Sodium, Rosuvastatin Calcium and Simvastatin.

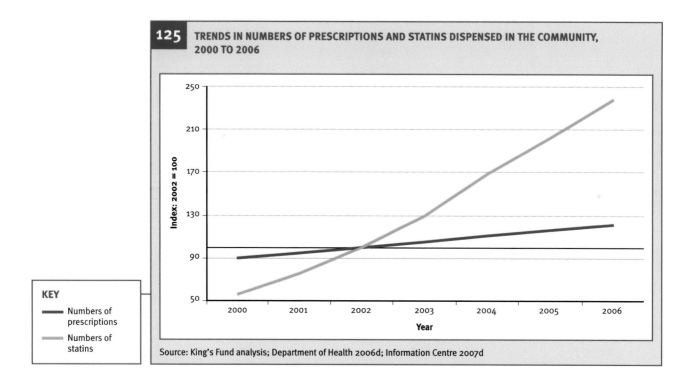

125 TRENDS IN NUMBERS OF PRESCRIPTIONS AND STATINS DISPENSED IN THE COMMUNITY, 2000 TO 2006

KEY
— Numbers of prescriptions
— Numbers of statins

Source: King's Fund analysis; Department of Health 2006d; Information Centre 2007d

representing an average annual increase of around 15 per cent (Wanless 2002). These projections are highly sensitive to assumptions about how many people currently have heart disease, how many might develop it in the future (which depends on preventive strategies relating to such lifestyle factors as diet, exercise and smoking), whether people take the drugs they are prescribed and, of course, the cost of the drugs (which partly depends on when their patents expire). Encouragingly, the actual cost to the NHS of prescribing statins has diverged from the 2002 review's projections since 2004. The cumulative saving compared with the projected spend on statins is around £944 million in the four years since 2002 (*see* Figure 124, p 241).

There are five statins currently approved for use within the United Kingdom for the treatment of high cholesterol: atorvastatin, fluvastatin, pravastatin, rosuvastatin and simvastatin. Since 2002 the number of statins dispensed has risen by 137.7 per cent to 39.7 million (*see* Table 84, p 241). This compares with an increase of only 22 per cent in the total number of prescriptions dispensed in England, as Figure 125, above, demonstrates.

The actual cost of prescribing statins rose then fell, so that in 2006 total costs were only 0.3 per cent higher than in 2002. However, the real cost to the NHS has actually fallen by almost 10 per cent (*see* Figures 124 and 125). This reduction resulted from a significant increase in the volume of low-cost statins (such as simvastatin and pravastatin) prescribed in England. In May 2003 the patent on Zocor (simvastatin) expired, resulting in the introduction of new generic products. Between 2002 and 2006 the volume of simvastatin prescribed rose by 216 per cent, compared with a 138 per cent rise in the volume of all statins. In consequence, simvastatin as a proportion of all statins prescribed in England rose from 43 per cent to 57 per cent. More importantly, over this period the cost per simvastatin prescription fell from £35.83 to £4.21, a reduction of almost 90 per cent. These savings are in line with Department of Health estimates of potential savings to be made by prescribing lower-cost statins (Department of Health 2006i).

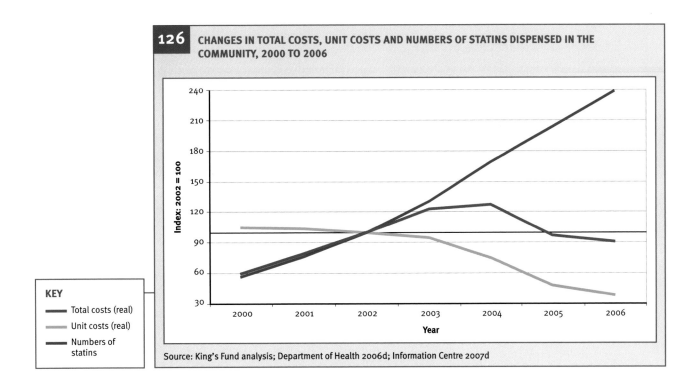

126 CHANGES IN TOTAL COSTS, UNIT COSTS AND NUMBERS OF STATINS DISPENSED IN THE COMMUNITY, 2000 TO 2006

KEY
— Total costs (real)
— Unit costs (real)
— Numbers of statins

Source: King's Fund analysis; Department of Health 2006d; Information Centre 2007d

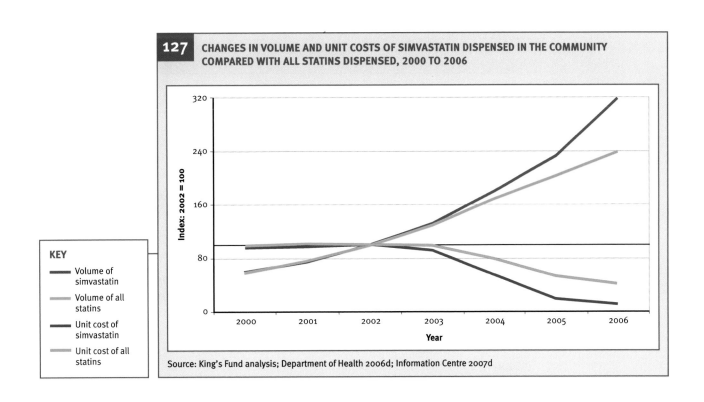

127 CHANGES IN VOLUME AND UNIT COSTS OF SIMVASTATIN DISPENSED IN THE COMMUNITY COMPARED WITH ALL STATINS DISPENSED, 2000 TO 2006

KEY
— Volume of simvastatin
— Volume of all statins
— Unit cost of simvastatin
— Unit cost of all statins

Source: King's Fund analysis; Department of Health 2006d; Information Centre 2007d

- While official indicators and efficiency measures provide one view of NHS productivity, the 2002 review emphasised the importance of unit cost reduction and quality improvement in its assumptions underlying NHS productivity in the future.
- Elective and non-elective activity accounted for around £15 billion of NHS spending in 2005/6. Between 1998/9 and 2005/6 there has been an overall real rise in combined spending on elective and emergency services of 56 per cent. However, activity increased by only 12 per cent, with unit costs rising by 39 per cent – from £849 to £1,179. Since 2002/3, real unit costs have risen by 10 per cent.
- Changes in case-mix account for only 0.3 per cent of the increase in elective and emergency unit costs since 1998/9.
- Had unit costs decreased in line with the 2002 review's assumptions, then in 2005/6 the same level of activity (of around 11.8 million finished consultant episodes) would have cost £1 billion less than the actual spend of £13.9 billion (at 2002/3 prices) – equivalent to treating an additional one million emergency and elective patients.
- In 2005/6, total expenditure on outpatient services (excluding mental health) amounted to around £5.8 billion. Trends for an aggregate of first, subsequent and 'undefined' outpatient appointments show that between 1999/2000 and 2005/6 real unit costs increased by 28 per cent. Since 2002/3, real unit costs have risen by 6.1 per cent, although in 2005/6 they actually fell by 3.4 per cent.
- Mental health and general practitioner services account for a significant proportion of the total NHS budget, yet virtually no conclusions can be drawn about productivity changes in these sectors since 2002, mostly because of the lack of routine and consistent data from which to calculate unit costs.
- Some 752 million prescription items were dispensed in the community in England in the year to December 2006, at a cost of £8.2 billion. Although the total cost has increased by 20 per cent since 2002, the cost per prescription has fallen by around 1.8 per cent. However, in real terms the cost per prescription has fallen by 12 per cent, largely because of reduced unit costs for statins between 2004 and 2006. The unit cost of statins prescribed has fallen substantially since 2003.

Quality: changes in health outcomes

Another of the 2002 review's key assumptions about productivity was that the nature of the health care 'product' would change. In particular, the review assumed that the quality of health care would improve over time and that basic measures of output, and hence productivity, would need to reflect this. The 2002 review broadly assumed that changes in quality would add as much as reductions in unit costs to productivity. As Figure 128, opposite, shows, the projected annual value of improvements in quality range from £700 million to £1.3 billion by 2022 (at 2002 prices) and represent between 0.75 per cent and 0.93 per cent of total NHS spend under the fully engaged scenario.

Cumulatively, by 2022/3, the value of quality improvements assumed by the 2002 review under the fully engaged/solid progress scenarios was projected to be around £20 billion.

While there is extensive published material exploring definitions of quality in health care, here it is taken primarily to mean improvements in health outcome – meaning length or (health-related) quality of life. Such a definition goes to the heart of the purposes of health

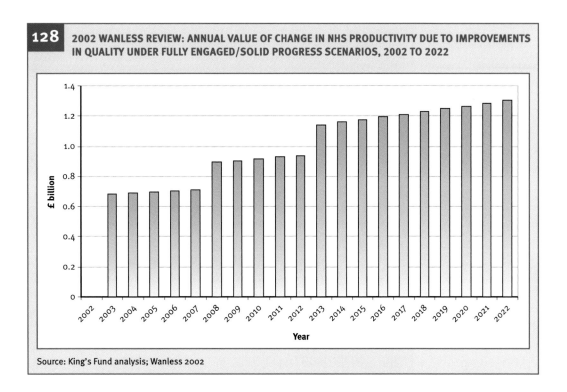

128 2002 WANLESS REVIEW: ANNUAL VALUE OF CHANGE IN NHS PRODUCTIVITY DUE TO IMPROVEMENTS IN QUALITY UNDER FULLY ENGAGED/SOLID PROGRESS SCENARIOS, 2002 TO 2022

Source: King's Fund analysis; Wanless 2002

care, yet the dearth of data or evidence about changes in quality is startling. Although important reports – such as the Atkinson review of 2005 and a follow-up report from the Department of Health (2005e) – set out the main principles of how to account for quality, there are no comprehensive measures of health available for the NHS (*see* box, overleaf). Even if such measures could be agreed, it would still be difficult to attach a *value* to them.

However, there are other measures, or indicators, that reflect the quality of health care – measures that are also valued by patients and that may contribute to eventual health outcomes or have their own intrinsic value. Progress on a selection of these other quality measures – patient safety, patient experience of care, waiting times and others – is summarised below, drawing on the more detailed assessment of health outcomes in the previous chapter.

First, however, it is worth noting the attempt by the Department of Health to quantify a particular quality improvement: the use of statins to lower cholesterol as part of a programme to prevent coronary heart disease.

STATINS: AN EXAMPLE OF QUALITY IMPROVEMENT

The 2002 review noted that a significant cost of improving quality in the treatment and prevention of coronary heart disease involved new and more effective drug treatments, such as lipid-regulating statins. The review estimated that expenditure on statins would increase from around £700 million in 2002/3 to £2.1 billion by 2010 (Wanless 2002).

Table 84 on p 241 shows volume and cost information for statins dispensed between 2000 and 2006 and reflects the unit price reductions from 2004. Assuming that the use of statins is an example of improved quality, what, in the light of their increased use, has been their contribution to NHS productivity gains?

The value of productivity gain due to quality assumed by the 2002 review was, as noted, around £700 million a year, at 2002 prices, for each year between 2002 and 2007. Setting this in the context of improvements in health, using NICE's current cost per quality adjusted life year (QALY) 'acceptability range' of £20,000–£30,000, suggests that such quality improvements are equivalent to an additional 23,000–35,000 QALYs per year.

Work by the Department of Health on assigning 'value weights' to NHS outputs (2005f) adds a further dimension to this calculation. Its conclusions suggest that in one year (2003), with around 21.6 million statin prescriptions, there were total life year gains of around 83,000 which, the Department argued, could be taken as equivalent to the same number of quality adjusted life years after taking account of various quality gains and losses. This was equivalent to a gain of 0.0038 QALYs (83,000/21,600,000) per prescription; using the upper end of NICE's cost per QALY range (£30,000), the Department then estimated the value of each prescription to be £115 (30,000 × 0.0038).

Using this *value* weight (rather than the *cost* weight of £27), the Department estimates that overall output of the NHS rose by 0.81 per cent on average over the years 1998/9 to 2002/3 as a result of increased use of statins. These are substantial gains. For example, again using NICE's cost per QALY acceptability range, the gain of 83,000 QALYs in one year

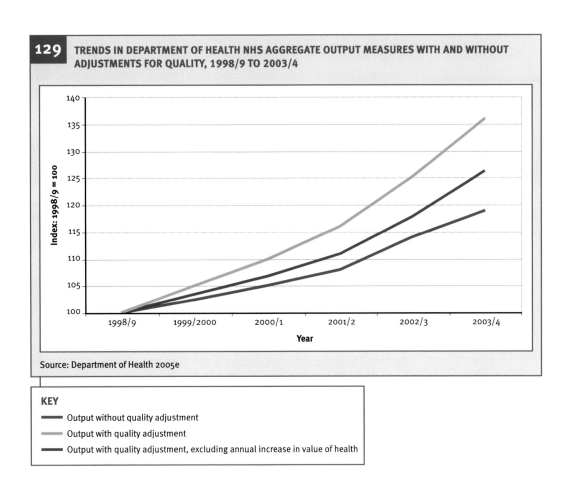

129 TRENDS IN DEPARTMENT OF HEALTH NHS AGGREGATE OUTPUT MEASURES WITH AND WITHOUT ADJUSTMENTS FOR QUALITY, 1998/9 TO 2003/4

Source: Department of Health 2005e

KEY
— Output without quality adjustment
— Output with quality adjustment
— Output with quality adjustment, excluding annual increase in value of health

TABLE 85: BENEFITS OF PRESCRIBING STATINS IN TERMS OF QALYS GAINED AND VALUE OF THESE TO THE NHS, 2000 TO 2007

Year	Prescriptions	Total cost (£ million)	Total QALYs[1]	Change in QALYs	Total benefit[2] (£ million)
2000	9.4	308	35,720	0	1,072
2001	12.6	421	47,880	12,160	1,436
2002	16.7	552	63,460	15,580	1,904
2003	21.6	694	83,000	19,540	2,490
2004	28.1	738	106,780	23,780	3,203
2005	33.8	578	128,440	21,660	3,853
2006	39.7	544	150,860	22,420	4,566
2007[3]	45.0	617	171,000	20,140	5,175

Source: King's Fund analysis
[1] Total QALYs = Number of prescriptions x 0.0038
[2] Total benefit = Prescriptions x £115
[3] Prescription figures for 2007 are estimates based on log trend since 2000; total costs are estimates based on 2006 unit cost of £13.70.

translates into a monetary equivalent of between £1.7 billion and £2.5 billion (against the actual prescription cost of around £700 million). Bearing in mind a degree of qualification surrounding these estimates due to necessary assumptions made in the calculations, this would imply that the use of statins alone just about meets the original 2002 review's assumptions about productivity gains due to quality improvements.

Although stretching the example somewhat, it is also possible to estimate the contribution statins have made (and will make) to the value of productivity gains attributable to quality improvements for the period 2000 to 2007. Based on current prescribing trends, the number of statin prescriptions for 2007 will be of the order of 45 million. Using the benefit value per prescription of £115 and the QALY gain per prescription of 0.0038, Table 85, p 247, sets out QALYs gained and the value of these to the NHS.

While a degree of uncertainty will necessarily surround these estimates, given various assumptions underlying the amount of QALY gain and value of the QALY benefits, significant productivity gains are likely to flow from the use of statins.

OTHER MEASURES OF QUALITY

As already noted, other measures apart from health outcomes are also generally accepted as indicators of health care quality. The previous chapter explored a number of key process outcome measures, including patient safety, choice and privacy, access and waiting times, and patients' satisfaction with their experience of care.

Patient safety

In broad terms, patient safety, including reports of hospital-acquired infections, seems to have improved over the last few years; however, the quality of data in some areas – for example, reports by staff witnessing potentially harmful errors, near misses or incidents – make it difficult to be certain about such improvements.

Patient choice

Although the national patient choice programme continues to roll out, with patients needing a referral to hospital due to be offered a choice of any hospital by 2008, the current evidence is that most patients don't recall being offered any choice by their GPs (Department of Health 2007u).

Although surveys suggest a desire for choice of hospital (for example Appleby and Alvarez 2005), it remains to be seen to what extent patients will not only exercise choice but, through such choices, improve their health and/or experience of health care. In theory, and with the right sort of information, choice of hospital could be expected to improve health and the patient experience. However, the nature of the choice currently on offer (of hospital only) may need to be extended much further into the patient pathway – to choice of clinical team, for example – and widened to include more active patient participation in decision-making before significant benefits are realised and/or patients begin to attach significant value to this aspect of quality.

Waiting times

The last five years have seen substantial improvements in waiting times, as noted in the previous chapter, and this represent an obvious improvement in quality. However, it is less clear what *value* is attached to these quality improvements; and, in the absence of any evaluation of the costs and benefits of reducing waiting times, the cost-effectiveness of these improvements is even *less* clear. Estimates by economists at the University of York (Dawson *et al* 2005) suggest that the value of waiting time reductions achieved add very little to a quality-weighted measure of NHS output. This conclusion needs to be considered in the light of what must have been a considerable NHS cash investment in reducing waiting times.

Analysis of the planned costs of moving towards the government's 18 week maximum waiting time target (from background analysis underpinning part of the 2004 Spending Review (Freedom of Information Act response to query reference DE-00000167126) suggests that £1.4 billion was earmarked for extra activity to help achieve the target in 2006/7, and a further £2.7 billion in 2007/8. Setting these sums in context, they amount to around a fifth and a third respectively of the total cash increase for the NHS in England in these years.

Patient experience
Patients' views can be difficult to interpret, given possible changes in public expectations of the NHS; nevertheless, survey evidence (such as the British Social Attitudes Survey) suggests some improvements not just in overall satisfaction but also in satisfaction with particular services (*see* p 30). Through its involvement with the national patient survey programme in England, the Picker Institute has concluded that the quality of NHS care and the patient experience has improved over time, particularly in those areas of the NHS that have been subject to co-ordinated action. There are, however, considerable variations in the quality of care in different sectors and institutions across England. As with other measure of quality, while the national patient survey programme suggests improvements in quality, quantifying the *value* to patients of that improvement (or lack of it) is very difficult.

Improving patients' experience and satisfaction with NHS services has been a key government objective – but such a policy is not without cost. As with efforts to reduce waiting times, much more work is needed to establish the costs of the policy and, importantly, the *value* to patients of the benefits. The failure by government to evaluate policies that absorb billions of pounds contrasts strongly with the efforts made by NICE to evaluate new health care technologies.

SUMMARY: QUALITY

- Improvements in the quality of NHS outputs were assumed by the 2002 review to contribute as much as reductions in unit costs to productivity improvements – a cumulative total of around £20 billion by 2022/3 (at 2002/3 prices).
- Despite recent attempts by the Department of Health and ONS to quantify the contribution of improvements in the quality of NHS outputs, there is no agreed overall measure of quality.
- Some attempts to quantify changes in quality over time (in relation to the increased use of statins, for example) suggest significant gains in quality. However, the lack of routinely-collected data on the change in patients' health status arising from NHS interventions hampers development of NHS output and productivity measures.
- Other metrics of quality, such as patient safety, waiting times and satisfaction with the experience of care, show broad improvements over the last few years, particularly in areas that have been subject to targets. However, without data on the costs and monetary valuations of these changes, it is impossible to assess the value to patients of, for example, recent reductions in waiting times.
- Changes in health as a result of changes in the quality of NHS care could be significant, and much more work is needed to accurately quantify this contribution. Ongoing work – by ONS and others – on public service output measurement and valuation is strongly encouraged.

Appendix 1
Key drivers of overall spending paths in the 2002 review scenarios

Cost drivers	Solid progress	Slow uptake	Fully engaged
Health system cost drivers			
Implementing current National Service Frameworks (NSFs)	*Involves:* • delivering best practice in the five NSF disease areas (coronary heart disease, cancer, renal disease, mental health and diabetes) • extending the NSF approach to other areas of the NHS over the next 20 years. *Implications* Delivering best practice in these five disease areas represents an average real terms increase in spending approaching 8% a year. These (and the new NSFs) are key to the NHS Plan's quality strategy for 'catching up' with other European countries. Costs are over and above the impact of demographic change, and 'quality' is defined in terms of access, technology and other aspects of service delivery and outcome.		
Implementing new NSFs	*Involves:* • extrapolating the costs of improvements in existing NSF areas to other specific diseases. *Implications* To achieve this, spending may need to increase by 6–8% a year in real terms over a period of 10 years. New NSFs are to be rolled out across other areas in phases, at an average rate of two per year, ensuring complete coverage by the end of the 20 years of the Review. Future NSFs are to include estimates of the resources necessary for their delivery; be supported by improved information and information collection; and take account of the fact that patients may have co-existing conditions.		
... and medical technology	Contributes around 3 percentage points a year to growth in health spending.	Contributes around 2 percentage points a year to growth in health spending.	Contributes around 3 percentage points a year to growth in health spending.
Improving access by reducing waiting times	*Involves:* • reducing maximum inpatient waiting time from 15 to 6 months by 2005/6, to 3 months by 2008/9, and to 2 weeks by 2022/3 • reducing the maximum outpatient waiting time (excluding cancer treatment) from 6 to 3 months by 2005/6, maintained until 2008/9, and to 2 weeks by 2022/3. *Implications* For all three scenarios, the additional cost of reducing waiting times to 2 weeks is estimated to be around £10 billion a year (at 2002 prices) by 2022/3.		

continued on next page

Cost drivers	Solid progress	Slow uptake	Fully engaged
Health system cost drivers *continued*			

Improving clinical governance	*Involves:*
	• increasing clinical governance time for medical staff in hospitals and primary care from 5–10% by 2010/11
	• increasing clinical governance time for nursing and other professional staff from 2–10% by 2010/11
	• realising the following benefits after 5 years:
	  – 15% reduction in hospital acquired infections (HAI) in acute care by 2012/13 (could lead to fall of 2.8% in all inpatient activity)
	  – 10% reduction in other adverse incidents in acute care by 2012/13 (could lead to an additional 0.6% reduction in inpatient activity)
	  – improvement in avoidable emergency admissions in the worst performing 25% of health authorities on this measure by 2012/13
	  – 25% reduction in clinical negligence bill from reduction in number of incidents in obstetrics and gynaecology by 2005.
	
	Implications
	The additional cost of improved clinical governance is estimated to be around £1.4 billion a year by 2022/3, with most of this incurred in the first five years.		

Modernising the NHS estate	*Involves:* • replacing one-third of NHS hospital estates over the next 20 years • replacing all equipment (excluding ICT) every 8 years • in new hospitals, ensuring that 75% of beds are in single en-suite rooms and that there are a maximum of 4 beds per room • upgrading or replacing the entire primary care estate over the next 10 years.		
...and ICT	Spending doubles in real terms by 2003/4 to 3% of total spend.	Spending doubles in real terms by 2007/8 to 3% of total spend.	Spending doubles in real terms by 2003/4 to 3% of total spend.

Increasing pay and prices	*Involves:*
	• pay rising by 2.4% a year in real terms (over and above GDP deflator inflation) for total hospital and community health services.
	
	This percentage is based on the following assumptions:
	  – price inflation remains at 2.5% throughout the 20-year period
	  – pay in GMS sector rises by 2.2% a year in real terms
	  – pay in the PSS sector rises by 2.3% a year in real terms
	  – pay and productivity assumptions include Agenda for Change programme – covering nurses, the GP contract and the consultant contract
	  – pay modernisation is important in order to increase capacity and create a more flexible workforce with greater scope for team working and facilitating changes in skill mix.		

continued on next page

Cost drivers	Solid progress	Slow uptake	Fully engaged
Health system cost drivers *continued*			

Changes in workforce patterns	*Involves:*
	 • reducing the working hours of hospital doctors to 48 hours a week in line with the EU Working Time Directive
	 • changes to staffing driven by changes in throughput and activity – specifically, a fall in the average length of stay in hospital in line with estimates in the National Beds Enquiry:
	  – for emergency admissions – 7.76 days (2000), 7.27 days (2005), 6.35 days (2010) and 5.43 days (2015)
	  – for elective admissions – 4.86 days (2000), 4.37 days (2005), 3.88 days (2010) and 3.38 days (2015).		

Increasing productivity	*Involves:* • increasing productivity from 2–2.5% a year in the first decade to 3% a year in the second.	*Involves:* • increasing productivity from 1.5% a year in the first decade to 1.75% a year in the second.	*Involves:* • increasing productivity from 2–2.5% a year in the first decade to 3% a year in the second.
Population health and health-seeking behaviour cost drivers			
UK life expectancy at birth	Men 80.0; Women 83.8	Men 78.7; Women 83.0	Men 81.6; Women 85.5
Long-term ill health among the elderly	No change in rates of ill health	Increase in long-term ill health (age-specific rates of physical dependency increase by 1% a year)	Healthy life expectancy increases broadly in line with life expectancy
Acute ill health among the elderly	5% reduction by 2022	10% increase by 2022	10% reduction by 2022
Use and impact of health promotion strategies (smoking, exercise, diet, etc)	Current public health targets met, leading to reductions in hospital admissions and GP visits	No change in public health measures	Progress beyond current public health targets – leading to greater reductions in hospital admissions and GP visits – combined with higher spending on health promotion
	Health promotion expenditure grows in line with expenditure on GP and hospital care	Health promotion expenditure grows in line with population growth and inflation	Health promotion expenditure grows in line with GP and hospital care, plus an additional £250 million a year by 2007/8 (ie, a doubling of spending)
	Less than 24% of adults smoke (baseline: 27%)	Prevalence of smoking remains the same	Prevalence of smoking achieves solid progress reduction ahead of target and then reduces further

continued on next page

Cost drivers	Solid progress	Slow uptake	Fully engaged
Population health and health-seeking behaviour cost drivers *continued*			
Use and impact of health promotion strategies (smoking, exercise, diet, etc) *continued*	Less than 15% of pregnant women smoke (baseline: 18%)	Prevalence of smoking remains the same	Prevalence of smoking achieves solid progress reduction ahead of target and then reduces further
	Number of babies born to teenage mothers in England and Wales reduces to 41,000 in 2005 and to 24,000 by 2010 (baseline: 48,000)	No change	Number of babies born to teenage mothers achieves the solid progress reduction ahead of target and then reduces further
	5% reduction in births requiring special or intensive care	No change	5% reduction in births requiring special or intensive care
	Trends in obesity slow and ultimately reverse, going from 21% for women, and 17% for men, to 8% and 6%, respectively	Levels of obesity remain the same	Trends in obesity achieve solid progress aims ahead of target and then continue further
	10% reduction in hospital admissions, GP visits and prescriptions related to coronary heart disease and stroke for 15–64 year olds. Reductions largely due to reductions in prevalence of smoking, plus higher levels of physical activity and better diet	No change	25% reduction in hospital admissions, GP visits and prescriptions related to coronary heart disease and stroke for 15–64 year olds. Reductions largely due to reductions in prevalence of smoking, plus higher levels of physical activity and better diet
	5% reduction in all other hospital admissions, GP visits and prescriptions for 15–64 year olds. Reductions partly due to reductions in prevalence of smoking, plus higher levels of physical activity and better diet	No change	15% reduction in all other hospital admissions, GP visits and prescriptions for 15–64 year olds. Reductions partly due to reductions in prevalence of smoking, plus higher levels of physical activity and better diet

continued on next page

Cost drivers	Solid progress	Slow uptake	Fully engaged
Population health and health-seeking behaviour cost drivers *continued*			
Health seeking behaviour among under 65s	By 2022, hospital and GP care use per head among over 75s matches current patterns of use among 65–74 year olds	No change in utilisation rates	By 2012, hospital and GP care use per head among over 75s matches current patterns of use among 65–74 year olds
	One additional GP visit per person per year on average by 2022	No change	One additional GP visit per person per year on average by 2022
Levels of self-care	Switch of 1% of GP activity to pharmacists; reduction of 17% in outpatient attendances among 225,000 people using self-care	Switch of 1% of GP activity to pharmacists; reduction of 17% in outpatient attendances among 225,000 people using self-care	Switch of 2% of GP activity to pharmacists; reduction of 17% in outpatient attendances among 450,000 people using self-care (result of a step-change in public engagement)
	Higher patient expectations	No change	Dramatic improvement in public engagement via ICT
Extent of inequalities	Reduced age discrimination	No change	Successes demonstrated under solid progress scenario are achieved more quickly and are then exceeded
	Reduction in socio-economic inequalities in health	Inequalities in health between socio-economic groups remain unchanged	Considerable reductions in socio-economic inequalities in health
	Gap in life expectancy between those in the poorest areas and the average falls by at least 10%	No change	Gap in life expectancy reached under solid progress scenario is achieved more quickly and then reduced further
	Smoking among adults in manual socio-economic groups falls from 30–26% by 2010	No change	Reduction in smoking among adults in manual socio-economic groups under solid progress scenario is achieved more quickly and then exceeded

Appendix 2
2002 Review recommendations

- The Review welcomes the government's intention to extend the National Service Framework (NSF) approach to other disease areas and recommends that NSFs, and their equivalents in the Devolved Administrations, are rolled out in a similar way to the diseases already covered.

- The Review recommends that the NHS workforce planning bodies should examine the implications of this Review's findings for their projections over the next 20 years.

- While the Review considered it vital to extend its Terms of Reference to begin to consider social care, it has had neither the information nor the resources to be able to develop a 'whole systems' model, nor indeed to build up projections for social care in the same level of detail as for health care. It is recommended that future reviews of this type should fully integrate modelling and analysis of health and social care. Indeed, it is for consideration whether a more immediate study is needed of the trends affecting social care.

- The Review recommends that the National Institute for Clinical Excellence (NICE), in conjunction with similar bodies in the Devolved Administrations, also has a major role to play in examining older technologies and practices that may no longer be appropriate or cost effective.

- It will also be important to ensure that recommendations from NICE – particularly its clinical guidelines – are properly integrated with the development of NSFs.

- The Review welcomes the proposed extension of the NSFs to other areas of the NHS. It recommends that NSFs should in future include estimates of the resources – in terms of the staff, equipment and other technologies and subsequent cash needs – necessary for their delivery.

- The Review's projections incorporate a doubling of spending on ICT to fund ambitious targets of the kind set out in the NHS Information Strategy. To avoid duplication of effort and resources and to ensure that the benefits of ICT integration across health and social services are achieved, the Review recommends that stringent standards should be set from the centre to ensure that systems across the United Kingdom are fully compatible with each other.

- To ensure that resources intended for ICT spending are not diverted to other uses and are used productively, the Review recommends that budgets should be ring fenced and achievements audited.

continued on next page

- In thinking about the level of detail to which objective setting should be taken, the Review was interested in work currently being undertaken by RAND Health to develop a new approach to assessing the quality of care given to children and adults in the United States. The Review recommends that the results of this and any similar research about comprehensive measurement of performance should be examined.

- The Review believes that the scope for greater future co-operation between the NHS and the private sector in the delivery of services should be explored, building on the concordat set out in the NHS Plan.

- The Review recommends that there should be a mechanism in place to ensure regular and rigorous independent audit of all health care spending and arrangements to ensure that it is given maximum publicity.

- The Review recommends that the government should examine the merits of employing financial incentives such as those used in Sweden to help reduce the problems of bed blocking.

- The Review believes that the present structure of exemptions for prescription charges is not logical, nor rooted in the principles of the NHS. If related issues are being considered in future, it is recommended that the opportunity should be taken to think through the rationale for the exemption policy.

- The Review believes that there is an argument for extending out-of-pocket payments for non-clinical services and recommends that they should be kept under review.

- The Review recommends that a more effective partnership between health professionals and the public should be facilitated, for example, by:
  - the setting of standards for the service to help give people a clearer understanding of what the health service will, and will not, provide for them
  - the development of improved health information to help people engage with their care in an informed way
  - in parallel with improved information, the use of pro-active policies driven by evidence of cost-effectiveness, to encourage reductions in key health risk factors
  - reinforcing patient involvement in NHS accountability arrangements, through measures such as patients' forums, the English National Commission on Patient and Public Involvement and better patient representation on trust boards, including the new primary care trusts
  - finding effective ways to provide the public with a better understanding of how their local health services are performing.

- The Review recommends that the boards of strategic health authorities (SHAs) should include local patient and business representatives.

- The Review recommends that, as part of improved public engagement, the Department of Health (with SHA involvement) and the Devolved Administrations should consider how a greater public appreciation of the cost of common treatments and appointments could best be achieved.

continued on next page

- The Review believes that, as an early step down this road towards better engagement of patients in thinking about the health service, there may be an argument for charging for missed appointments.

- The Review's final recommendation is that a further review should be conducted in, say, five years' time to re-assess the future resource requirements for both health and social care. It should be able to draw upon the better information, research findings and international knowledge base; and have the benefit of accumulated knowledge from the bodies charged with auditing the success of the service and its change programme.

RECOMMENDATIONS ABOUT EFFECTIVE USE OF RESOURCES

Standards	Well defined and transparent clinical standards should be set by the departments and agencies of the government, which oversee and regulate the health system. In some cases, there may also be a role for the central setting of non-clinical standards (for example, in the case of ICT). The role of NICE is crucial and will become increasingly significant over the next 20 years. NICE should also have a role in examining older technologies and practices. Together with various stakeholders, it should have an input into the technology assessment selection process, with greater focus on topics of importance to patients and professionals. Recommendations from NICE must be properly integrated with the development of NSFs.
Processes	The way resources and information flow around the system and the use of incentives and targets to encourage efficient and effective delivery of care is crucial. Appropriate processes must be in place to ensure that nationally set standards are delivered by the health service. These must be designed to ensure that they achieve the required results rather than distort resource allocation. Targets must be designed to minimise the risks of perverse incentives, and where targets are not met, the reasons must be examined, with sanctions deployed or targets redesigned as appropriate.
Delivery	There will need to be enhanced local discretion, with appropriate sensitivity to local circumstances. To support delivery, resources must be allocated in a transparent way, that takes account of local needs and does not create perverse incentives. Stability and certainty of funding is also important to facilitate long-term planning and investment decisions. New structures must work effectively and involve a high degree of accountability and public involvement at local level. There is significant scope to give more local discretion to those delivering care to nationally set standards. There is greater scope for future co-operation between the NHS and private sector in the delivery of services, and this should be explored, building on the concordat set out in the NHS Plan. There should be a mechanism in place to ensure regular and rigorous independent audit of all health care spending and arrangements to ensure that it is given maximum publicity.
Balance of care	Care needs to be provided in the right place and at the right time and this requires finding an appropriate balance between primary and secondary care and between treatment and prevention. The current balance between health and social care is wrong – in particular, care is too focused on the acute hospital setting. Effective integration between health and social care, using appropriate incentives, is an important strand for achieving balance.
Financing of care	There is little evidence to suggest that there is an alternative financing method to that currently in place in the United Kingdom that would deliver a given level and quality of health care either at lower cost to the economy or in a more equitable way.
Public engagement	Effective public engagement will require an active partnership between those who provide care and those who receive it. A more sophisticated partnership will need to develop over the next 20 years. Ensuring an appropriate role for community representatives on the boards of the new SHAs will also be important and the Review recommends that these boards should include local patients and business representatives. Additional resources will need to be directed to public health, targeted at those interventions where the long-term impact will be greatest in terms of health gains. Interventions that successfully target population groups who currently suffer the most ill health will need to be identified and scaled up appropriately. The desirable health outcomes depicted in the fully engaged scenario are only likely to come about with a step-change in the way public health is viewed, resourced and delivered nationally.

Appendix 3
Achieving full engagement: securing good health for the whole population

RECOMMENDATIONS OF THE 2004 REVIEW

1: Public health policy principles	All new public health policy should be considered against a 'checklist' before implementation to assist in the development of targeted interventions that increase both health and welfare. The following principles are suggested for adoption by government:
	• Interventions should tackle public health objectives and the causes of any decision-making failures as directly as possible.
	• Interventions should be evidence-based, although the lack of conclusive evidence should not, where there is a serious risk to the nation's health, block action proportionate to that risk.
	• The total costs of an intervention to the government and society must be kept to a minimum and be less than the expected benefits over the life of the policy: interventions should be prioritised to select those that represent best value.
	• The distributional effects of any programme of interventions should be acceptable.
	• The right of the individual to choose their own lifestyle must be balanced against any adverse impacts those choices have on the quality of life of others.
2: Public health policy-making	HM Treasury should provide a framework for the use of economic instruments to guide government interventions in relation to public health and a consistent framework should be used to evaluate the cost-effectiveness of interventions and initiatives across both health care and public health.
	Future National Service Frameworks should be fully costed, including information about the cost-effectiveness of interventions, and corresponding research programmes should be established to allow them to be reviewed and continually updated in the light of emerging evidence.
	Productivity measures should be developed that move away from narrow definitions of output to overall measures of health outcomes, and allow comparisons of effectiveness of prevention and cure.
	The government needs to engage stakeholders and seek advice about what quantified objectives it should set for progress in tackling all major determinates of health and health inequalities. Where appropriate, important sub-group objectives should be set, in particular to achieve objectives to reduce health inequalities. Objectives should have set time-frames, and these should be monitored and reassessed regularly. The Secretary of State for Health should be given the role of ensuring that the Cabinet assesses the impact on the future health of the population of any major policy development.
	Based on these national objectives, there needs to be joint-working at local level to determine shared local objectives based on local needs. Local objectives should be considered in the planning and performance management of both primary care trusts (PCTs) and local government – through the Priorities and Planning Framework and the Comprehensive Performance Assessment.

continued on next page

3: Review of arm's length bodies	The Department of Health review of arm's length bodies should ensure that identified gaps within public health activity are filled and that defined responsibilities are assigned for a range of areas. This includes:
	• responsibility for developing the cost-effectiveness evidence base in public health
	• researching the practical effectiveness of current activities and interpreting findings for future implementation
	• the educational role at a time when full engagement requires the public and the health workforce to have more support
	• reassessing periodically national objectives for all major determinants of health and health inequalities; and the regulation of nicotine and tobacco.
	The review of arm's length bodies should also examine their relationships with PCTs. Finally, the efforts of arm's length bodies should be co-ordinated at a local level.
4: Research and evaluation programmes	When planning any national programme of action to tackle the key determinants of health, there should be a commitment for adequate resources for monitoring and feedback.
	An experiment, directed towards areas of inequality, should be established across primary care to assess the benefits of additional resource in information systems, in monitoring risk and in services. This will produce evidence about the effectiveness of information to assist personalised risk management and disease prevalence in local populations.
	There is a need for an overall public health research strategy that would, *inter alia*, identify the roles of the various research bodies in relation to public health, and how they might best work together to identify and address gaps in public health research. This will ensure a structured and coherent development of the public health research requirements for England.
	In addition, the public health White Paper should address the possible threat to public health research, which arises from the difficulty of obtaining access to data because of the need to strike a balance between individual confidentiality and public health research requirements.
5: Full engagement	The consultation ahead of the public health White Paper provides a good opportunity to engage the population on the issue of their own health and the balance between an individual's 'right to choose' and the impact that individual behaviour has on the well-being of others.
	The consultation should consider the acceptability of different ways of tackling smoking.
	Feedback should also be sought regularly from the population and important sub-groups to provide an indication of their degree of awareness of issues and of the current best advice, as well as the acceptability to them of possibly controversial state interventions. An annual report about the state of people's health and of the major determinants of health should be made available at national and local authority levels to encourage understanding.
	There is a need for a programme of research to be undertaken to identify what forms of intervention best improve health literacy, ensuring that messages are personalised for population sub-groups. Further, to assist in the full engagement of the population, advice should be made available, freely, in formats all find accessible, including development of internet and telephone services; the NHS Direct brand should be considered as a route to deliver this.

References

Abacus (2005). *A Survey Measuring the Impact of NICE. Guideline 11. Survey 1 PCT Commissioning Managers*. Available at: www.nice.org.uk/download.aspx?o=279254 (accessed on 2 August 2007).

Appleby J, Alvarez A (2005). 'Public responses to NHS reform' in Park A, Curtice J, Thomson K, Bromley C, Phillips M and Johnson M (eds), *British Social Attitudes*. Two terms of New Labour: the public's reaction. 22nd Report. London: Sage.

Appleby J, Boyle S, Devlin N, Harley M, Harrison A, Thorlby R (2004). *What is the Impact of Waiting Times Targets on Clinical Treatment Priorities?* Second stage report to the Department of Health. London: King's Fund.

Atkinson T (2005). *Atkinson Review: Final report. Measurement of government output and productivity for the national accounts*. London: HMSO.

Audit Commission (2005). *Early Lessons from Payment by Results*. London: Audit Commission.

Bell J, Pike G (2006). *Impact of Agenda for Change: Results from a survey of RCN members working in the NHS/GP practices*. London: Royal College of Nursing.

Berrino F, Capocaccia R, Esteve J, Gatta G, Hakulinen T, Micheli A, Sant M, Verdecchia A (eds) (1999). *Survival of Cancer Patients in Europe: The EUROCARE-2 study*. Lyon: World Health Organization, International Agency for Research on Cancer (IARC Scientific Publication, No. 151).

Bolling K (2006). *Infant Feeding Survey 2005: Early results*. Leeds: The Information Centre.

Brewer M, Goodman A, Muriel A , Sibieta L (2007). *Poverty and Inequality in the UK: 2007*. London: The Institute for Fiscal Studies.

British Computer Society Health Informatics Forum Strategic Panel (2006). *The Way Forward for NHS Health Informatics: Where should NHS Connecting for Health (NHS CFH) go from here?* Swindon: British Computer Society.

British Medical Association (2007). *A Rational Way Forward for the NHS in England*. London: BMA.

Brown G (2002). *Budget 2002: The strength to make long-term decisions: Investing in an enterprising, fairer Britain*. Economic and Fiscal Strategy Report and Financial Statement and Budget Report. London: The Stationery Office.

Buchan J, Evans D (2007). *Realising the Benefits? Assessing the implementation of Agenda for Change*. London: King's Fund.

Bury M (2007). 'Self-care and the English National Health Service'. *Journal of Health Services Research and Policy*, vol 12, no 2, pp 65–66.

Cabinet Office (2007). *Capability Review of the Department of Health*. London: Cabinet Office.

Calman K, Hine D (1995). *A Policy Framework for Commissioning Cancer Services: A report by the Expert Advisory Group on Cancer to the Chief Medical Officers of England and Wales. Guidance for providers and purchasers of cancer services*. London: Department of Health.

Capability Reviews Team (2007). *Capability Review of the Department of Health* [online]. Available at: www.civilservice.gov.uk/reform/capability_reviews/publications/pdf/Capability_Review_DfH.pdf (accessed on 30 July 2007).

Coleman MP, Gatta G, Verdecchia A, Estève J, Sant M, Storm H, Allemani C, Ciccolallo L, Santaquilani M, Berrino F (2003). 'EUROCARE-3 summary: cancer survival in Europe at the end of the 20th century'. *Annals of Oncology*, vol 14 (suppl 5), pp v128–49.

Construction Products Association (2006). *Achievable Targets: Is government delivering?* London: Construction Products Association.

Construction Products Association (2005). *Achievable Targets: Is government delivering?* London: Construction Products Association.

Cooksey D (2006). *A Review of UK Health Research Funding*. London: HM Treasury.

Coulter A (2005). *Trends in Patients' Experience of the NHS*. Oxford: Picker Institute Europe.

Curry N (2006). 'Predicting the risk of readmission: The PARR tool'. *Health Care Risk Report*, vol 12, no 6, pp 14–15.

Darzi A (2007). *Healthcare for London: A framework for action*. London: NHS London.

Davies H, Powell A, Rushmer R (2007). *Healthcare Professionals' Views on Clinical Engagement in Quality Improvement*. London: The Health Foundation.

Dawson D, Gravelle H, Kind P, O'Mahony M, Street A and Weale M (2005). *Developing New Approaches to Measuring NHS Outputs and Activity*. CHE Research Paper 6. York: University of York.

Delpierre C, Cuzin l, Fillaux J, Alvarez M, Massip P, Lang T (2004). 'A systematic review of computer-based patient record systems and quality of care: more randomized clinical trials or a broader approach?' *International Journal for Quality in Health Care*, vol 16, no 5, pp 407–16.

Department for Education and Skills (2006). *Schools Racing Ahead of Sport Targets*. London: Department for Education and Skills. Available at: www.dfes.gov.uk/pns/DisplayPN.cgi?pn_id=2006_0148 (accessed 30 July 2007).

Department of Health (2007a). '£10m boost to improve safety and quality for patients'. Press release, 6 April. Available at: www.gnn.gov.uk/environment/fullDetail.asp?ReleaseID=277066&NewsAreaID=2&NavigatedFromDepartment=False (accessed on 2 August 2007).

Department of Health (2007b). *Choosing Health Progress Report*. London: Department of Health.

Department of Health (2007c). 'Clean Hospitals'. Department of Health website. Available at: www.dh.gov.uk/en/Policyandguidance/Organisationpolicy/Healthcareenvironment/DH_4116447 (accessed on 30 July 2007).

Department of Health (2007d). 'Clinical Leadership Health Summit'. Department of Health website. Available at: www.dh.gov.uk/en/Policyandguidance/Organisationpolicy/Healthreform/DH_073231 (accessed on 30 July 2007).

Department of Health (2007e). *Explaining NHS Deficits 2003/4 to 2005/6*. London: Department of Health.

Department of Health (2007f). *Getting it Right for People with Cancer: Clinical case for change*. Report by Professor Mike Richards. London: Department of Health.

Department of Health (2007g). 'GP reforms improve NHS referrals'. Press release, 26 January. Available at: www.gnn.gov.uk/content/detail.asp?ReleaseID=259600&NewsAreaID=2 (accessed on 2 August 2007).

Department of Health (2007h). 'Health Risk and Costs of Obesity'. Department of Health website. Available at: www.dh.gov.uk/en/Policyandguidance/Healthandsocialcaretopics/Obesity/DH_4133949 (accessed on 30 July 2007).

Department of Health (2007i). 'Helping patients to take control of long-term illnesses'. Press release, 2 April. Available at: www.gnn.gov.uk/Content/Detail.asp?ReleaseID=275719&NewsAreaID=22007/0076 (accessed on 2 August 2007).

Department of Health (2007j). 'Hi-tech home healthcare'. Press release, 23 May. Available at: www.gnn.gov.uk/environment/fullDetail.asp?ReleaseID=286491&NewsAreaID=2&NavigatedFromDepartment=True (accessed on 2 August 2007).

Department of Health (2007k). *Initial Regulatory Impact Assessment: Good doctors, safer patients*. London: Department of Health.

Department of Health (2007l). *Keeping it Personal*. Clinical case for change: report by David Colin-Thome, National Director for Primary Care. London: Department of Health.

Department of Health (2007m). *Making it Better: For children and young people*. London: Department of Health.

Department of Health (2007n). *Making it Better: For mother and baby*. London: Department of Health.

Department of Health (2007o). 'Mapping the Success of NHS Building Schemes'. Department of Health website. Available at: www.dh.gov.uk/en/Policyandguidance/Organisationpolicy/Healthreform/DH_072391 (accessed on 30 July 2007).

Department of Health (2007p). *Maternity Matters*. London: Department of Health.

Department of Health (2007q). 'New network widens access to cutting-edge studies'. Press release, 1 March 2007. Available at: www.gnn.gov.uk/Content/Detail.asp?ReleaseID=267902&NewsAreaID=2 (accessed on 2 August 2007).

Department of Health (2007r). *NHS Financial Performance: Quarter 4*. London: Department of Health.

Department of Health (2007s). *Options for the Future of Payment by Results: 2008/9 to 2010/11*. London: Department of Health.

Department of Health (2007t). *Quarterly Waiting Time Statistics.* London: Department of Health. Available at: www.performance.doh.gov.uk/waitingtimes/index.htm (accessed on 30 July 2007).

Department of Health (2007u). *Report on the National Patient Choice Survey – November 2006 England.* London: Department of Health.

Department of Health (2007v). *Review of the Health Inequalities Infant Mortality PSA Target.* London: Department of Health.

Department of Health (2007w). *Saws and Scalpels to Lasers and Robots – Advances in Surgery.* Clinical case for change: report by Professor Sir Ara Darzi, National Advisor on Surgery. London: Department of Health.

Department of Health (2007x). 'Scan and Save – NHS to save £ millions and improve patient safety with bar codes'. Press release 16 February. Available at: www.gnn.gov.uk/environment/fullDetail.asp?ReleaseID=264567&NewsAreaID=2&NavigatedFromDepartment=False (accessed on 22 August 2007).

Department of Health (2007y). 'Tsar announces £1m in new research funding'. Press release 7 March. Available at: www.gnn.gov.uk/environment/fullDetail.asp?ReleaseID=269413&NewsAreaID=2&NavigatedFromDepartment=True (accessed on 22 August 2007).

Department of Health (2007z). 'Total time in A&E'. Department of Health website. Available at: www.performance.doh.gov.uk/hospitalactivity/data_requests/total_time_ae.htm (accessed on 30 July 2007).

Department of Health (2007aa). 'Your doctor will never look at you in the same way again'. Press release 21 May. Available at: www.gnn.gov.uk/environment/fullDetail.asp?ReleaseID=289202&NewsAreaID=2&NavigatedFromDepartment=False (accessed on 22 August 2007).

Department of Health (2006a). *Autumn Performance Report.* London: Department of Health.

Department of Health (2006b). *Best Research for Best Health: A new national health research strategy: the NHS contribution to health research in England.* London: Department of Health.

Department of Health (2006c). *Care and Resource Utilisation: Ensuring appropriate care.* London: Department of Health.

Department of Health (2006d). *Chief Executive's Report to the NHS.* London: Department of Health.

Department of Health (2006e). *Departmental Report 2006.* London: Department of Health.

Department of Health (2006f). 'Expert Patients Programme'. Department of Health website. Available at: www.dh.gov.uk/en/Aboutus/MinistersandDepartmentLeaders/ChiefMedicalOfficer/ProgressOnPolicy/ProgressBrowsableDocument/DH_5380885 (accessed on 30 July 2007).

Department of Health (2006g). 'Go-ahead for billion pound-plus wave of new NHS hospitals'. Press release 18 August. Available at: www.gnn.gov.uk/environment/fullDetail.asp?ReleaseID=221563&NewsAreaID=2&NavigatedFromDepartment=False (accessed on 30 July 2007).

Department of Health (2006h). 'Investing in Facilities'. Department of Health website. Available at: www.dh.gov.uk/en/PolicyAndGuidance/HealthAndSocialCareTopics/Cancer/DH_4063777 (accessed on 30 July 2007).

Department of Health (2006i). 'NHS could save millions through smarter prescribing of cholesterol-busting drugs'. Press release 28 December. Available at: www.gnn.gov.uk/environment/fullDetail.asp?ReleaseID=252781&NewsAreaID=2&NavigatedFromDepartment=False (accessed on 30 July 2007).

Department of Health (2006j). *Our Health, Our Care, Our Say.* London: Department of Health.

Department of Health (2006k). *Supporting People with Long Term Conditions for Self Care: A guide to developing local strategies and good practice.* London: Department of Health. Available at: www.dh.gov.uk/en/Publicationsandstatistics/Publications/PublicationsPolicyAndGuidance/DH_4130725 (accessed on 30 July 2007).

Department of Health (2006l). *Tackling Health Inequalities: 2003–05 data update for the National 2010 PSA Target.* London: Department of Health.

Department of Health (2005a). *Choosing a Better Diet: A food and health action plan.* London: Department of Health.

Department of Health (2005b). *Departmental Report 2005.* London: Department of Health.

Department of Health (2005c). *Gershon Efficiency Programme 2004–2008: Efficiency technical note.* London: Department of Health.

Department of Health (2005d). *Healthcare Output and Productivity: Accounting for quality change.* London: Department of Health.

Department of Health (2005e). *Measurement of Healthcare Output and Productivity: Use of statins and calculation of value weight. Technical paper No 2.* London: Department of Health.

Department of Health (2004a) 'Arm's length bodies review'. Department of Health website. Available at: www.dh.gov.uk/en/AboutUs/DeliveringHealthAndSocialCare/OrganisationsThatWorkWithDH/ArmsLengthBodies/DH_4105578 (accessed on 22 August 2007).

Department of Health (2004b). *Agenda for Change: Final agreement.* London: Department of Health.

Department of Health (2004c). *Choosing Health: Making healthier choices easier.* London: Department of Health. Available at: www.dh.gov.uk/en/Publicationsandstatistics/Publications/PublicationsPolicyAndGuidance/DH_4094550 (accessed on 30 July 2007).

Department of Health (2004d). *At Least Five a Week.* London: Department of Health.

Department of Health (2004e). *Reconfiguring the Department of Health's Arm's Length Bodies.* London: Department of Health.

Department of Health (2004f). *The Configuring Hospitals Evidence File: Part one.* London: Department of Health.

Department of Health (2004g). *The Configuring Hospitals Evidence File: Part two.* London: Department of Health.

Department of Health (2004h). *The 'Experimental' NHS Cost Efficiency Growth Measure.* London: Department of Health.

Department of Health (2004i). *The NHS Improvement Plan*. London: Department of Health.

Department of Health (2003a). *A Code of Conduct for Private Practice: Guidance for NHS medical staff*. London: Department of Health. Available at: www.dh.gov.uk/en/Publicationsandstatistics/ Publications/PublicationsPolicyAndGuidance/DH_4100689 (accessed on 20 August 2007).

Department of Health (2003b). *Investing in General Practice: The new general medical services contract*. London: Department of Health. Available at: www.dh.gov.uk/en/Publicationsandstatistics/ Publications/PublicationsPolicyAndGuidance/DH_4071966 (accessed on 20 August 2007).

Department of Health (2003c). 'New joint task force to promote growth and performance of UK healthcare industry'. Press release 17 October. Available at: www.dh.gov.uk/en/ Publicationsandstatistics/Pressreleases/DH_4062748 (accessed on 30 July 2007).

Department of Health (2002). *Delivering the NHS Plan: Next steps on investment, next steps on reform*. London: Department of Health.

Department of Health (2001a). *NHS Plan Implementation Programme*. London: Department of Health.

Department of Health (2001b). *Shifting the Balance of Power within the NHS: Securing delivery*. London: Department of Health.

Department of Health (2001c). *The Expert Patient: A new approach to chronic disease management*. London: Department of Health.

Department of Health (2000a). *An Organisation with a memory*. London: Department of Health.

Department of Health (2000b). *Shaping the Future: Long term planning for hospitals and related service*. London: Department of Health. Available at: www.dh.gov.uk/en/Consultations/ Closedconsultations/DH_4102910 (accessed on 1 August, 2007).

Department of Health (2000c). *The NHS Plan: A plan for investment, a plan for reform*. London: Department of Health.

Department of Health (2000d). *The NHS Cancer Plan: A plan for investment, a plan for reform*. London: Department of Health.

Department of Health (1999a). *Clinical Governance in the New NHS*. Health Service Circular HSC 1999/065. London: Department of Health.

Department of Health (1999b). 'Up To £30 million to develop 20 NHS fast access walk-in centres'. Press release, 13 April. Available at: www.dh.gov.uk/en/Publicationsandstatistics/Pressreleases/ DH_4025471 (accessed on 30 July 2007).

Department of Health (1998a). *A First Class Service: Quality in the NHS*. London: The Stationery Office.

Department of Health (1998b). *Smoking Kills: A White Paper on tobacco*. London: The Stationery Office. Available at: www.archive.official-documents.co.uk/document/cm41/4177/4177.htm (accessed on 30 July 2007).

Department of Health (1997). *The New NHS: Modern, dependable*. London: The Stationery Office.

Department of Health (1996). *A Service with Ambitions*. London: The Stationery Office.

Department of Health (1995a). *The Calman/Hine Report: A policy framework for commissioning cancer services*. London: Department of Health.

Department of Health (1995b). *The Patient's Charter and You: A charter for England*. London: Department of Health.

Department of Health (1993). *Report of An Independent Review of Specialist Services in London*. London: HMSO.

Department of Health (1992). *An Information Management and Technology Strategy for the NHS in England*. London: Department of Health and NHS Executive.

Department of Health Strategy Unit (2002). *Game Plan: A strategy for delivering Government's sport and physical activity objectives*. A Joint DCMS/Strategy Unit Report. London: Department of Health Strategy Unit.

Derrett S, Paul C, Morris JM (1999). 'Waiting for elective surgery: effects on quality of life'. *International Journal for Quality in Health Care*, vol 11, no 1, pp 47–57.

Donaldson L (2006). *The Chief Medical Officer on the State of Public Health: Annual Report 2005*. London: Department of Health.

ESRC (2007). 'UKCRC Public Health Research Centres of Excellence'. ESRC website. Available at: www.esrcsocietytoday.ac.uk/ESRCInfoCentre/opportunities/current%5Ffunding%5Fopportunities/ukcrc.aspx (accessed on 30 July 2007).

European Antimicrobial Resistance Surveillance System (2007) Interactive database [online]. Available at: www.rivm.nl/earss/database/ (accessed on 2 April 2007).

European Antimicrobial Resistance Surveillance System (2005). *EARSS Annual Report 2005*. Available at: www.rivm.nl/earss/Images/EARSS%202005_tcm61-34899.pdf (accessed on 22 August 2007).

Farrar S, Ikenwilo D, Chalkley M, Sussex J, Yuen P, Scott A (2006). *National Evaluation of Payment by Results. Interim report: Quantitative and qualitative analysis*. OHE/University of Aberdeen. Available at: www.aberdeen.ac.uk/heru/documents/PbR%20interim%20report%20feb%2007.pdf (accessed on 30 July 2007).

Foresight Programme (2007). *Tackling Obesity: Future choices project*. Available at: www.foresight.gov.uk/Obesity/Obesity.htm (accessed on 30 July 2007).

Fulop N, Protopsaltis G, Hutchings A, King A, Allen P, Normand C, Walters R (2002). 'Process and impact of mergers of NHS trusts: multicentre case study and management cost analysis'. *British Medical Journal*, vol 325, pp 243–6.

Gershon P (2004). *Releasing Resources to the Front Line. Independent review of public sector efficiency*. London: HM Treasury.

Glover G, Arts G, Babu KS (2006). 'Crisis resolution/home treatment teams and psychiatric admission rates in England'. *British Journal of Psychiatry*, vol 189, pp 441–45.

Goddard E (2006). *Smoking and Drinking Among Adults, 2005*. London: Office for National Statistics.

Godden S, McCoy D, Pollock A (2007). 'Can we tell if government policies are working? Interpreting government data on delayed discharges from hospitals'. *Discussion Paper 0703. The Public Services Programme: Quality, performance and delivery.* London: ESRC.

Government Actuary's Department (2006). *Period and Cohort Expectations of Life.* London: Government Actuary's Department. Available at: www.gad.gov.uk/Life_Tables/ Period_and_cohort_eol.htm (accessed on 30 July 2007).

Gravelle H, Dusheiko M, Sheaff R, Sargant P, Boaden R, Pickard S, Parker S, Roland M (2007). 'Impact of case management (Evercare) on frail elderly patients: controlled before and after analysis of quantitative outcome data'. *British Medical Journal*, vol 334, pp 31–33.

Ham C, Kipping R, McLeod H (2003). 'Redesigning work processes in health care: lessons from the National Health Service'. *Milbank Quarterly*, vol 81, no 3, pp 415–39.

Hansard (House of Commons Debates) (2007a). 6 March 2007 col 1972W. Available at: www.publications.parliament.uk/pa/cm200607/cmhansrd/cm070306/text/70306w0035.htm#colu mn_1972W (accessed on 1 August 2007).

Hansard (House of Commons Debates) (2007b). 23 January 2007 col 1737W. Available at: www.publications.parliament.uk/pa/cm200607/cmhansrd/cm070123/text/70123w0026.htm#colu mn_1736W (accessed on 1 August 2007).

Hansard (House of Commons Debates) (2007c). 4 June 2007 col 326W. Available at: www.publications.parliament.uk/pa/cm200607/cmhansrd/cm070604/text/70604w0073.htm#colu mn_326W (accessed on 1 August 2007).

Hansard (House of Commons Debates) (2007d) 19 February 2007 col 31W. Available at: www.publications.parliament.uk/pa/cm200607/cmhansrd/cm070216/text/70219w0006.htm#0702 1932001686 (accessed 17 August 2007)

Hansard (House of Commons Debates) (2004). 4 March 2004 col 1128W. Available at. www.publications.parliament.uk/pa/cm200304/cmhansrd/vo040304/text/40304w18.htm#40304w 18.html_sbhd3 (accessed on 1 August 2007).

Harrison A (2002). *Public Interest: Private decisions: health related research in the UK.* London: King's Fund.

Harvey S, McMahon L, Liddell A (2007). *Windmill 2007: The future of health care reforms in England.* London: King's Fund.

Healthcare Commission (2007a) *Independent sector treatment centres. A review of the quality of care.* London: The Healthcare Commission

Healthcare Commission (2007b). *Inpatients: The views of hospital inpatients in England. Key findings from the 2006 survey.* London: The Healthcare Commission.

Healthcare Commission (2006a). *Living Well in Later Life: A review of progress against the National Service Framework for Older People.* London: The Healthcare Commission.

Healthcare Commission (2006b). *National Survey of NHS Staff 2005: Summary of key findings.* London: The Healthcare Commission.

Healthcare Commission (2006c). *State of Healthcare 2006*. London: The Healthcare Commission.

Healthcare Commission (2005a). *A Snapshot of Hospital Cleanliness in England. Findings from the Healthcare Commission's rapid inspection programme*. London: The Healthcare Commission.

Healthcare Commission (2005b). *Getting to the Heart of It. Coronary heart disease in England: A review of progress towards the national standards*. London: The Healthcare Commission.

Healthcare Commission (2005c). *Survey of Patients 2005, Primary Care Trusts*. London: The Healthcare Commission.

Healthcare Industries Task Force (HITF) (2007). *Innovation for Health: Making a difference*. HITF. Report of the Strategic Implementation Group (SIG). London: Department of Health.

Health Protection Agency (2007). *Quarterly Reporting Results for* Clostridium difficile *Infections and MRSA Bacteraemia April 2007*. London: Health Protection Agency.

Health Protection Agency (2006). *Mandatory Surveillance of Healthcare Associated Infections Report 2006*. London: Health Protection Agency.

HM Treasury (2007). 'GDP deflator data'. HM Treasury website. Available at: www.hm-treasury.gov.uk/economic_data_and_tools/gdp_deflators/data_gdp_fig.cfm.(accessed on 2 August 2007).

HM Treasury (2006). *Public Expenditure Statistical Analyses (PESA)*. Cm 6811. London: HM Treasury.

HM Treasury (2004). *2004 Spending Review: Public Service Agreements*. London: HM Treasury.

HM Treasury (2002a). *2002 Spending Review: Opportunity and security for all: Investing in an enterprising, fairer Britain*. London: HM Treasury.

HM Treasury (2002b). *Tax and the Environment: Using economic instruments*. London: HM Treasury.

Hirvonen J, Blom M, Tuominen U, Seitsalo S, Lehto M, Paavolainen P, Hietaniemi K, Rissanen P, Sintonen H. (2006). 'Health-related quality of life in patients waiting for major joint replacement: A comparison between patients and population control'. *Health and Quality of Life Outcomes*, vol 4, p 3.

Hospital Episodes Statistic (2007). HES Online. Available at: www.hesonline.nhs.uk (accessed on 30 July 2007).

House of Commons Health Committee (2007). *Workforce Planning*. Vol 1. Fourth Report, session 2006. HC 171-1. London: The Stationery Office.

House of Commons Health Committee (2006a). *Changes to Primary Care Trusts*. HC 646. London: The Stationery Office.

House of Commons Health Committee (2006b). *Independent Sector Treatment Centres*. Fourth Report of Session 2005–06. HC 934-I. London: The Stationery Office.

House of Commons Health Committee (2006c). *NHS Charges*. Third Report of Session 2005–06 Volume I. HC 815-1. London: The Stationery Office.

House of Commons Health Committee (2006d). *NHS Deficits*. Sixth Report of Session 2005/06, Vol 1. HC 1204-1. London: The Stationery Office.

House of Commons Health Committee (2006e). *Public Expenditure on Health and Social Services 2006. Memorandum received from the Department of Health containing personal replies to a written questionnaire from the committee*. HC 1692i. London: The Stationery Office.

House of Commons Health Committee (2005). *The Use of New Medical Technologies within the NHS*. Fifth Report of Session 2004-05. Available at: www.publications.parliament.uk/pa/cm200405/cmselect/cmhealth/398/39802.htm (accessed on 20 August 2007).

House of Commons Public Accounts Committee (2007a). *Department of Health: The National Programme for IT in the NHS. Twentieth Report of Session 2006–07. Report, together with formal minutes, oral and written evidence*. HC 390. London: The Stationery Office.

House of Commons Public Accounts Committee (2007b). *Tackling Child Obesity – first steps*. London: The Stationery Office.

House of Commons Public Accounts Committee (2007c). *The Provision of Out-of-Hours Care in England*, Sixteenth Report of Session 2006–07. HC 360. London: The Stationery Office.

House of Commons Public Accounts Committee (2006). *A Safer Place for Patients: Learning to improve patient safety*. London: The Stationery Office.

House of Lords (1988). *Priorities in Medical Research : third report of the Select Committee on Science and Technology, session 1987–88*. London: HMSO

Information Centre (2007a). *Ambulance Services, England*. Available at: www.ic.nhs.uk/statistics-and-data-collections/audits-and-performance/ambulance/ambulance-services-england-2006-07 (accessed on 30 July 2007).

Information Centre (2007b). *NHS Maternity Statistics: England 2005-06*. Leeds: The Information Centre.

Information Centre (2007c). *NHS Staff 1996–2006*. Available at: www.ic.nhs.uk/statistics-and-data-collections/workforce/nhs-staff-numbers/nhs-staff-1996–2006 (accessed on 30 July 2007).

Information Centre (2007d). *Prescription Cost Analysis: England 2006*. Leeds: The Information Centre.

Information Centre (2007e). *Technical Note on Updating of 2004–05 GP Earnings and Expenses Enquiry Results*. Leeds: The Information Centre.

Information Centre (2006a). *Health Survey for England 2005*. Leeds: The Information Centre.

Information Centre (2006b). *MHMDS Data 2003/04*. Information Centre website. Available at: www.ic.nhs.uk/our-services/improving-data-collection-and-use/datasets/dataset-list/mental-health/report-library/mhmds-data-2003-04 (accessed on 30 July 2007).

Information Centre (2006c). *MHMDS Data 2004/5*. Available at: www.ic.nhs.uk/our-services/improving-data-collection-and-use/datasets/dataset-list/mental-health/report-library/mhmds-data-2004-05 (accessed on 30 July 2007).

Information Centre (2006d). *Statistics on Smoking*. Available at: www.ic.nhs.uk/statistics-and-data-collections/health-and-lifestyles/smoking/statistics-on-smoking-england-2006 (accessed on 1 August 2007).

Information Centre (2006e). *Three Month NHS Staff Vacancy Results*. Available at: www.ic.nhs.uk/statistics-and-data-collections/workforce/nhs-vacancies/nhs-workforce-vacancy-survey-results-as-at-31-march-2006 (accessed on 30 July 2007).

Institute for Fiscal Studies (2007). *Briefing Note No. 73, Poverty and inequality in the UK*. London: IFS.

International Association for the Study of Obesity (IASO) (2007). *Prevalence of Adult Obesity*. Available at: www.iotf.org/database/GlobalAdultTableJune07.htm (accessed on 30 July 2007).

Johnston RL, Sparrow JH, Canning CR, Tole D, Price NC (2005). 'Pilot national electronic cataract surgery survey 1. Method, descriptive and process features'. *Eye*, vol 19, pp 788–94.

Judge Institute of Management Studies (2002). *Evaluating the Impact of the NHS Clinical Governance Support Team's Clinical Governance Development Programme*. Cambridge: Judge Institute of Management Studies. Available at: www.jbs.cam.ac.uk/research/health/downloads/project-evaluation_summary.pdf (accessed on 22 August 2007).

King's Fund (2007). 'Predictive Risk Project'. King's Fund website. Available at: www.kingsfund.org.uk/current_projects/predictive_risk/index.html (accessed on 30 July 2007).

King's Fund (2006). Written submission to Health Committee.

Kjekshus LE, Hagen TP (2005). 'Ring fencing of elective surgery: does it affect hospital efficiency?' *Health Services Management Research*, vol 18, pp 186–97.

Le Grand J, Mays N, Mulligan J-A (1998). *Learning from the NHS Internal Market: A review of the evidence*. London: King's Fund.

Maheswaran R, Pearson T, Munro J, Jiwa M, Campbell MJ, Nicholl J (2007). 'Impact of NHS walk-in centres on primary care access times: Ecological study'. *British Medical Journal*, vol 334, p 838.

Mahon JL, Bourne RB, Rorabeck CH, Feeny DH, Stitt L, Webster-Bogaert S (2002). 'The effect of waiting for elective total hip arthroplasty on health-related quality of life'. *Canadian Medical Association Journal*, vol 167, pp 1115–21.

Malhotra N, Jacobson B (2007). *Save to Invest: Developing criteria-based commissioning for planned health care in London*. London: London Health Observatory.

Martin S, Rice N, Smith P (2007). *The Link Between Health Care Spending and Health Outcomes: Evidence From English Programme Budgeting Data, CHE Research Paper 24*. York: University of York, Centre for Health Economics.

McCoy D, Pollock A, Bianchessir C, Godden S (2007). *Survey on the Implementation of the Community Care (Delayed Discharges) Act (2003)*. ESRC Public Services Programme Discussion Paper Series no 0702. London: ESRC.

Medix (2006). 'Doctors' Survey: NHS computer system'. BBC website. Available at: news.bbc.co.uk/1/hi/programmes/file_on_4/5019636.stm (accessed on 30 July 2007).

Modernisation Agency (2005). *PACS Benefits Realisation and Service Redesign Opportunities*. London: Department of Health.

Modernisation Agency (2003). *NHS Modernisation: Making it mainstream*. London: Matrix Research and Consultancy.

National Audit Office (2007a). *Pay Modernisation: A new contract for NHS consultants in England*. Report by the Comptroller and Auditor General. HC 335 Session 2006–07. London: National Audit Office.

National Audit Office (2007b). *The Efficiency Programme: A second review of progress report by the comptroller and auditor general*. HC 156-I Session 2006–07. London: National Audit Office.

National Audit Office (2006). *The National Programme for IT in the NHS*. Report by the Comptroller and Auditor General. HC 1173 Session 2005–2006. London: National Audit Office.

National Audit Office (2003). *Achieving Improvements through Clinical Governance*. A progress report on implementation by NHS trusts. HC 1055. London: The Stationery Office.

National Centre for Social Research (2006). *An Assessment of Dietary Sodium Levels among Adults (Aged 19–64), in the General Population, Based on Analysis of Dietary sodium in 24 hour Urine Samples*. London: Food Standards Agency.

NHS Connecting for Health (2007a). *Latest Deployment Statistics and Information*. London: NHS Connecting for Health. Available at: www.connectingforhealth.nhs.uk/newsroom/latest/factsandfigures/deployment (accessed on 30 July 2007).

NHS Connecting for Health (2007b). *NHS Connecting for Health NHS IM&T Investment Survey 2006*. London: NHS Connecting for Health.

NHS Connecting for Health (2005a). *A Guide to the National Programme for Information Technology*. London: NHS Connecting for Health.

NHS Connecting for Health (2005b). *National Programme for IT Implementation of Choose and Book*. London: NHS Connecting for Health. Available at: www.connectingforhealth.nhs.uk/newsroom/news-stories/310105/ (accessed on 30 July 2007).

NHS Direct (2007). 'Background and Statistics: General information about NHS Direct'. NHS Direct website. Available at: www.nhsdirect.nhs.uk/articles/article.aspx?articleId=2168 (accessed on 30 July 2007).

NHS Education for Scotland (2006). *Second National Survey of Non-training Grade Doctors in NHS Scotland: Changes in job satisfaction, work commitments and attitudes to workload following contractual reform*. Aberdeen: NHS Education for Scotland and Health Economics Research Unit, University of Aberdeen.

NHS Estates (2007). 'Clean Hospitals'. NHS Estates website. Available at: patientexperience.nhsestates.gov.uk/clean_hospitals/ch_content/national_results/introduction.asp (accessed on 30 July 2007).

NHS Institute for Innovation and Improvement (2006). *Delivering Quality and Value: Focus on productivity and efficiency*. London: Department of Health.

NHS Institute for Innovation and Improvement (1996). 'No Delays Essentials'. NHS Institute for Innovation and Improvement website. Available at: www.nodelaysachiever.nhs.uk/Essentials (accessed on 30 July 2007).

NHS Litigation Authority (2007). *Data on damages payments made on settled claims and number of claims received by incident year for Clinical Negligence Scheme for Trusts (CNST). Obstetrics claims as at 28/02/07.* Personal communication – 15 May 2007.

NHS National Institute for Health and Clinical Excellence (2005). 'Evaluation and review of NICE implementation evidence (ERNIE)'. NHS National Institute for Health and Clinical Excellence website. Available at: www.nice.org.uk/page.aspx?o=ernie (accessed on 20 August 2007).

NHS Reference Costs (2007). *NHS Reference Costs.* London: Department of Health. Available at: www.dh.gov.uk/en/Policyandguidance/Organisationpolicy/Financeandplanning/DH_076912 (accessed on 1 August 2007).

National Patient Safety Agency (2007). NPSA Announces Continued Improvement in Hospital Food and Cleanliness. London: NPSA. Available at: www.npsa.nhs.uk/npsa/display?contentId=5218 (accessed on 30 July 2007).

National Patient Safety Agency (2006). *Quarterly National Reporting and Learning System data summary: Autumn 2006.* London: National Patient Safety Agency.

National Prescribing Centre (2007). *Community Pharmacy Framework Collaborative: Final report.* Liverpool: National Prescribing Centre.

National Primary Care Research and Development Programme (2007). *National Evaluation of the Expert Patients Programme.* Executive Summary 44 [online]. Available at: www.npcrdc.ac.uk/ Publications/National_Evaluation_of_EPP_-_Shanleys.pdf (accessed on 20 August 2007).

National Primary Care Research and Development Centre (2006). *The National Evaluation of the Pilot Phase of the Expert Patient Programme: Final report.* Manchester: NPCRDC.

OECD (2007). Health Data file. Paris: OECD.

Ofcom (2006). *Ofcom Own-initiative Investigation into the Price of Making Telephone Calls to Hospital Patients.* A case closure document issued by the Office of Communications Case: CW/00844/06/05. London: Ofcom. Available at: www.ofcom.org.uk/bulletins/comp_bull_index/ comp_bull_ccases/closed_all/cw_844/ (accessed on 20 August 2007).

Office of Fair Trading (2007). *The Pharmaceutical Price Regulation Scheme.* London: Office of Fair Trading.

Office for National Statistics (2007a). *Cancer Survival in England by Strategic Health Authority.* London: ONS. Available at: www.statistics.gov.uk/StatBase/Product.asp?vlnk=11991&Pos= 4&ColRank=1&Rank=160 (accessed on 30 July 2007).

Office for National Statistics (2007b). *Gini Coefficients, 1980 to 2004–05 (per cent): The effects of taxes and benefits on household income, 2004–05.* London: ONS. Available at: www.statistics.gov.uk/StatBase/ssdataset.asp?vlnk=9295&Pos=1&ColRank=2&Rank=1000 (accessed on 30 July 2007).

Office for National Statistics (2006a). *General Household Survey 2005.* London: ONS.

Office for National Statistics (2006b). *Public Service Productivity: Health, Economic Trends 628*. London: ONS.

Opinion Leader Research (2006). *Your Health, Your Care, Your Say: Research report*. London: Department of Health.

Osprey (2006). *The Training Programme for Clinical System Engineers*. Available at: www.steyn.org.uk/OSPREY.pdf (accessed on 2 August 2007).

Palmer K (2006). *NHS Reform: Getting back on track*. London: King's Fund.

Palmer K (2005). *NHS Reform: Will it deliver the desired health outcomes?* London: King's Fund.

Palmer G, MacInnes T, and Kenway PI (2006). *Monitoring poverty and social exclusion in the UK 2006*. York: The Joseph Rowntree Foundation.

Park A (2007). *British Social Attitudes Survey*. The 23rd Report, National Centre for Social Research. London: Sage.

Pathology Service Improvement (2005). *Challenges and Top Tips for Pathology Service Improvement*. Leicester: Pathology Service Improvement. Available at: www.pathologyimprovement.nhs.uk/View.aspx?page=/publications.html (accessed on 30 July 2007).

Patient Power Review Group (2007). *Report to the Department of Health by the Patient Power Review Group*. London: Department of Health.

Pharmacy Practice Research Trust (2007). *Community Pharmacy Contractual Framework: Delivering its Promise?* Evaluation of the Implementation of the Community Pharmacy Contractual Framework in England and Wales [online]. Available at: www.rpsgb.org/pdfs/pprtcommpharmbrief.pdf (accessed on 20 August 2007).

Picker Institute Europe (2005). *Is the NHS Getting Better or Worse? An in-depth look at nearly a million patients between 1998 and 2004*. Oxford: The Picker Institute Europe.

Poissant L, Pereira J, Tamblyn R, Kawasumi YJ (2005). 'The impact of electronic health records on time efficiency of physicians and nurses: a systematic review'. *Journal of the American Medical Informatics Association*, vol 12, pp 505–16.

Redshaw M, Hamilton K (2006). *Networks, Admissions and Transfers: The perspectives of networks, neonatal units and parents*. Oxford: University of Oxford, National Perinatal Epidemiology Unit.

Review Body for Nursing and Other Health Professions (2007). *Twenty-second Report on Nursing and Other Health Professions*. Cm 7029. London: The Stationery Office.

Review Body on Doctors' and Dentists' Remuneration (2007). *Thirty-sixth Report*. Cm 7025. London: The Stationery Office.

Richards M (2007). *Getting it Right for People with Cancer: Clinical case for change* [online].London: Department of Health. Available at: www.cancer.nhs.uk/documents/getting_it_right_for_people_with_cancer.pdf (accessed on 20 August 2007).

Richards M (2006). *Cancer Ten Years On: Improvements across the whole care pathway* [online]. Available at: www.dh.gov.uk/en/Publicationsandstatistics/Publications/ PublicationsPolicyAndGuidance/DH_074240 (accessed on 20 August 2007).

Robertson R, Dixon A (2007). *Building a Business Case for Self Care*. King's Fund unpublished report for Proprietary Association of Great Britain.

Rogers PG (2006). 'RAID methodology: the NHS Clinical Governance Team's approach to service improvement'. *Clinical Governance: An International Journal*, vol 11, No 1, pp 69–80.

Royal College of Physicians (2007). *National Sentinel Stroke Audit Phase 1(organisational audit) 2006. Phase 2 (clinical audit) 2006*. London: Royal College of Physicians.

Royal College of Physicians (2006). *NHS Services for People with Multiple Sclerosis: A national survey*. London: Royal College of Physicians.

Sant M, Aareleid T, Berrino F, Bielska Lasota M, Carli PM, Faivre J, Grosclaude P, Hédelin G, Matsuda T, Møller H, Möller T, Verdecchia A, Capocaccia R, Gatta G, Micheli A, Santaquilani M, Roazzi P, Lisi D (2003). 'EUROCARE-3: survival of cancer patients diagnosed 1990–94 – results and commentary'. *Annals of Oncology*, vol 14 (suppl 5), v61–118.

Science and Technology Committee House of Lords (1988). *Medical Research*. London: HMSO.

Secretary of State for Health (2007a). *Darzi Review of the NHS*. Available at: www.dh.gov.uk/en/News/Speeches/DH_076534 (accessed on 30 July 2007).

Secretary of State for Health (2007b). *The Government's Response to the Health Select Committee's Report on NHS Deficits*. Cm 7028. London: The Stationery Office.

Secretary of State for Health (2007c). *Trust, Assurance and Safety – The regulation of health professionals in the 21st century*. Cm 7013. London: The Stationery Office.

Secretary of State for Health (2006). *The Government's Response to the Health Select Committee's Report on Changes to Primary Care Trusts*. Cm 6760. London: The Stationery Office.

Secretary of State for Health (1999). *Health Act 1999*. Available at: www.opsi.gov.uk/acts/ acts1999/19990008.htm (accessed on 30 July 2007).

Secretary of State (1992). *The Health of the Nation. A strategy for health in England*. Cm 1986. London: HMSO.

Sheldon T, Cullum N, Dawson D, Lankshear AJ, Lowson K, Watt I, West P, Wright D, Wright J (2004). 'What's the evidence that NICE guidance has been implemented? Results from a national evaluation using time series analysis, audit of patients' notes, and interviews'. *British Medical Journal*, vol 329, pp 999–1007.

Sibbald B, McDonald R, Roland M (2007). 'Shifting care from hospital to the community; a review of the evidence on quality and efficiency'. *Journal of Health Services Research and Policy*, vol 12, no 2, pp 110–17.

Simpkins A (2007). *Measuring Quality as Part of Public Service Output: Strategy following consultation*. London: UKCeMGA. Available at: www.statistics.gov.uk/cci/article.asp?id=1831 (accessed 3 July 2007).

Smith J, Lewis R, Harrison A (2006). *Making Commissioning Effective in the Reformed NHS in England*. London: Health Policy Forum, available at: www.npa.co.uk/news_uploads/HPF_Effective_Commissioning_Report_Dec_2006.pdf (accessed on 30 July 2007).

Steel N, Maisey S, Clark A, Fleetcroft R, Howe A (2007). 'Quality of clinical primary care and targeted incentive payments: an observational study'. *Journal of General Practice*, vol 57, no 539, pp 449–54.

Strategic Implementation Group (2007). *Innovation for Health: Making a difference*. London: Department of Health.

Sutherland K, Leatherman S (2006) . *Regulation and Quality Improvement: A review of the evidence*. London: The Health Foundation.

Taylor K, Dangerfield B, Le Grand J (2005). 'Simulation analysis of the consequences of shifting the balance of care: a systems dynamics approach'. *Journal of Health Services Research and Policy*, vol 10, no 4, pp 196–202.

TNS (2006). *2005/06 School Sport Survey*. London: Department for Education and Skills.

Walshe K, Cortvriend P, Mahon A (2003). *The Implementation of Clinical Governance: A survey of NHS trusts in England*. Manchester: Centre for Healthcare Management.

Wanless D (2006). *Securing Good Care for Older People*. London: King's Fund.

Wanless D (2004). *Securing Good Health for the Whole Population. Final report*. London: HM Treasury.

Wanless D (2002). *Securing our Future Health: Taking a long term view. A final report*. London: HM Treasury.

Wanless D (2001). *Securing our Future Health: Taking a long term view. An interim report*. London: HM Treasury.

Wilkin D, Bojke C, Coleman A, Gravelle H (2003). 'The relationship between size and performance of primary care organisations in England'. *Journal of Health Services Research and Policy*, vol 8, no 1, pp 11–17.

Williams S, Buchan J (2006). *Assessing the New NHS Consultant Contract: A something for something deal?* London: King's Fund.

World Health Organization (2007) 'Tobacco Control Database'. World Health Organization Regional Office for Europe website. Available from: http://data.euro.who.int/tobacco/ (accessed on 3 August 2007).

Zaninotto P, Wardle H, Stamatakis E, Mindell J and Head J (2006). *Forecasting Obesity to 2010*. London: Department of Health.

Index